1806300870
WITHDRAWN FROM STOCK

PC ABERYSTWYTH
LLYFRGELL

AF616304

COMPARATIVE NUTRITION

International Symposium organized by the Rank Prize Funds
and held at The Dormy Hotel, Ferndown, Dorset, UK
during 15–18 November, 1987

COMPARATIVE NUTRITION

Editors

SIR KENNETH BLAXTER FRS

IAN MACDONALD

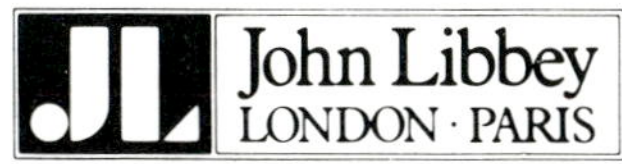

First published 1988 by
John Libbey & Company Limited
80–84 Bondway, London SW8 1SF, England

British Library Cataloguing in Publication Data

Comparative nutrition
1. Man. Nutrition. Compared with animal nutrition 2. Animals. Nutrition. Compared with human nutrition
I. Blaxter, *Sir* Kenneth, *1919–*
II. Macdonald, Ian
613.2

ISBN 0086196-169-2

Phototypeset by Dobbie Typesetting Limited, Plymouth, Devon
Printed and bound in Great Britain by
Whitstable Litho Ltd., Whitstable, Kent

Foreword

This volume records the proceedings of the 9th International Symposium sponsored by the Nutrition Committee and the Trustees of the Rank Prize Funds. The first of these symposia was held in 1974 and, looking back, I am surprised that comparative nutrition did not figure as a topic earlier. Comparative studies have been extremely powerful in giving greater insight in a variety of intellectual fields; it is certainly not too much to say that comparative anatomy has been the bedrock of all evolutionary theory leading indeed to a revolution in many branches of philosophy, and that comparative physiology, which started in earnest early this century (followed rapidly by comparative biochemistry), was the start of a great leap forward in that subject. Anthropology, sociology and indeed religion all use comparative studies as an integral part of their research activities and scholarship.

Comparative nutrition cannot, of course, be considered to start with this symposium, but this collection of papers, given at Ferndown in 1987, gives us some new insights to help research into nutrition on its way.

A few words about the origin of these meetings.

The Rank Prize Funds were established by the late Lord J. Arthur Rank shortly before his death in 1972 at the age of 84. He set up the Funds to encourage scientific work in two broad subjects which indirectly had been the bases of his personal fortune, namely nutrition (including crop husbandry) on the one hand and opto-electronics on the other. The first theme reflected Lord Rank's involvement with the flour milling industry as chairman of the family business started by his father, and the second with the film and electronics industries as chairman of a business he set up himself. A substantial sum of money was divided equally to establish a fund for each of these subjects.

It is of historical interest that Lord Rank died before he had been able to indicate in any detail the objectives of the funds. Trustees were appointed from among his closest friends and they endeavoured to interpret what they believed would have been his wishes; Lord Rank was a religious man and they were helped by the guideline that the outcome should be of special benefit to mankind. The trustees established two expert committees of eminent scientists, one in each subject, to advise them.

Although the Funds were dedicated to two very different areas of science, the original Trustees decided that the wishes of the founder would best be met, first by awarding substantial prizes to individuals in recognition of significant advances in the fields of science with which the Funds are concerned, secondly by sponsorship of research in key areas identified by the advisory committees, and thirdly by sponsorship of international symposia in each of the two subject areas. The proceedings of the symposia are always published and so made available to other research workers and students.

This volume is dedicated to the memory of the late Lord Rank without whose benefaction the symposium on comparative nutrition which it records would not have taken place.

J. Edelman CBE

Contents

1

The relevance of allometric comparisons to growth, reproduction and nutrition in primates and man

R. H. PETERS

Introduction

For a biologist, the world is often so rich and intriguing that it simply bewilders. One response to such complexity is scientific specialization: we choose a part of the universe which is small enough to be apprehended and understood, and study that. Regrettably, such choices often narrow our fields-of-view, sacrifice the contexts in which phenomena occur, and concentrate expertise in so few individuals that it is difficult for the population at large to gain access to science or to use it. The disadvantages of specialization can be reduced if a set of general theories provide the perspective and scope which were sacrificed for depth. To be useful, such a body of theory must be sufficiently known that experts are aware of it and sufficiently simple that experts can use it without diverting much effort from their speciality.

Allometry, the study of how biological structures and functions scale with body size, is one such body of general theory. This essay uses examples from the allometry of growth, reproduction, and nutrition to characterize allometry, to explore some of its shortcomings, and to show that general allometric patterns can provide a context for the study of primates and man.

The general area has been the subject of several recent reviews (Peters, 1983a; McMahon & Bonner, 1983; Calder, 1984; Schmidt-Nielsen 1984), and some of its problems of method or statistics have been examined there and elsewhere (Harvey & Mace, 1982; Harvey, 1982; Smith, 1984; Harvey & Clutton-Brock, 1985; Prothero 1986). This paper adds to that literature by providing new examples and a self-consciously practical, empirical view of the difficulties allometry presents.

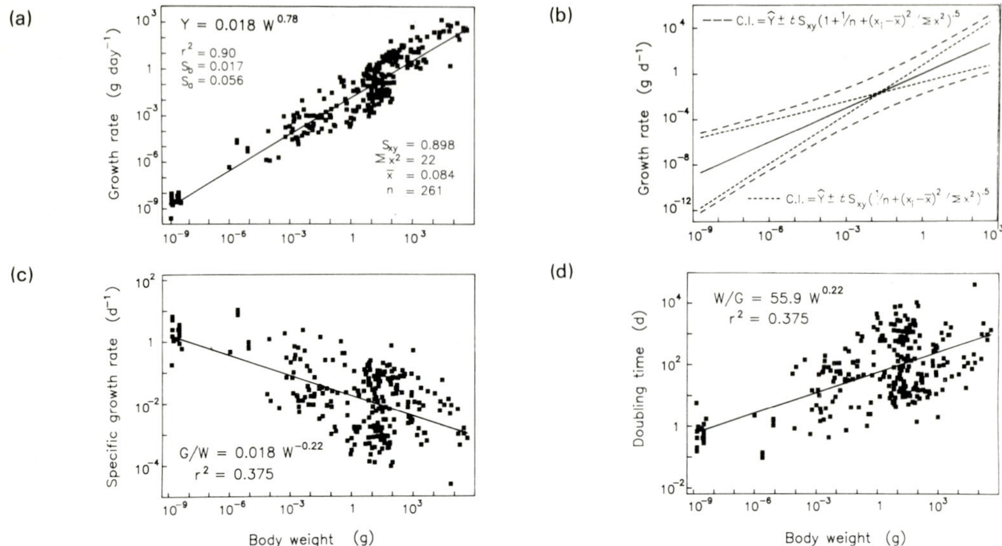

Fig. 1. *A general relation between growth rate and body size for a wide range of living organisms expressed as (a) a scatter diagram, regression line and statistics for individual growth rates, (b) 95% confidence intervals around the mean and around individual values, scatter diagrams (c) for specific growth rates, and (d) for doubling times.* With the exception of the mean line and r^2, regression statistics for panels a, c and d are identical.

Fundamentals of allometric analysis: growth

Figure 1 exemplifies allometric relations with data for growth rate. These data, which will be described in detail elsewhere (Peters, in prep.), were collected as part of a broad survey of allometric data in 1980 (Peters & Wassenberg, 1983). They represent organisms from protozoans to mammals, and growth in its broadest sense, including population production, reproductive output and somatic growth. In this analysis, body size is the average size over the interval when production was measured. For reproduction or population production, each point represents the value of growth extracted for each species in each study and its average size. When somatic growth data were available, they were divided into three equal time intervals and growth rate estimated as the difference in initial (W_o) and final (W_f) weights divided by the time interval (t), ie. $G = (W_f - W_o)/t$. The data were collected to estimate the productivity of similar sized organisms of many species and ages, given only their number and size. For example, relations based on these data might be used to make a quick estimate of the productivity of the contents of a plankton net dragged through the sea or a lake during the growing season (Platt, 1985).

Statistics in allometry

Like many large sets of biological data, the growth rates in Fig. 1a are not normally distributed unless they are logarithmically transformed to stabilize and normalize variance in the dependent variable. The independent variable is also log-transformed to linearize the relation and to even out the distribution of data along the X-axis. As a result of these transformations, the regression analysis which describes growth (G, g/d) as a function of body weight (W, g), actually fits the equation

$$\log G = \log a + b \log W \tag{1}$$

All regression statistics refer to this form and all scatter diagrams of the data use logarithmic axes. When the regressions are back-transformed to arithmetic units, they take the familiar form of a power equation

$$G = aW^b \tag{2}$$

where a is the intercept or elevation and the exponent, b, is the slope. Solutions to Equation 2 give the medians or geometric means (not the arithmetic means) at a particular body size. Miller (1984) provides simple corrections to back-transform values to allow for this bias, but no such correction was applied in the present paper.

The regression model used to erect these equations is a matter of dispute. Most authors use ordinary least squares. In part, this is because it is familiar and available in most computer statistical packages and programmed calculators. However, least squares regression is also preferred because it maximizes predictive power (Gujarati, 1978) and because there is little unanimity in favour of alternative models (Kermack & Haldane, 1950; Jolicoeur & Heusner, 1971; Harvey & Mace, 1982; Ricker, 1984; Seim & Saether, 1983). In my experience, when alternative models give very different equations, the uncertainty associated with the statistics of least squares regression are so high that one would be foolish to give a functional interpretation to the regression coefficients. Moreover, regressions based on body weight are usually intended as descriptions and predictions not depictions of causal connection and so alternate 'functional' regressions are not appropriate. For convenience, for applicability, for principle and for tradition, the present paper considers only least square regressions.

Of the series of statistics that should accompany a regression equation; only the coefficient of determination (r^2) is almost always provided. This is an index of the 'goodness of fit' and estimates the proportion of the variance in the dependent variable which is explained by reference to size. In practice, r^2 is a measure of how strong the pattern in the scatter diagram appears, and tends to increase with the range of the data, the steepness of the slope, the appropriateness of the transformation, and the reduction in residual error.

The main problem with r^2 is that it is often used to the exclusion of other statistics (Smith, 1984). Among the most important of these is the standard error associated with the mean, S_{xy}, calculated as the root of the mean squared error. S_{xy} is a measure of the uncertainty associated with the description of the trend represented by equation 1 and gives a good measure of the effectiveness of the relation's predictive power. S_{xy} is used with the sample size (n), the mean of the independent variable ($\bar{X}$, ie log W) and the sum of squared deviations in X (Σx^2) to calculate the confidence limits around the mean. Allometricians who are primarily interested in average trends usually calculate the confidence limits around the mean. These are narrow and deeply bowed and become more so as sample size increases. Confidence limits around individual estimates are much broader, less bowed, and less dependent on sample size (Fig. 1b). Unfortunately, few studies provide the information necessary to estimate either type of confidence limits.

There are a number of other statistics available to describe the regressions (Draper & Smith, 1981; Montgomery & Peck, 1982), including the standard errors associated with the slope (S_b) and intercept (S_a), the F-value, and the probability level, but those mentioned above are the minimum to describe the regression, its effectiveness in describing the data in hand, and its power in prediction.

Figure 1a provides a regression of growth rate on body size because this seems more straightforward and yields effective figures. Other workers prefer to plot specific rates (ie fractional growth rate, G/W in d^{-1}) against weight (Fig. 1c). Although this introduces an autocorrelation (because W appears on both axes), there is nothing intrinsically wrong with the use of specific rates: the slope of the relation is exactly 1 less than that of the individual rate equation and r^2 is depressed, but the other statistics are unchanged and predictive power is unimpaired.

One can also regress the inverse of G/W (doubling time, W/G in d) against body size (Fig. 1d), and the regression is exactly that which would be determined by algebraic manipulation of Eq. 1. Again r^2 is less than that for individual rates, but it is identical in both regression of G/W and W/G against W.

Empirical regularities in allometry

Although regression statistics are particular to each set of data, there are patterns in the slopes, the elevations, and the unexplained variations among regressions that deserve wide recognition.

There are literally hundreds of regressions which analyse individual rates as functions of body size, like Fig. 1a. Among these are relations for rates of respiration, including air flow, blood flow and oxygen consumption, for rates of production, including somatic growth, milk production and reproductive output, for rates of elimination including defecation, evaporative water loss and creatine excretion, and for rates of ingestion including caloric intake, N intake and vitamin requirements (Peters, 1983a). Remarkably, all these different regressions for various animal groups have slopes with values close to ¾ (Kleiber, 1961). The mean for 297 such estimates (Peters, 1983a,b) is 0.736 and the dispersion around this value is small (SE = 0.0071).

Specific rates are consistent with this pattern and therefore decline approximately as $W^{-1/4}$ (Fig. 1c), implying that the rate of flux through a unit of tissue is lower in larger animals. The same exponent applies to a number of fractional rates, including population growth rate (Blueweiss *et al.*, 1978; Hennemann, 1983), rate constants of uptake and release (Smith & Kalff, 1982), pulse rates, and the turnover rates of the tissues (Vachá & Znojil, 1981).

The characteristic slope associated with physiological times, like population doubling time (Fig. 1d), red blood cell life span (Vachá & Znojil, 1981) or biological half-time of radio-contaminants (Di Gregorio *et al.*, 1978), is ¼ (Lindstedt & Calder, 1981) as should be expected, since physiological times are the inverses of fractional or specific rates which have a slope of − ¼. However, many physiological times that are not obviously the inverse of a specific rate also rise as $W^{1/4}$. These include many aspects of life history (gestation times, incubation times, time to sexual maturity and life span [Calder, 1984]), of behaviour (eg, the length of the sleep cycle [Peters, 1983a]), and of physiology (eg, breath time, gut beat time [Adolph, 1949]).

The consistency of these slopes has several consequences. Because the slopes associated with individual rates rise as $W^{3/4}$, large individuals do more of any process per unit time. Because all rates have similar exponents, the relative size of these different processes is similar across the animal kingdom. As a result, flows of material and energy through living organisms are scaled similarly with size. Animals which eat twice as much tend to consume twice as much water, produce twice as much new tissue, and do twice as much of everything else per unit time. Because specific rates decline as $W^{-1/4}$, the tissues of larger organisms are less active than similar tissue in smaller organisms. Finally, because physiological times rise as $W^{1/4}$, large animals devote a longer time to any given task, but, since the slopes associated with times are similar, the proportion of the total available time required for similar tasks and phases is similar for all organisms, regardless of size.

Precision and generality

The patterns described by very general allometric regressions like those in Fig. 1a are extremely strong. The chance of such a trend occurring by chance is less than 1 in 100 000; the slope and intercepts are very well defined and over 90% of the variation in the dependent variable is explained by reference to body size. Nevertheless, the standard error (S_{xy}) associated with the estimate is so large that the 95% confidence limits around the individual estimates cover almost four orders of magnitude. These general relations are not very effective for precise prediction about particular cases.

The imprecision of general regressions is only one aspect of allometric relations that offend expert sensibilities. The collections are indiscriminate because they give equal weight to the careful measurements of the expert and the sloppy estimates of the dilettante. Because the analysis uses only one independent variable, the regressions ignore many factors which we know to be important. A similar objection is often raised because the regressions ignore established taxonomic boundaries. So much is wrong with the approach that no one would pay any attention to them if they did not work.

More precise relations can be produced by considering additional variables, like temperature (Robinson *et al.*, 1983; Andrews & Pough, 1985), but the imprecision of general relations is usually addressed by treating smaller, more taxonomically homogeneous groups. One of the most consistently effective subdivisions in allometry is the separation into 'metabolic groups': homeotherms, poikilotherms, and unicells (Hemmingsen, 1960). Homeotherms have rates 10 to 30 times greater than poikilotherms of similar size, which in turn perform at rates 5 to 10 times greater than unicells (once size effects are removed).

Figure 2 shows that the same pattern applies to the growth data under analysis here. There are highly significant differences among the growth rates of metabolic groups, and separate analysis yields more precise relations, as indicated by the decline in S_{xy}. Other statistics also change in these more restricted regressions, for the

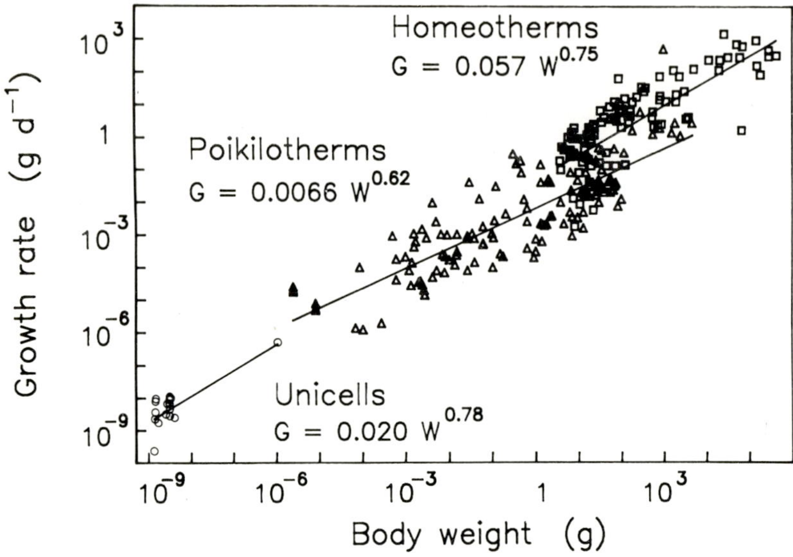

Fig. 2. *Division of the data in Fig. 1 into different metabolic groups sacrifices the generality of a single equation for improved predictive and descriptive power.* For unicells, $r^2 = 0.64$; $S_{xy} = 0.388$; $x^2 = 7.15$; $\bar{X} = 8.517$; $n = 18$; $S_b = 0.14$; for poikilotherms, $r^2 = 0.72$; $S_{xy} = 0.830$; $x^2 = 603$; $\bar{X} = -0.458$; $n = 136$; $S_b = 0.034$; and for homeotherms, $r^2 = 0.63$; $S_{xy} = 0.767$; $x^2 = 189$; $\bar{X} = 2.199$; $n = 107$; $S_b = 0.056$.

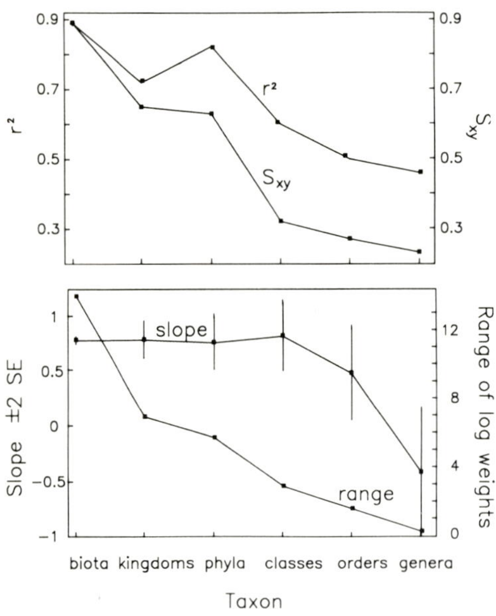

Fig. 3. *The effect of taxonomic level on allometric regression statistics.* The data in Fig. 1a were separated into increasingly smaller taxa and the median values calculated at each taxonomic level for the coefficient of determination (r^2), the standard error of the estimate (S_{xy}), the allometric slope (b), its standard error (SE) and the range of the logarithms of body weight. Only taxa for which at least 4 data pairs were available were used.

relations become less defined: r^2 declines, the standard errors around the regression coefficients rise, and the coefficients themselves vary more.

These patterns usually recur whenever the data are divided into more homogeneous taxa. To illustrate this, the data in Fig. 1 were divided into progressively smaller taxa, regressed, and the median values for r^2, b, S_{xy} and S_b determined at each

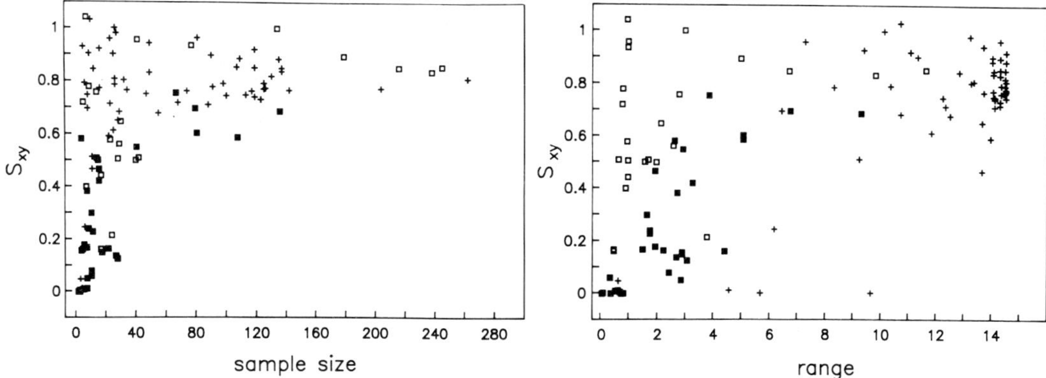

Fig. 4. *The interaction of sample size, the range of the independent variable, and taxonomic level on the precision of the estimate (S_{xy}).* Solid squares represent statistics from different taxa used in Fig. 3, and represent the combined effects of variation in taxon, sample size and range. Open squares were derived from regressions of all data in Fig. 1 lying in a series of subsets of arbitrarily restricted range; as a result, those regressions are largely determined by the effects of varying sample size and range, but not the effects of taxon. Crosses represent samples of different sample size drawn at random from the data in Fig. 2 in which sample size has a larger effect than the range in weight or taxon. Because taxonomically defined regressions are more precise than either artificial set, it appears that taxonomic diversity contributes significantly to the imprecisions in both artificial data sets and, by extension, to those in Fig. 1.

taxonomic level. Figure 3 shows that r^2 steadily declines as progressively smaller taxa are considered, while S_b rises. The median slope is less affected but eventually it is depressed. Although these trends show that the regressions are more poorly defined in smaller taxa, the precision of the relation improves, for S_{xy} declines across the comparisons. These patterns suggest that allometry becomes less effective at defining functional relationships as smaller taxa are considered (Gould, 1966, 1975; Harvey & Clutton-Brock, 1985), but more effective in making predictions. Reducing the size of the taxa also reduces the range of both variables (Fig. 3) and the sample size. It is difficult to distinguish the relative importance of these various factors in the aggregate response illustrated in Fig. 3.

In an attempt to sort out the relative contributions of range, sample size, and taxonomic diversity, I selected two data sets, one varying primarily in sample size and range, and the other primarily in sample size, but neither varying much in taxonomy. One data set consisted of 68 subsets of different sample size (n) selected at random from the entire data set in Fig. 1a. These subsets tended to have high taxonomic diversity, wide ranges in body size, and variable sample sizes. The other data set consisted of 33 subsets with different ranges in body size, generated by dividing Fig. 1a along the X axis into one to 14 size classes, varying over 14 to 1 orders of magnitude, respectively. These subsets tended to vary both in range and sample size, but less in taxonomy. The regression statistics for each subset were calculated and S_{xy}, r^2, and S_b plotted as functions of range and sample size. Data generated by 34 different taxa within the data set (ie, those used to generate Fig. 3) were then plotted on the same figure. I hypothesize that if the regressions are more affected by taxonomy than by sample size and range, then the taxonomically-derived set would occupy different positions in the plots than those created artificially.

The precision of the regression is reflected in the standard error of the estimate (S_{xy}). For both artificial data sets, variation in sample size affects this statistic when n is so small (<30) that the error in the data is not effectively estimated. Regressions based on smaller ranges of the artificial data sets also yield variable values of S_{xy}, which probably reflect low sample sizes. The similar shapes in the scatter diagrams (Fig. 4) suggest that range and sample size also affect the precision of the estimates based on different taxa. However, regressions based on narrowly defined taxa are more precise than those based on artificial sets with similar ranges and sample sizes. Estimates of S_{xy} for different taxa are only about 2/3 those based on artificial data sets. It appears that the variance (which varies as S_{xy}^2) in regressions based on taxonomically defined groups is only about half as large as that in more broadly-based regressions of similar sample size and range.

In contrast, the definition of the regression line, as reflected by r^2, b, and S_b, is not greatly affected by either taxonomic diversity or sample size. Instead, scatter diagrams using range as the independent variable seem similar in all three data sets (Fig. 5). These figures also suggest that a range of six orders of magnitude is sufficient to define the regression line in this case. This critical range depends on the relative variation in the dependent and independent variables, but because these data are quite variable, six orders of magnitude are likely to be sufficient in most cases involving individual rates.

We can tease several rules of thumb from these patterns. Always work with a data set of at least 30 values, but sample sizes much above 100 are not necessary; when the point of the study is to generate a general curve, the widest possible range in the data is most effective; if the point of the study is to generate the most precise prediction, then regressions based on narrow taxa are most effective. In the latter case, smaller sample sizes can be used; in either case, both the predicted value and its associated uncertainty should be reported. This is the most effective representation of the regression and the most useful tool for prediction and for comparison of the regressions with data and each other.

The interdependence of slopes and intercepts

The patterns and interdependencies apparent in Figs 4 and 5 are not surprising; they reflect similarities in the algorithms used to derive regression statistics from the raw data. The algorithms of least squares regression minimize the sum of the squared deviations between the observed values of the dependent variable ($d_{xy}^2 = S_{xy}^2[n-2]$), subject to the constraint that the line must go through the means of all the data ($\bar{X}$, $\bar{Y}$). Given the inevitable stochastic differences in collections of essentially similar biological data, this is achieved by balancing the effects of slope against those of elevation. In consequence, slopes and intercepts interact to describe the regression line, and regressions which differ markedly in slope and elevations may make very similar predictions.

This interdependence yields particularly surprising results when the intercept lies to either side of the mean of the data (Zar, 1967). For example, when regressions describing the allometry of homeotherm metabolic rate are based on weight measured in grams, there is a negative relation between slope and intercept (Peters, 1983a).

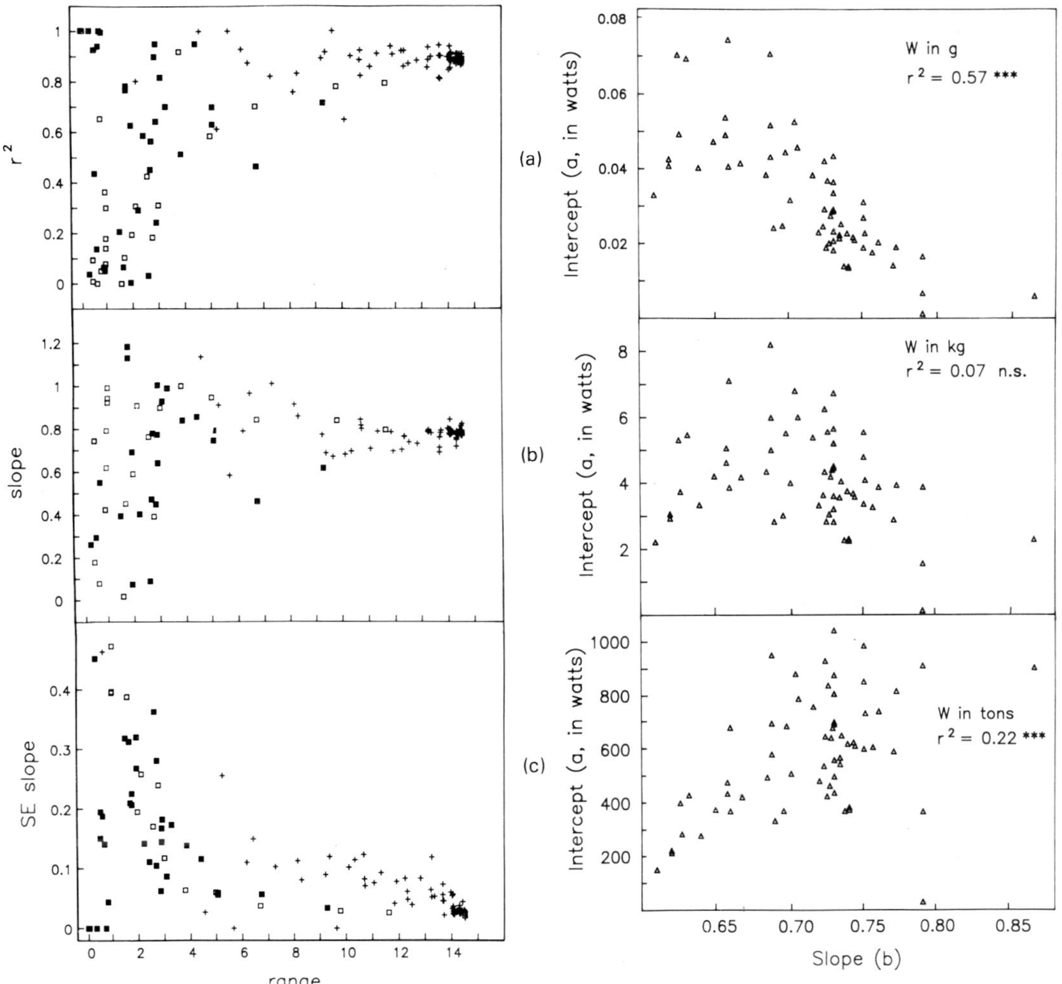

Fig. 5. *The effect of the range of the independent variable (log body weight) on regression statistics describing mean responses and scatter diagrams when the data are divided into the different groupings described in Fig. 4.* Because all divisions are similarly affected by range, it appears that sample size and taxonomic diversity have only small consistent additional effects. Some extreme values for slope and its standard error generated when sample sizes are small were eliminated in the two lower panels. These gave the high values of r^2 at low range in upper panels.

Fig. 6. *The interrelationship of slope and intercept in 63 allometric relations describing the basal or standard metabolic rates of homeotherms (data from Peters, 1983a) when body weight is expressed in (a) g, (b) kg, or (c) tons.*

If instead the equations are re-expressed with weight in kg, the intercept at W = 1 kg is closer to the mean weight and the interdependence of slope and intercept disappears. If weight is expressed in tons, the two statistics are again interrelated but the relation is positive (Fig. 6). This is easily explained (Fig. 7), but rarely appreciated. Similar data can yield apparently different regression statistics and therefore such statistics

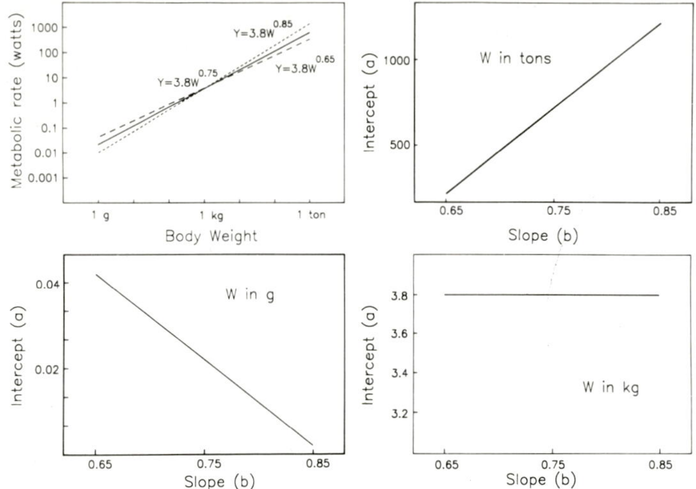

Fig. 7. *A graphical explanation for the patterns in Fig. 6 using three simulated plots differing in slope but intersecting at 1 kg.* When slope is steep, the value at 1 g is low; when slope is shallow, values at 1 g are high. As a result, there is a negative relation between slope and intercept when the units are such that the intercept lies to the left of the data swarm (ie, when weight is expressed in g). The opposite is true when the intercept lies to the right of the data swarm (when weight is expressed in tons) and the two are independent when W is in kg.

should always be accompanied by estimates of error and we should examine their composite effect. The statistics associated with each regression form a unit that describes an abstraction of the data set. Individual statistics ought to be seen as parts of the description of a larger whole, and as a corollary, isolated statistics do not merit close examination.

Growth and reproduction in primates

Despite the pitfalls and limitations mentioned above, allometric relations are essential to comparative biology, for they answer the need for a standard basis of comparison when specific information is available, and provide one of the few tools for quantitative estimation when we are confronted with ignorance.

The comparative use of allometric relations can be illustrated by comparing the predictions of a series of general relations with specific information for a smaller taxon. For example, Fig. 8 compares the somatic growth rates for a series of primates with predictions from equation 1. Although each primate datum lies within the very broad 95% confidence limits for individual points (Fig. 1b), the primate relation is more precise, in the sense that it has lower residual error (F-test; Snedecor & Cochran, 1980), and less biased, because there is a significant trend with size in residuals around the general line. This could also be confirmed by non-parametric sign tests over different ranges in the data. Finally, F-tests could be used to compare the slopes (which differ significantly) and the elevations (which differ in variance but do not differ at the means). These comparisons involve standard statistical tests and are unequivocal

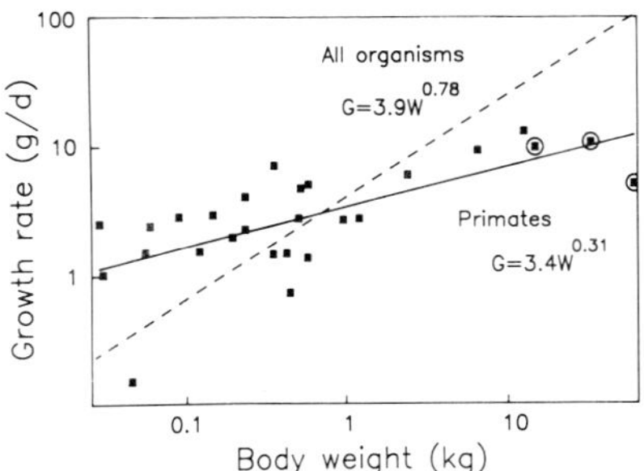

Fig. 8. *A comparison of the effects of size on observed somatic growth rates of primates with those predicted by the general regression line in Fig. 1.* Data are drawn from sources listed by Case (1978): Altman & Dittmer (1972), Asdell (1964), Clewe (1969), Fleagle & Simonds (1975), Gucwinska & Gucwinska (1968), Jewall & Oates (1969), Lorenz & Heinemann (1967), Petter-Rousseaux (1984), and Snow (1967). Human data are circled. For primates $r^2 = 0.46$; $S_{xy} = 0.307$; $x^2 = 21.2$; $\bar{X} = -0.28$, $n = 25$, $S_b = 0.067$.

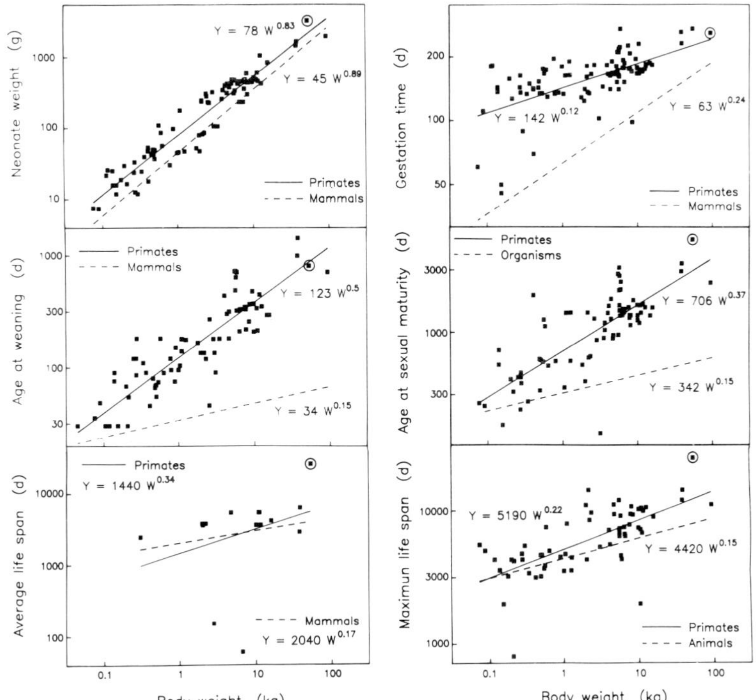

Fig. 9. *A comparison of primate data and their regression lines with taxonomically more general regression lines predicting life history phenomena.* The point representing man is circled in each panel. Data from Altman & Dittmer (1962), Leutenegger (1973), Western (1979), Eisenberg (1981), Millar (1981), Harvey & Clutton-Brock (1985), Lefebvre (1985). Regression statistics in Table 1.

in showing differences and similarities between the regressions and therefore in the data. Unfortunately, few of us have time to complete such analyses, the necessary data and statistics are rarely available, and most audiences find the summaries about F-values and significance unilluminating. Moreover, the bald fact that these two equations are statistically different obscures their similarity. Although the general equation is an imperfect estimator of primate growth rate, it is much better than no information at all.

Table 1. *Regression statistics for growth and life history phenomena for primates and other animals.* Subscript numbers refer to (1) primates, averaging for each species, (2) primates without averaging and (3) other animals. The independent variables are weight at birth (W_b, g), time for gestation (T_G), weaning (T_W), sexual maturity (T_S), average life span (L_{AVG}), maximum lifespan (L_{MAX}), all in days. The independent variable, adult body weight (W_b) is expressed in kg throughout. Sources for general relations are: (1) Millar, 1981; (2) Blaxter, 1971; (3) Blueweiss *et al.*, 1978.

	W_b	T_G	T_W	T_S	L_{AVG}		L_{MAX}
a_1	1.890	2.153	2.090	2.851	3.158		3.702
a_2	1.874	2.147	2.100	2.840	—		3.731
a_3	1.655	1.799	1.530	2.640	1.826		3.645
b_1	0.835	0.167	0.495	0.374	0.341	(NS)	0.218
b_2	0.830	0.130	0.486	0.386	—		0.218
b_3	0.888	0.238	0.150	0.260	0.170		0.150
S_{a1}	0.0223	0.0121	0.0246	0.0273	0.288		0.0243
S_{a2}	0.0175	0.0084	0.0214	0.0216	—		0.0180
S_{a3}	—	—	—	—	—		—
S_{b1}	0.0291	0.0154	0.0313	0.0343	0.282		0.0301
S_{b2}	0.0209	0.0097	0.0257	0.0247	—		0.0205
S_{b3}	0.015	0.032	—	—	—		—
r_1^2	0.908	0.383	0.787	0.617	0.101		0.457
r_2^2	0.904	0.471	0.756	0.676	—		0.600
r_3^2	0.94	0.72	—	0.96	0.56		0.56
S_{xy1}	0.188	0.103	0.207	0.203	0.634		0.179
S_{xy2}	0.211	0.106	0.217	0.204	—		0.138
S_{xy3}	—	—	—	—	—		—
$\bar{x}_1$	0.308	0.269	0.238	0.417	0.839		0.321
$\bar{x}_2$	0.307	0.446	0.296	0.492	—		0.381
$\bar{x}_3$	—	—	—	—	—		—
n_1	85	95	78	76	15		64
n_2	168	200	116	119	—		78
n_3	250	250	11	63	67		—
Sources	(1)	(1)	(2)	(3)	(3)		(3)

Whereas full comparisons need statistics, the simple visual comparison of data swarms or regression lines of particular groups with the general patterns is also essential. Figure 8 shows clearly that, although primate growth rates are consistent with observations from other organisms, small primates tend to grow more rapidly than other animals of similar size and that larger primates grow more slowly. While one could make a rough estimate of primate growth rates from the general relation, more precise predictions are possible if one uses a regression specific to primates. In such comparisons, statistical analysis serves largely to protect us from overinterpretation by discussing differences which are not real. The choice of which differences to compare, however, is not a matter of statistics, but of scientific intuition and purpose. This graphical approach works equally well in comparing other aspects of primate growth and reproduction with general regressions for the same processes (Fig. 9). Primate life history has such a special allure that a number of authors have studied its allometry. The primate data in Fig. 9 were extracted from these compilations

(Eisenberg, 1981; Harvey & Clutton-Brock, 1985; Lefebvre, 1985; Leutenegger, 1979; Millar, 1981; Western, 1979). The statistics (Table 1) differ somewhat from those presented by these authors because final data sets used here contain some few amendments and omissions reflecting the availability of the data at McGill University. The general regression chosen for these comparisons is that involving the largest taxonomic diversity and, for equally general relations, that based on the most data. The available comparisons show clearly where primates differ from other animals and where they do not.

At birth, both large and small primates tend to weigh somewhat more than other mammals. The difference is small and reflects a tendency for primates to bear litters of one or two individuals (Leutenegger, 1973), whereas most mammals have more ($\bar{X} = 3$; Peters, 1983a). The consistency of the pattern across all mammals is likely to reflect the architectural constraints of internal gestation: females can only carry a certain amount of fetal tissue and only offspring below a certain size can pass through the pelvic canal. The existence of such constraints is clearly identified by consistencies in allometric regressions. These patterns are therefore receiving belated, but increasing, attention in evolutionary biology (Gould & Lewontin, 1979).

The remaining panels in Fig. 9 deal with the times required to complete phases of development. Data swarms and regressions both show that body size influences physiological times in primates. The general relations again provide crude estimates of the observed values, but there are obvious biases in their predictions. Small primates have longer gestation times than other mammals but are similar in age at weaning, at maturation, and at death. Larger primates have only moderately long gestation times in relation to other mammals of similar size, but these primates are older when they are weaned, when they mature, and when they die.

Incidentally, the data for average life span differ from those in the other panels because each point represents a different species. In the other panels, each point represents a different study and one species may be represented by two or more points. Harvey & Mace (1982) suggest that this may be a form of pseudoreplication which is inappropriate because the two points for one species are not independent. I believe that this is a misapprehension. Statistical independence results because the measurements are taken independently and it is not prejudiced if a theory links the two measurements. Moreover, I suspect that as much or more error enters our data through differences among sites or investigators or years as through species differences. Certainly one would be suspicious if most of the data came from any single species, site, scholar, method, etc. because these other factors may induce more variation than is represented in the data and hence the data are unrepresentative. Such dominance of the data is rare in allometry. In any case, the effect of multiple points from a single species is not a matter for debate but for empirical test. In the examples of Fig. 9, the regression statistics for species averages differ little from those generated by the unaveraged data (Table 1). If one suspects that any taxon dominates the data, Harvey & Mace (1982) provide methods to assess its effect. The most practical advice in this regard is to be very circumspect in analysing any pattern which changes with the degree of taxonomic amalgamation of the data (T. H. Clutton-Brock, personal communication).

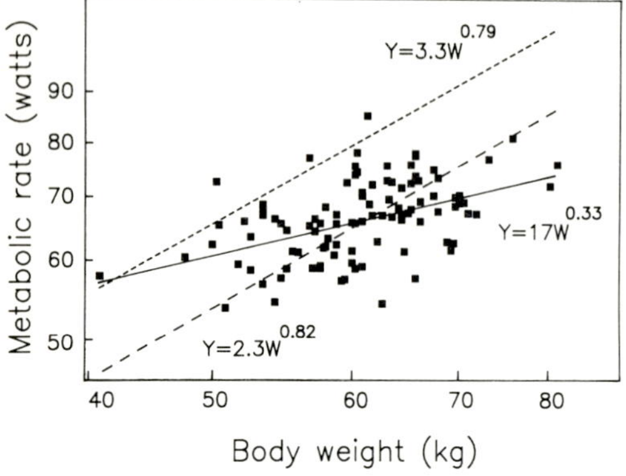

Fig. 10(above). *A comparison of data describing the basal metabolic rate of individual women (McKittrick, 1933) and the regression through those data with an apparently very different relation for women (Durnin & Passmore, 1967) and a regression for animals (Robinson* et al.*, 1983).*

(a)

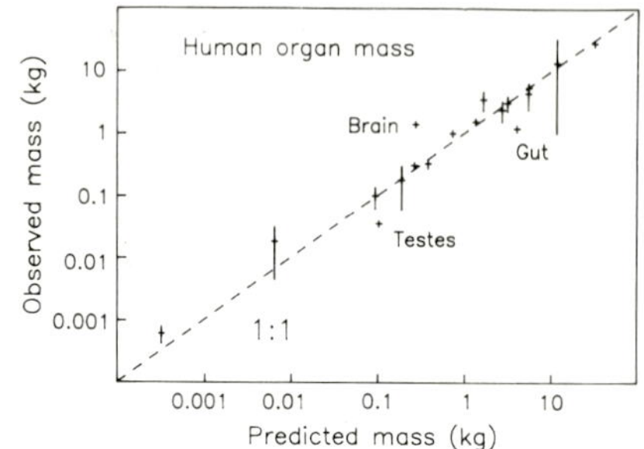

(b)

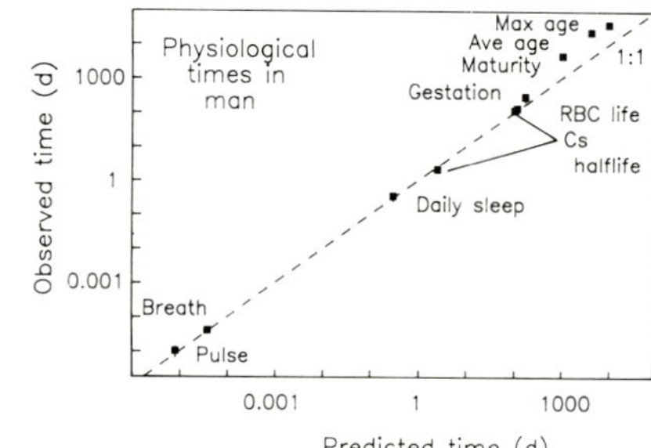

(c)

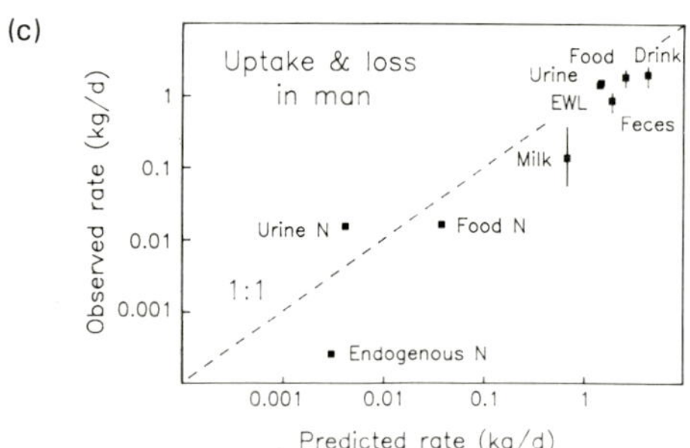

Fig. 11(right). *The effectiveness of general regression lines in predicting (a) body composition, (b) physiological times, and (c) individual rates for man.* Data are those for 'reference man' (ICRP 1975) except for those dealing with lactation and breast size (Linzell, 1972). General regressions are drawn from those listed in Peters 1983a, except for that for testes weight (Kenagy & Trombulak, 1986). The order of the data points in panel a is from left to right, pituitary, thyroid, testes, pancreas, spleen, kidney, heart, lungs, gut, breasts, brain, red blood cells, plasma, neonate, skeleton, blood, and fat.

Man

It will not have escaped the reader that humans, like other larger primates, are eccentric in their reproductive behaviour. One might, therefore, be tempted to consider man (and perhaps his close relatives) as exceptions and therefore to consider that general allometric relations have little application to man.

This view has considerable support. Obviously each species, including man, is distinctive in many ways. Figure 9 demonstrates some. An early study (McKittrick, 1933) of the most classical allometric relationship, that between metabolism and size, established that the slope for man was half that for other animals (Fig. 10). This has helped confirm the belief that a general relation has little application for particular species.

Figure 10 shows that this is not so. McKittrick's relation is an extreme case in which a lower slope is balanced by a higher elevation. This is made possible by the narrow range and relatively large scatter in the data. However, a regression based on more modern 'best estimates' of metabolic rate in adult women (Durnin & Passmore, 1967) has a much higher slope (and much lower elevation) yet fits the data almost as well. Even a general protozoan to whale regression (Robinson *et al.*, 1983) provides a good approximation of the data.

Basal metabolic rate is, in many ways, the least interesting of all metabolic rates because it is so standardized that it has little application outside the laboratory. However, multispecific allometric relations are also available to predict the metabolic rate of man in other more dynamic situations. For example, the equations of Taylor *et al.* (1981) for non-human mammals predict maximum rates of oxygen consumption that are only 4 to 18% lower than the mean value measured in man by Astrand (1952) and only 15 to 30% higher than the mean values reported by Hoppeler *et al.* (1973). One can calculate the metabolic rate of animals moving at other speeds as the sum of postural costs, associated with maintaining an erect posture, and transport costs, associated with moving a unit of body mass over a unit of distance at a given speed. Both costs can be predicted from interspecific allometry relations and both sets of relations appear to apply to man (Fedak & Seeherman, 1979; Paladino & King, 1979) despite early evidence to the contrary (Taylor *et al.*, 1970). Thus the predicted metabolic rate of man walking at 4.8 km/h is about 420 W; rates tabulated by Astrand & Rodahl (1970) vary between 210 and 350 W. Still other allometric relations consider the additional costs of carrying a load (Taylor *et al.*, 1980) or climbing a grade (Taylor, 1973), but these need not be detailed further. The available examples are sufficient to show that approximate values for human metabolic rates are available from allometric relationships.

Figure 11 compares a number of other measures for man with values predicted from general regressions. These suggest that, in the main, man is not much different from other organisms of similar size. His brain is larger (and his gut and testes smaller) than expected, but allometric regressions usually give a reasonable estimate of the organ and tissue mass (Fig. 11a). This is also true of a range of physiological times (Fig. 11b), although different phases of human life history are relatively prolonged. Individual rates (Fig. 11c) are predicted somewhat more erratically. Part of this seems to reflect low ingestion rates in contemporary man (as measured by recommended daily energy requirements [Altman & Dittmer, 1968]). Our sedentary habits have so lowered our energy requirements that we need eat only about 50% more energy than is needed to fuel basal metabolism. Energy demand in free-living animals is about twice as high (Nagy, 1987) and much closer to the predicted ingestion rate. Men working actively, like postmen or miners, have energy demands much more similar to expectation (Durnin & Passmore, 1967). Lower ingestion rates also seem to be reflected in defecation and N metabolism. Other differences, like endogenous N release rates, are harder to explain, but I would be unwilling to accept that the general line is necessarily wrong on the basis of this information. The past success of allometry is impressive enough to suggest that disagreements between individual estimates and general curves reflect errors in the specialists' estimates.

Even the failure of the general regression to predict ingestion rate is not complete. To illustrate this, I used growth data from several countries (Altman & Dittmer, 1968) to estimate the body weight for men of different age and these estimates were then used in an allometric relation to predict the ingestion rate. The predicted values and the recommended daily food requirements are both plotted as a function of age (Fig. 12). This plot shows that the food demands of children and adolescents are effectively predicted by the general equation and that it is only after ingestion rates decline in

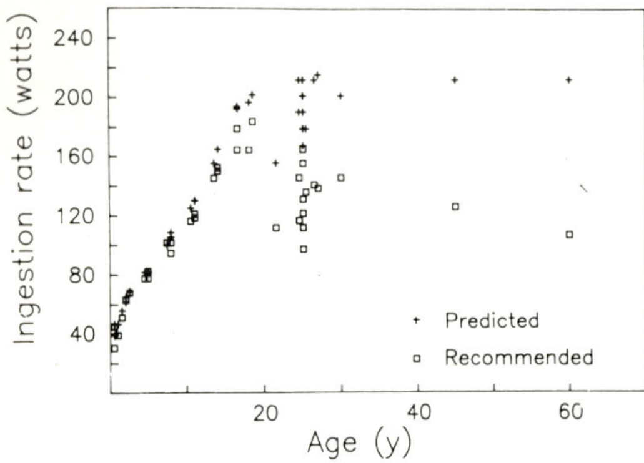

Fig. 12. *Predicted and recommended ingestion rates for man at different ages.* For this calculation, predicted $I = 10.8\ W^{.708}$, where W is in kg and I in watts (Farlow, 1976, recalculated in Peters, 1983a). Recommended energy intake and weight at age were taken from Altman & Dittmer, 1968).

adulthood that man differs from other animals. The inability of allometry to predict the inactivity of civilized man is scarcely damning. Instead, the success of Fig. 12 suggests that allometry may be effective in dealing with the ontogeny of nutrition within species.

In summary, general allometric relations provide an effective context for specialized studies and a tool that can be used to make predictions outside one's area of expertise, and so to evaluate expert opinion when necessary. Allometry requires a small battery of techniques and access to appropriate regressions. Fortunately, the former are simple and easy to learn, and the latter are available (Peters, 1983a; Calder, 1984). It is important to recognize that allometry provides only probabilistic estimates, that predictions are best when areas of application are narrowly defined, and that full statistics are essential if the potential of the approach is to be achieved.

I want to end by considering briefly how allometry could interact with human biology. As a generalist, I am frustrated by having to compare my regressions with dubious data from poorly investigated organisms. Man provides well defined means, with good estimates of the associated error for many processes. This sort of information could be used to determine the extent of variation within a species and to test the predictive power of the regressions more adequately. Such data could be used to determine whether the proportionalities suggested by the regressions are maintained within a species. Moreover, they could be used to determine if the proportions are maintained under a range of conditions, and if certain characteristics move together as a syndrome. If such patterns exist in one species, they may also exist across species. Recognition of such syndromes might allow more precise estimates than are now possible from weight alone. In short, human biology offers a splendid opportunity to allometry to evaluate present regressions and uncover new patterns.

I hope that allometry can provide a modest opportunity for human biology too. Allometry should serve as a check against spurious values in particular cases. I think it also provides a context for human values which highly focussed specific studies often lack. Finally, it may suggest syndromes of linked traits. For example, small testes in primates are often related to lower levels of sexual activity and increased monogamy (Kenagy & Trombulak 1986). In short, good specific biology has a great deal to contribute to allometry and can also extract something in return. We should try to make the most of this interaction.

References

Adolph, E. F. (1949): Quantitative relations in the physiological constitutions of mammals. *Science* **109**, 579–585.

Altman, P. L. & Dittmer, D. S. eds (1962): *Growth, including reproduction, and morphological development*. Washington, DC: Fed. Amer. Soc. Exp. Biol.

Altman, P. L. & Dittmer, D. S. (1968): *Metabolism*. Bethesda, MD: Fed. Amer. Soc. Exp. Biol.

Altman, P. L. & Dittmer, D. S. (1972): *Biology data book*, Vol. I. Bethesda, MD: Fed. Am. Soc. Exp. Biol.

Andrews, R. M. & Pough, F. H. (1985): Metabolism of squamate reptiles: Allometric and ecological relationships. *Physiol. Zool.* **58**: 214–215.

Asdell, S. A. (1964): *Patterns of mammalian reproduction*. Ithaca, NY: Cornell Univ. Press.

Astrand, P.-O. (1952): *Experimental studies of physical working capacity in relation to sex and age*. Copenhagen: Ejnar Munksgaard.

Astrand, P.-O. & Rodahl, K. (1970): *Textbook of work physiology*. New York: McGraw-Hill.

Blaxter, K. C. (1971): The comparative biology of lactation. In *Lactation*, ed E. R. Falconer, pp. 51–59. London: Butterworth.

Blueweiss, L., Fox, H., Kudzma, V., Nakashima, D., Peters, R. & Sams, S. (1978): Relationships between body size and some life history parameters. *Oecologia* **37**, 257–272.

Brody, S. (1945): *Bioenergetics and growth*. Baltimore, MD: Reinhold.

Calder, W. A. III. (1984): *Size, function and life history*. Cambridge, Mass: Harvard University Press.

Case, T. J. (1978): On the evolution and adaptive significances of postnatal growth rates in the terrestrial vertebrates. *Quart. Rev. Biol.* **53**, 243–282.

Clewe, T. H. (1969): Observations on reproduction of squirrel monkeys in captivity. *J. Reprod. Fert.* (Suppl.) **6**, 151–156.

Di Gregorio, D., Kitchings, T. & van Voris, P. (1978): Radionuclide transfer in terrestrial animals. *Hlth Phys.* **34**, 3–31.

Draper, N. R. & Smith, H. (1981): *Applied regression analysis*, 2nd ed. New York: Wiley.

Durnin, J. V. & Passmore, R. (1967): *Energy, work, and leisure*. London: Heineman.

Eisenberg, J. F. (1981): *The mammalian radiations. An analysis of trends in evolution, adaptation, and behavior*. Chicago: The University of Chicago Press.

Farlow J. O. (1976): A consideration of the trophic dynamics of a late Cretaceous large-dinosaur community (Oldman Formation). *Ecology* **57**, 841–857.

Fedak, M. A. & Seeherman, H. J. (1979): Reappraisal of energetics of locomotion shows identical costs in bipeds and quadrupeds including ostrich and horse. *Nature* (London) **282**, 713–716.

Fleagle, J. G. & Simonds, K. W. (1975): Physical growth of Cebus monkeys (*Cebus albifrons*) during the first year of life. *Growth* **39**, 35–52.

Gould, S. J. (1966): Allometry and size in ontogeny and phylogeny. *Biol. Rev.* **41**, 587–640.

Gould, S. J. (1971): Geometric similarity in allometric growth: a contribution to the problem of scaling in the evaluation of size. *Am. Nat.* **105**, 113–136.

Gould, S. J. (1975): Allometry in primates with an emphasis on the scaling and evolution of the brain. In *Approaches to primate paleobiology*, ed F. Szalay, pp. 244–292. Basel: Karger.

Gould, S. J. & Lewontin, R. C. (1979): The spandrels of San Marco and the Panglossion paradigm: a critique of the adaptationist program. *Proc. Roy. Soc. London Ser. B.* **205**, 581–598.

Gucwinska, H. & Gucwinska, A. (1968): Breeding the Zanzibar galago. *Int. Zoo. Yb.* **8**, 111–114.

Gujarati, D. (1978): *Basic econometrics*. New York: McGraw-Hill.

Harvey, P. H. (1982): On rethinking allometry. *J. Theor. Biol.* **95**, 37–41.

Harvey, P. H. & Clutton-Brock, T. H. (1985): Life history variation in primates. *Evolution* **39**, 559–581.

Harvey, P. H. & Mace, G. M. (1982): Comparisons between taxa and adaptive trends: problems in methodology. In *Current problems in sociobiology*, ed King's College Sociobiology Group, pp. 343–361. Cambridge: Cambridge Univ. Press.

Hemmingsen, A. M. (1960): Energy metabolism as related to body size and respiratory surfaces, and its evolution. *Rep. Steno. Mem. Hosp.* (Copenhagen) **9**, 1–110.

Hennemann, W. W. (1983): Relationships among body mass, metabolic rate, and intrinsic rate of natural increase in mammals. *Oecologia* **56**, 104–108.

Heusner, A. A. (1982): Energy metabolism and body size. I. Is the 0.75 mass exponent of Kleiber's equation a statistical artefact? *Resp. Physiol.* **48**, 1–12.

Hoppeler, H., Lüthi, P., Glassen, H., Weibel, E. R. & Howald, H. (1973): The ultrastructure of the normal human skeletal muscle. A morphometric analysis on untrained men, women, and well-trained orienteers. *Pflügers Arch.* **344**, 217–232.

ICRP—International Commission on Radiological Protection. (1975): *Report of the task force on men.* ICRP publ. 23. Oxford: Pergamon Press.

Jewall, P. A. & Oates, J. F. (1969): Breeding activity in prosimians and small rodents in West Africa. *J. Reprod. Fert.* (Suppl.) **6**: 23–28.

Jolicoeur, P. & Heusner, A. A. (1971): The allometric equation in the analysis of the standard oxygen consumption and body weight of the white rat. *Biometrics* **27**, 841–855.

Kenagy, G. L. & Trombulak, S. C. (1986): Size and function of mammalian testes in relation to body size. *J. Mammal.* **67**, 1–22.

Kermack, K. A. & Haldane, J. B. S. (1950): Organic correlation and allometry. *Biometrika* **37**: 30–41.

Kleiber, M. (1961): *The fire of life.* New York: John Wiley.

Lefebvre, L. (1985): Parent-offspring food sharing: a statistical test of the early weaning hypothesis. *J. Human Evol.* **14**, 255–261.

Leggett, R. W. (1986): Predicting the retention of Cs in individuals. *Health Phys.* **50**, 741–760.

Leutenegger, W. (1973): Maternal fetal weight relationships in primates. *Folia Primat.* **20**, 280–293.

Leutenegger, W. (1979): Evolution of litter size in primates. *Am. Nat.* **114**, 525–531.

Lindstedt, S. L. & Calder, W. A. III. (1981): Body size, physiological time and longevity of homeothermic animals. *Quart. Rev. Biol.* **56**, 1–16.

Linzell, J. L. (1977): Milk yield and energy loss in milk and mammary gland weight in different species. *Dairy Sci. Abs.* **34**, 351–360.

Lorenz, R. & Heinemann, H. (1967): Beitag zur Morphologie und korperlichen Jugendentwicklung des Springtamarin *Callimico goeldii*. *Folia Primatol.* **6**, 1–27.

McKittrick, E. J. (1933): Basal metabolism of Wyoming University women. *J. Nutr.* **11**, 219–223.

McMahon, T. A. & Bonner, J. T. (1983): *On size and life.* New York: Freeman.

Millar, J. S. (1981): Post-partum reproductive characteristics of eutherian mammals. *Evolution* **35**, 1149–1163.

Miller, D. M. (1984): Reducing transformation bias in curve fitting. *Amer. Stat.* **38**, 124–126.

Montgomery, D. C. & Peck, G. A. (1982): *Introduction to linear regression analysis.* New York: John Wiley and Sons.

Nagy, K. (1987): Field metabolic rate and food requirement scaling in mammals and birds. *Ecol. Monogr.* **57**, 111–128.

Paladino, F. V. & King, J. R. (1979): Energy cost of terrestrial locomotion: Biped and quadruped runners compared. *Rev. Can. Biol.* **38**, 321–323.

Peters, R. H. (1983a): *The ecological implications of body size.* New York: Cambridge Univ. Press.

Peters, R. H. (1983b): Size structure of the plankton community along the trophic gradient of Lake Memphremagog. *Can. J. Fish. Aquat. Sci.* **40**, 1770–1778.

Peters, R. H. & Wassenberg, K. (1983): The effect of body size on animal abundance. *Oecologia* **60**, 89–96.

Petter-Rousseaux, A. (1964): Reproductive physiology and behaviour of the Lemuroidea. In *Evolutionary and genetic biology of the primates* II, ed J. Buettner-Janusch, pp. 92–132. New York: Academic Press.

Platt, T. (1985): Structure of the marine ecosystem: Its allometric basis. *Bull. Can. Fish. Aquat. Sci.* **213**, 55–64.

Prothero, J. (1986): Methodological aspects of scaling in biology. *J. Theor. Biol.* **118**, 258–286.

Ricker, W. E. (1984): Computation and uses of central trend lines. *Can. J. Zool.* **62**, 1897–1905.

Robinson, W. R., Peters, R. H. & Zimmerman, J. (1983): The effects of body size and temperature on metabolic rate of organisms. *Can. J. Zool.* **61**, 281–288.

Schmidt-Nielsen, K. (1984): *Scaling: Why is animal size so important?* Cambridge: Cambridge Univ. Press.

Seim, E. & Saether, B.-E. (1983): On rethinking allometry: Which regression model to use. *J. Theor. Biol.* **104**, 161–168.

Smith, R. E. & Kalff, J. (1982): Size-dependent phosphorus uptake kinetics and cell quota in phytoplankton. *J. Phycol.* **18**, 275–294.

Smith, R. J. (1984): Allometric scaling in comparative biology: Problems of concept and method. *Am. J. Physiol.* **246**, R152–R160.

Snedecor, G. W. & Cochran, W. G. (1980): *Statistical methods*, 7th ed. Ames, Iowa: Iowa State Univ. Press.

Snow, C. G. (1967): Some observations on the growth and development of the baboon. In *The baboon in medical research*, Vol. II, ed H. Vagtborg, pp. 187–201. Austin, Texas: Univ. Texas Press.
Taylor, C. R. (1973): Energy cost of animal locomotion. In *Comparative Physiology*, eds L. Bolis, K. Schmidt-Nielsen and S. H. P. Maddrell, pp. 23–42. Amsterdam: North Holland.
Taylor, C. R., Hegland, N. C., McMahon, T. A. & Looney, T. R. (1980): Energy cost of generating muscular force during running: A comparison of large and small mammals. *J. Exper. Biol.* **86**, 9–18.
Taylor, C. R., Maloiy, G. M. O., Weibel, W. R. *et al.* (1981): Design of the mammalian respiratory system. III. Scaling maximal aerobic capacity to body mass: Wild and domestic animals. *Resp. Physiol.* **44**, 25–37.
Taylor, C. R., Schmidt-Nielsen, K. & Raab, J. L. (1970): Scaling of energetic cost of running to body size in mammals. *Amer. J. Physiol.* **219**, 1104–1107.
Vachá, J. & Znojil, V. (1981): The allometric dependence of the life span of erythrocytes on body weight in mammals. *Comp. Biochem. Physiol. A*. **69**, 357–362.
Western, D. (1979): Size, life history and ecology in mammals. *Afr. J. Ecol.* **17**, 185–204.
Zar, J. (1967): The effects of changes in units of measurement on least squares regression lines. *BioScience* **17**, 818–819.

* * * * *

Discussion

Dr Speakman noted the extent of the scatter of points in some of the allometric plots which had been presented and wondered whether these were due to differences in technique used to make the measurements. *Dr Peters* replied that he thought some of the differences could certainly be due to differences among laboratories; however in *Daphnia* he had not found any technical basis for the scatter in regressions describing feeding rates.

Sir Kenneth Blaxter commented that *Dr Peters* had deliberately not given any causal explanation for the fact that the power of weight with which many variables are associated was 0.75 and wondered whether he would be able to give an opinion on this. *Dr Peters* replied that he regarded the relationship as purely statistical and probabilistic and that while a number of explanations had been given none of these was other than retrospective conjecture.

Professor Webster said that studies by Dr Kirkwood at the London Zoo had shown that the growth rates of sub-groups of primates were best described by a series of parallel lines each with a slope close to $W^{0.75}$ but slowing progressively from prosimians to the great apes. He wondered whether Dr Peters would care to comment. *Dr Peters* said that this was quite possible but that he had not analysed the data in this way, beyond the division into gross metabolic classes.

Professor Garrow queried the slide which Dr Peters had shown which indicated that the food intake of man should decline with increasing age whereas that predicted for an average mammal showed stability after maturity had been reached, and wondered whether this arose from lack of non-human animals of comparable age for comparisons. *Dr Peters* replied that the relationship could well be an artifact due to the long life of man and he agreed that the assumption that an animal had constant metabolism after it reached mature weight was not necessarily well founded.

Professor Forbes asked how the growth rates of the various animal species were selected to give the general allometric relationship which Dr Peters had described. *Dr Peters* replied that he had largely used data culled from the ecological literature. These were based on rates of production as well as individual growths and could well be biased towards wild species in their growing season. He stated that zero growth rate data had not been included.

Professor Waterlow asked if, with increasing body weight, most organs increase more slowly than the whole body. There must be some tissue that increases more rapidly. *Dr Peters* replied that the 'missing tissue' appeared to be fat, as had been demonstrated by the analysis [Calder (1984)]. *Professor Gurr*, continuing this part of the discussion, stated that another component could well be the bone mass of the body, to which *Dr Peters* replied that the allometric coefficient for the growth of bone was slightly above one and that, therefore, the bone would contribute to the missing mass but that bone formed a smaller proportion of the body than did fat.

Dr Andrew Prentice pointed out that discussion of generalised allometric relationships fails to account for possible 'grade shifts' in which specific adaptations are represented by changes in the intercept, but not the slope of regressions. This has been well illustrated by Oftedal's work demonstrating that milk output in primates lies on a separate regression substantially below that derived for other mammals.

Mr Payne commented in respect of the statistical methods used, that there were some differing schools of thought. In particular, many people consider that the standard least squares regression is not appropriate for allometric studies in so far as it requires one or other of the two variables to be nominated as being independent and the other dependent. Not only does this entail the kind of causal implication which Dr Peters is anxious to avoid, it introduces a bias into the assessment of the gradient of the line, since all of the variance of both parameters is reflected upon that chosen as the independent variable. Alternative procedures such as the 'major axis' method advocated by R. D. Martin effectively avoid these problems.

2

Comparative physiology of the vertebrate digestive system

C. E. STEVENS

Introduction

Studies of comparative physiology of the digestive system furnish information necessary for the proper care and maintenance of domesticated and captive wild animals, and for the preservation of wild and sometimes endangered species. Another major contribution is the information that studies of structural and functional adaptations to the diet and environment provide for the understanding of basic mechanisms that are involved. This discussion will deal with the general characteristics and major adaptations of the digestive system in each class of vertebrates. Much of this information can be found in books or chapters on the digestive system of fish (Barrington, 1957; Harder, 1975a,b; Kapoor *et al.*, 1975), amphibians (Reeder, 1964), reptiles (Luppa, 1977; Parsons & Cameron, 1977; Skoczylas, 1978), and birds (Ziswiler & Farner, 1972), and the comparative physiology of the vertebrate digestive system (Stevens, 1988).

General characteristics of the digestive system

Although the digestive systems of all vertebrates show many similarities in structure and function, various parts of this system are not always homologous, analogous, or even present. Therefore, broad comparisons can be most easily made under the heading of headgut (mouth parts and pharynx), foregut (oesophagus and stomach), midgut, pancreas, biliary system, and hindgut.

Comparative Nutrition, ed K. Blaxter & I. Macdonald. ©John Libbey 1988.

Headgut and feeding practices

The 43 200 surviving species of vertebrates can be divided into four classes of fish (Myxini, Cephalaspidomorphi, Chondrichthyes, and Osteichthyes) and four classes of tetrapods (Amphibia, Reptilia, Aves, and Mammalia). Cloudsley-Thompson (1972) described the mouthparts of animals in relation to feeding habits. The first two classes of fish are primitive vertebrates that lack articulating jaws, and are often referred to as cyclostomes. The Myxini or hagfish are marine animals. Although a few species are scavengers, most species feed on larger fish by burrowing into their mouth or body. The Cephalaspidomorphi or lampreys include both marine and fresh water species that attach to other fish and feed on their body fluids. However, the larval forms are generally filter-feeders and some lampreys spend most of their life as larvae. Class Chondrichthyes contains the cartilagenous fish (chimeras, sharks, skates, and rays). Osteichthyes consists of the teleosts or bony fish including the lungfish, lobe-finned fish, gar, sturgeon, paddle fish, bowfin, and the most predominant subclass, the ray-finned fish. Fish in these two classes include carnivores, omnivores, and herbivores. They may be micro- or macrophagous and feed on dead or living material. Jaws and teeth are generally used for grasping and tearing, but the mouth parts or pharynx of some species serve to grind food into smaller particles and the mouth parts, pharynx, and gills of a few such as the whale shark, basking shark, and paddle fish have elaborate adaptations for the filtering or sorting of food particles. The tongue of fish is usually relatively immobile. One exception is the archer fish (*Toxotes jaculator*), which uses the tongue to eject a stream of water at its prey.

Larval amphibians include carnivores, omnivores and herbivores, and many of these are microphagous filter-feeders. However, the adult amphibians are all carnivores with weak dentition and in some, such as the frogs and toads, a highly mobile tongue is used for the procurement of prey. The deglutition or swallowing of food is aided by the secretions of mucous cells in the mouth of fish and salivary glands in higher vertebrates. Most reptiles are either carnivores or omnivores, and even the few species of chelonians (turtles, tortoises, and terrapins) and lizards that are herbivores become so only after they reach an advanced stage of maturation. The chelonians use a horny beak for the grasping and tearing of food, but other reptiles have teeth, which are generally used for grasping and/or tearing and continuously replaced throughout life. Some herbivorous reptiles have fairly well-developed molars, which are used for the trituration or grinding of food.

The birds include carnivorous, omnivorous, and herbivorous species. A bill substitutes for the teeth of other vertebrates (except the chelonians). It can be used for grasping, tearing, or breaking down food, and the lateral processes of the flamingo bill are used for filter feeding. The tongue is highly mobile in some species such as the woodpecker.

The original mammals are believed to have been small carnivores that fed principally on insects, other invertebrates, and the eggs or young of other vertebrates (Crompton, 1980). Thirteen of the twenty mammalian orders consist of or include carnivorous species (Table 1). Ten orders include species that are either omnivores or feed on the portion of plants (seeds, nuts, fruit, roots, nectar, pollen), in which nutrients are highly concentrated. Eleven orders include species that can subsist largely on the

Table 1. *Mammalian orders listed according to diets of inclusive species.*

Mammalian order	*Animal*	*Principal diet* *Animal + plant or plant concentrates*	*Plant*
Monotremata (Echidna and duck-billed platypus)	+		
Pholidota (Pangolins)	+		
Tubulidentata (Aardvarks)	+		
Cetacea (Whales, porpoise, dolphins)	+		
Macrocelidea (Elephant shrews)	+		
Scandentia (Tree shrews)	+	+	
Insectivora (Shrews, moles, etc.)	+	+	
Chiroptera (Bats)	+	+	
Carnivora (Dogs, cats, mink, bears, etc.)	+	+	+
Marsupialia (Kangaroos, opposums, etc.)	+	+	+
Edentata (Anteaters, armadillos, sloths)	+	+	+
Rodentia (Rats, mice, squirrels, etc.)	+	+	+
Primates (Lemurs, monkeys, apes, humans)	+	+	+
Dermoptera (Flying lemurs)		+	
Artiodactyla (Cattle, sheep, pigs, etc.)		+	+
Lagomorpha (Rabbits, hares, pica)			+
Perissodactyla (Horses, tapirs, rhinoceros)			+
Proboscidea (Elephants)			+
Sirenia (Manatees, dugongs)			+
Hyracoidea (Conies)			+

Modified from Stevens (1988).

structural or fibrous portion of plants as a result of a highly efficient system for the production of nutrients by microbes endogenous to the gut. Five of these orders contain only this type of species.

The masticatory apparatus of mammals is advanced in its capacity for trituration of food (Davis, 1961; Crompton & Parker, 1978). Teeth erupt opposite one another; permanently in the adult. Most mammals have well-developed incisors and canine teeth, and the premolars and molars are large, with uneven occluding surfaces. The articulation of the jaw and the sling of muscles that attach to the mandible allow for its lateral movement during mastication. However, mammals also demonstrate variations in their feeding apparatus. The anteaters in orders Pholidota, Tubulidentata, Edentata, and Marsupialia tend to have weak jaws, simple teeth (absent in the edentate anteaters), and a highly mobile tongue adapted for this purpose. The filtering apparatus of baleen whales consists of two rows of horny baleen plate that hang from the upper jaws. Carnivorous mammals tend to have well-developed incisors and canine teeth. However, in herbivores the canine teeth are often absent, as are the upper incisors of most ruminants, and the molars tend to have an elaborate occluding surface. With a few exceptions, such as the anteaters and some nectivorous bats, the tongues of most mammals serve principally for the placing of food between the teeth and as aids to deglutition.

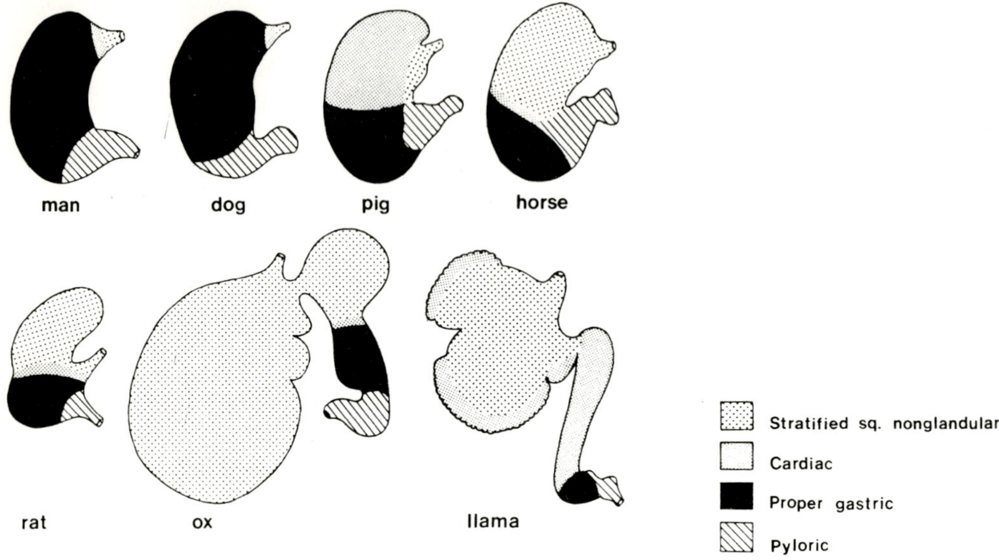

Fig. 1. *Some variations in the distribution of gastric mucosa.* The stomach of each species demonstrates regions of cardiac, proper gastric, and pyloric glandular mucosa. The pig and llama stomachs contain a relatively large region of cardiac glandular mucosa. The pig, horse, rat, llama, and ox also show increasingly large areas of stratified squamous, nonglandular epithelium. Stomachs are not represented on the same scale, eg, the volume capacity of the adult bovine stomach is approximately 70 times that of the human stomach, or 14 times the capacity per kg body weight (Adapted from Stevens 1973).

Foregut

The oesophagus serves as a conduit for the passage of food from the mouth and pharynx to the remainder of the digestive tract. It is used as a temporary storage area in some carnivorous fish and reptiles that swallow their prey whole. Although it does not generally function as an absorptive organ, the oesophagus of marine fish absorbs Na^+ and Cl^-, which decreases the osmolality and NaCl content of sea water before it reaches the stomach. The oesophagus of egg-eating turtles and snakes breaks the shells of these eggs against the vertebral column.

The stomach is absent from the digestive tract of cyclostomes and some advanced species of fish. In other vertebrates, it, or its analogous organs (crop, ventriculus, proventriculus) in birds, serves for the storage and masceration of food and, with few exceptions, for the initial process of protein digestion by HCl and pepsin. The stomach of some reptiles and the ventriculus (gizzard) of most birds is the major site for trituration of food. The stomach of vampire and some frugivorous and nectivorous bats, and that of the whales, provides a large sacculated or compartmentalized reservoir for food storage. The same is true for a few herbivorous species of marsupials (kangaroos), edentates (sloths), rodents (voles, hamsters), primates (colobus and langur monkeys), the sirenians (dugongs and manatees), and most artiodactyles (ruminants, hippopotamus, and some species of swine), where it provides a reservoir for the retention of plant material and microbial production of nutrients.

The epithelial lining of the vertebrate stomach can generally be divided into sequential zones of cardiac, proper gastric, and pyloric mucosa (Fig. 1). Cardiac and pyloric mucosa secrete mucus and an alkaline fluid. The proper gastric mucosa also secretes mucus, in addition to HCl and pepsinogen. The latter two are produced by the same cell in fish, amphibians, reptiles and birds, but by separate cells in mammals. An additional zone of non-glandular, stratified squamous epithelium is found in the stomach of many mammals, including the monotremes, scaley anteaters, whales, perissodactyles, pigs, and most herbivores that have large, complex stomachs (Fig. 1). It may serve as a protection against damage by ingested material. In the ruminants, it aids in the absorption of Na^+, Cl^-, and the volatile fatty acids, which are the principal end-products of carbohydrate fermentation.

Midgut, pancreas and biliary system

The intestine of vertebrates consists of a midgut and hindgut, which are separated by a sphincter or valve in teleosts, some adult amphibians, reptiles, birds, and most mammals. Due to a difference in their relative diameter, these are generally referred to as the small and large intestine in some adult amphibians, reptiles, and birds, and in many mammals.

The midgut of vertebrates is the principal site for the digestion of carbohydrates, lipids and protein by endogenous enzymes, and for absorption of the end-products. This segment of the tract shows numerous adaptations that increase the surface area available for digestion and absorption. Much of this can be attributed to the microvilli or brush border present at the lumen surface of intestinal absorptive cells in all vertebrates and some invertebrates. It is further increased by a spiral valve or pyloric caeca in some fish, by folds and ridges in reptiles, and by villi in the midgut of birds and mammals. The surface area is dependent also on the relative length of the midgut. For example, the length of the midgut of herbivorous lizards tends to be over twice that of carnivorous species in relation to their respective body lengths (Lönnberg, 1902).

The pancreas provides most of the enzymes responsible for extracellular (intraluminal) digestion of carbohydrate, lipid and protein, and an alkaline fluid that aids in the titration of the HCl in gastric effluent. Pancreatic tissue is dispersed along the digestive tract of cyclostomes and some of the more advanced species of fish, but it is formed into a compact organ in other vertebrates.

The biliary system consists of the liver cells that secrete bile, the biliary ducts, and the gallbladder, in which bile is stored and often concentrated prior to its episodic release into the midgut. A gallbladder is present in all but a few species. Exceptions are usually animals that feed almost continuously. The chemical structure of bile salts can vary between and even within classes of vertebrates (Haslewood, 1964, 1967), but they serve the common function of increasing the surface area of fat globules available for enzymatic attack and aiding in the formation of micelles, which are absorbed by the intestinal cells.

Hindgut

The hindgut of vertebrates shows major variations in structure. This segment of the digestive tract, which is short and often difficult to discern in many fish and some

Table 2. *Principal food components and endogenous digestive enzymes of vertebrates.*

Substrate	*Extracellular enzymes*		*Intestinal mucosal enzymes*	*Endproducts*
Carbohydrates				
Amylose Amylopectin Glycogen	α-Amylase		Maltase Isomaltase	Glucose
Chitin	Chitinase		Chitobiase	Glucosamine
Sucrose			Sucrase	Glucose Fructose
Lactose			Lactase	Glucose Galactose
Trehalose			Trehalase	Glucose
Lipids				
Triglycerides	Lipase Co-lipase			β-monoglyceride Fatty acids
Phospholipids	Phospholipase		Phosphatase	Alcohols Fatty acids Phosphate
Cholesterol Esters	Cholesterol Esterase			Cholesterol Fatty acids
Waxes	Lipase Esterase			Monohydric alcohol Fatty acids
Protein				
Protein	Pepsin Trypsin Chymotrypsin Elastase	Carboxypeptidase A Carboxypeptidase B	Aminopeptidase Tripeptidase Dipeptidase	Amino acids
Nucleoprotein	Protein Hydrolysis	Ribonuclease Deoxyribonuclease	Oligonucleotidase 5′ Nucleotidase Alkaline phosphatase Adenosine deaminase	Purine bases Pyrimidine bases Pentose-1-PO_4

Modified from Stevens (1988).

species of Insectivora, whales, bats and marsupials, can be a major site for the retention and recovery of electrolytes and water secreted into the upper digestive tract of other vertebrates. A cul-de-sac or caecum is present at the beginning of the hindgut in a few reptiles. The hindgut of most birds contains a pair of caeca and in a few birds such as the grouse, rhea, and ostrich these have evolved into voluminous organs which contain a major percentage of the total gut contents. In a few fish, the adult amphibians, and all reptiles and birds, the hindgut terminates, along with the urinary tract, in a cloaca. Therefore, urine and digesta are mixed prior to their evacuation from the body, and the hindgut serves as a site for the recovery of urinary electrolytes and water excreted into the cloaca of many reptiles and birds. It is also the major site for microbial production of nutrients in herbivorous reptiles and birds, and most herbivorous mammals.

The digestive and urinary tracts of most mammals exit separately from the body. The mammalian hindgut tends to be longer than that of lower vertebrates in relation to body length. A caecum is present in many species, and it contains a large percentage of the total gut contents in most small mammalian herbivores. In the larger mammalian herbivores, the colon is the most voluminous segment of the hindgut, and it is often sacculated due to haustral formations. The colon of perissodactyles and elephants is both sacculated and compartmentalized.

Endogenous digestive enzymes

Vonk & Western (1984) have recently reviewed the comparative biochemistry and physiology of enzymatic digestion. Table 2 lists the principal substrates that are available for digestion by endogenous enzymes, the principal enzymes that act upon these substrates, and the end-products of this activity. The predominant complex carbohydrates are the starches, which are the storage carbohydrates of plants (amylose and amylopectin) and animals (glycogen), and chitin, the structural carbohydrate present in the integument of insects and a number of other invertebrates. Sucrose is the most common disaccharide found in plants. The major disaccharides in animals are trehalose, the blood transport carbohydrate of insects, and lactose, the carbohydrate present in mammalian milk. The only free monosaccharides found in significant quantities are glucose and fructose in plants and glucose in animals.

The principal lipids are the triglycerides, phospholipids, glycolipids, and waxes. Triglycerides are the major components of animal fat and the seeds of plants, and phospholipids are major components of the cell and cell organelle membranes of animals. Glycolipids are found mainly in photosynthetic tissue of plants. The waxes of most general significance as a dietary source are the wax-esters. They constitute 20% of the lipids in planktonic crustaceans (Lee *et al.*, 1972), and it has been estimated that as much as 50% of the organic material synthesized by phytoplankton is temporarily stored as wax by marine animals (Benson & Lee, 1975).

Plant and animal protein consists of chains of L-amino acids linked together with peptide bonds to form a wide range of compounds of variable sensitivity to attack by endogenous enzymes. The nucleic acids, ribonucleic acid (RNA) and deoxyribonucleic acid (DNA), are found in the cells of plants and animals. Except in bacteria and viruses, they are mostly bound to protein.

The enzymes that hydrolyze these substrates consist of those that act within the gut lumen (extracellular) and those that act in the brush border or cytosol of intestinal cells. Extracellular enzymes, with the exception of α-amylase, pepsinogen and chitinase, are secreted solely by the pancreas. The salivary glands of some species produce additional amounts of α-amylase. Pepsinogen is secreted by the stomach of all vertebrates, with the exception of the stomachless fish, some larval amphibians, and a few mammals. Chitinase has been demonstrated in the gastric mucosa and pancreas of many fish, adult amphibians, reptiles, birds, and mammals. Chitobiase activity has been demonstrated in the gastric, pancreatic, and intestinal tissue of the horseshoe bat *Rhinolophus* (Jeuniaux, 1962) and the pancreas of chimaeras (Fänge *et al.*, 1979). It also has been found in the gastric and intestinal mucosa of fish, but Vonk & Western (1984) concluded that this may be of dietary or microbial origin. The other pancreatic enzymes have been demonstrated in species belonging to all classes of vertebrates with the exception of elastase and carboxypeptidase B, which do not appear to be present in cyclostomes, amphibians, or reptiles.

Digestive enzymes in the brush border or cytosol of intestinal cells have been examined in relatively few mammals and very few lower vertebrates. Maltase appears to be common to all vertebrates, but sucrase and trehalase are absent from the intestine of some. Lactase appears to be largely confined to neonate mammals, but is absent in pinnipeds (seals, sea lions, and walruses), which produce little or no lactose in their milk, and decreases or disappears in the adults of many species (Koldovsky, 1970).

The levels of enzymes that attack protein and polypeptides tend to be highest in carnivores and lowest in herbivores. Pancreatic ribonuclease levels tend to be much higher in herbivores that have a stomach populated with large colonies of bacteria. Enzyme activity also can vary with age. This is especially true if there is a marked change in the normal diet such as that seen between larval and adult amphibians and between neonate and adult mammals.

Intestinal absorption of carbohydrate is limited to glucose, galactose, xylose, fructose, mannose, and a few other monosaccharides. These are absorbed by mechanisms of active transport (glucose, galactose, xylose), facilitated diffusion (fructose), or passive diffusion that appear to be common to all vertebrates and some invertebrates. The same appears to be generally true for mechanisms responsible for the absorption of peptides and amino acids. Acetyl glucosamine absorption has been demonstrated in the cat shark *Scylinhinus* (Alliot, 1967). The end-products of lipid digestion appear to be passively absorbed by similar processes in all vertebrates.

Production of nutrients by endogenous microbes

Microbes indigenous to the forestomach of sheep and cattle convert a wide range of substances into utilizable nutrients (Hungate, 1968; Bryant, 1977; Phillipson, 1977). A large portion of most plants is composed of structural carbohydrates (cellulose, hemicellulose, pectin, galactan), which are not subject to digestion by endogenous enzymes of vertebrates. Microbes in the ruminant forestomach ferment sugars, starches, and the structural carbohydrates into volatile fatty acids (VFA), principally acetate, propionate, and butyrate, which are readily absorbed and utilized as a source of energy. These microbes also are capable of converting endogenous urea and a variety of dietary nitrogenous compounds into ammonia or into essential amino acids and microbial protein. Furthermore, they can synthesize the B-complex vitamins and vitamin K required by the host. A similar process of microbial fermentation has been observed in the stomach of kangaroos (Moir *et al.*, 1956; Hume, 1984), sloths (Denis *et al.*, 1967), and the colobus and langur monkeys (Bauchop & Martucci, 1968).

Microbial fermentation of carbohydrate into VFA also has been demonstrated in the hindgut of carnivores and herbivorous reptiles (Guard, 1980), and omnivorous and herbivorous birds (McBee & West, 1969; Clemens *et al.*, 1975), and these organic

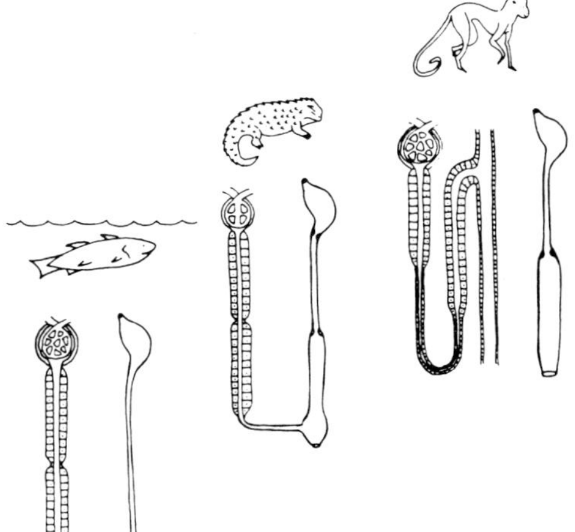

Fig. 2. *Development of the nephron and hindgut in relation to habitat.* The nephrons of the fish and reptile kidneys are limited in their ability to conserve fluid. However, urinary electrolytes and water also are recovered by the hindgut of reptiles and birds. A few mammals have retained the cloaca, but the majority excrete their digesta and urine separately, and conservation of urinary water is largely accomplished by the loop of Henle and countercurrent multiplier system of the nephron. (Modified from Smith, 1943, by Stevens, 1977).

acids appear to be the major anions present in the hindgut of most carnivorous, omnivorous, and herbivorous mammals (Argenzio & Stevens, 1984). The substrates for VFA production in the hindgut include starches that have escaped digestion in the midgut, the large carbohydrate portion of mucus, and the structural carbohydrates of plants. VFA are readily absorbed from the hindgut and their absorption is intimately tied to the secretion and absorption of other electrolytes (Stevens *et al.*, 1986). Bacteria in the hindgut of mammalian herbivores have been shown to also convert urea and other endogenous nitrogenous compounds into ammonia and microbial protein, and synthesize vitamins in a manner similar to that seen in the ruminant forestomach.

Secretion and absorption of electrolytes and water

Digestion of food requires the secretion of substantial quantities of Na^+, H^+, Cl^-, HCO_3^-, and water by the digestive tract and its accessory organs. Most of these ions are reabsorbed from the midgut and hindgut, and the mechanisms responsible for this absorption have recently been reviewed by Powell (1987). Water is absorbed as a result of osmotic gradients produced by the absorption of these and other substances. The hindgut also reabsorbs some of the urinary electrolytes and water excreted into the cloaca of reptiles and birds. Urine and digesta are refluxed the length of the hindgut and into the caecum, when present, by periodic waves of antiperistaltic contractions, which originate in the area of the cloaca (Fig. 2). This mechanism for the reflux of digesta is retained in mammals that lack a cloaca, but it is confined to the more proximal segments of the hindgut.

The daily salivary, gastric, pancreatic, biliary, and small intestinal secretions into the upper digestive tract of humans previously starved for 24 hours was equivalent to approximately 40% of the extracellular fluid volume and 30–40% of its Na^+, Cl^-, and HCO_3^- content (Soergel & Hofmann, 1972). Approximately 80% of the water was reabsorbed by the small intestine, principally the ileum and jejunum. The large intestine reabsorbed an additional 18% of these secretions, plus any secretions of its own. Feeding places a much larger absorptive load on the small and large intestine.

The gut of herbivores secretes and retains considerably higher volumes of fluid. The alimentary tract of sheep contains a much higher percentage of the total body water as compared to that of humans. Most of this is found in the voluminous forestomach, but the large intestine of many herbivorous mammals also contains a major fraction of the total body water. This is chiefly due to much greater volumes of secretory fluid. The daily resorptive load of the sheep large intestine, aside from any additional secretions by the caecum and colon, was found to be equivalent to approximately one-half of the extracellular fluid volume (Kay & Pfeffer, 1970). The daily reabsorptive load of the pony large intestine, including its own secretions, was greater than the total extracellular fluid volume of these animals (Argenzio *et al.*, 1974).

Evolution of herbivores

The adaptations of the reptilian and avian hindgut that retained digesta and urine for reabsorption of electrolytes and water also encouraged the multiplication of endogenous bacteria. These bacteria can aid in the conservation of nitrogen by converting either uric acid or urea or other nitrogenous compounds to ammonia or microbial protein. They convert endogenous and dietary carbohydrate to VFA, providing an additional energy source to carnivores and omnivores and the principal source of energy in herbivorous species.

As stated earlier, the mammalian hindgut tends to be longer than that of lower vertebrates and many species have a well-developed caecum. In most mammals that have been studied, the pacemaker for antiperistaltic contraction is located at a more proximal site in the colon, with the result that the caecum and proximal colon are the major sites for digesta retention. There is evidence in some herbivorous species that these proximal segments of the hindgut or large intestine secrete and retain fluids, and the more distal segments of colon and the rectum are the principal sites of electrolyte and water absorption (Stevens *et al.*, 1980).

Many mammals are herbivores that can derive a major portion of their nutritional requirements from the products of microbial fermentation and metabolism. Those of small body size, such as the lagomorphs, herbivorous rodents and small herbivorous marsupials, utilize the caecum as the major site for the retention of microbes and their substrates. The effectiveness of this process as a source of nutrients is improved in many of these species by coprophagy, which cycles unabsorbed VFA and the proteins and vitamins synthesized by bacteria into the upper digestive tract. It is further improved in some species by adaptations of the proximal colon and caecum that allow periodic passage and reingestion of essentially unaltered caecal contents (caecotrophy). The practice and advantages of caecotrophy have been reviewed by Hörnick & Björnhag (1979) and Björnhag (1987). In herbivores of larger body size, the proximal colon is the major site of microbial activity. This is true for most large primates, the perissodactyles and elephants. Microbial production of nutrients in the large intestine has the advantage of allowing for the more efficient extraction of readily available nutrients prior to their attack by gut microbes. It also allows for an increase in the transit time of plant material of low nutritive value through the gut.

The stomach is the major site for microbial digestion in sloths, kangaroos, colobus and langur monkeys, and all artiodactyles with the exception of some species of swine. Microbial production of nutrients in the stomach allows for the more efficient extraction of end-products, especially proteins and vitamins, in the absence of coprophagy. These microbes also aid in the destruction of plant toxins. Adaptations of the ruminant forestomach provide for the prolonged retention of large digesta particles, resulting in a very efficient system for the extraction of nutrients from plant fibre. Janis (1976) hypothesized that this efficiency could explain the replacement of perissodactyles by artiodactyles (principally ruminants) as the predominant ungulates following the replacement of much of the tropical forest with grasslands, during the Eocene Epoch of the Tertiary Period. However, Van Soest (1982) concluded that the ruminant type of forestomach is most efficient in animals with a body weight of 500 to 1800 kg. Therefore prolonged retention of digesta in the stomach also places constraints on the size of these animals, which gives rise to some interesting conjectures on where microbial digestion took place along the digestive tract of the giant sloth (*Megatherium*) and the largest herbivorous dinosaurs (*Apatosaurus*).

Conclusions

This brief review demonstrates some of the major adaptations of the vertebrate digestive system to the diet, environment, and other characteristics of these animals. As one would expect, the mouth parts and pharynx show a wide range of variations that often correlate with the diet. The same is true for adaptations of the stomach or large intestine to the diet of herbivores. However, some adaptations are related to the environment or other characteristics of the animal. For example, the necessity to pass ingested water through the gills of fish requires special structures such as the gill rakers to prevent the escape of food particles, and flight placed restrictions on both the total weight of the digestive tract and the distribution of this weight in birds. Variations in the foregut are chiefly limited to the relative size, the degree of compartmentalization, and the distribution of various types of epithelium. The midgut demonstrates a number of structural variations that affect the surface area of its lumen but, with some exceptions, its principal digestive and absorptive functions appear to have evolved prior to the appearance of vertebrates. Although there are some major variations in the complement and activity of digestive enzymes, most of these enzymes also appeared earlier in the phylogeny of animals. The hindgut of non-mammalian vertebrates shows many adaptations related to the recovery of electrolytes and water. These are expanded in a few reptiles and birds and in many mammals, to serve the additional function of providing an efficient system for microbial production of nutrients.

The culture, husbandry, and general care of animals is partly dependent on an understanding of the digestive systems. Many of the problems associated with the maintenance of domestic and wild herbivores stem from the fact that they have a digestive system designed for continuous feeding, rather than the episodic digestive and absorptive functions that result from the feeding of one or two meals a day. Many species of large African herbivores are endangered due to the restrictions of expanding farmlands or their confinement to an area that allows observation by tourists. They require extensive rangelands to obtain enough feed and take advantage of the interdependency between those that require succulent versus mature plant material, and to interfere with the life cycles of gut parasites. More information is needed on food chains such as the importance of the wax-esters to marine animals.

The use of comparative physiology for the better understanding of basic mechanisms is of special interest to physiologists and nutritionists. One of the major questions is what constitutes a good model for the study of a particular mechanism. One could argue that the rabbit, guinea pig, hamster and rat have developed special adaptations of the large intestine that severely limit their use in studies principally designed for the understanding of the human counterpart. This type of argument has been presented as evidence that human physiology should be studied in humans. However, aside from the fact that the cost or potential danger of research on human subjects tends to encourage either less rigidly controlled retrospective studies or prospective studies that are non-invasive and safe, the rodents and lagomorphs can be used if their adaptations are understood. Furthermore, they have provided some very useful information on the mechanisms responsible for antiperistaltic contractions and the secretory and absorptive mechanisms of the colon. The equine large intestine has proved to be an excellent model for compartmental analysis of secretion, absorption, and digesta transit. Due to ready access and a lack of glandular secretions, the rumens of sheep and cattle have provided much of the basic information on microbial fermentation of carbohydrate and the synthesis of protein and vitamins, as well as the mechanisms of VFA absorption.

A great deal of information on renal function was learned from studies of aglomerular fish and the separate blood supply to the glomerulus and renal tubules of birds. For similar reasons, much can be learned from animals that lack a stomach, a gallbladder, or the ability to produce lactase, as well as those that produce chitinase or very high levels of ribonuclease. Therefore the major requirement for selection of a good animal model is effective communication between those with a primary interest in basic mechanisms and those who are principally interested in the animals themselves.

References

Alliot, E. (1967): Absorption intestinale de l'N-acétyl-glucosamine chez la petite Roussette: *Scylliorhinus canicula*. *C. R. Soc. Biol. (Paris)* **161**, 2544–2546.

Argenzio, R. A., Lowe, J. E., Pickard, D. W. & Stevens, C. E. (1974): Digesta passage and water exchange in the equine large intestine. *Am. J. Physiol.* **226**, 1035–1042.

Argenzio, R. A. & Stevens, C. E. (1984): The large bowel — a supplementary rumen? *Proc. Nutr. Soc.* **43**, 13–23.

Barrington, E. J. W. (1957): The alimentary canal and digestion. In *The physiology of fishes*, Vol. 1: *Metabolism*, ed M. E. Brown, pp. 109–161. New York: Academic Press.

Bauchop, T. & Martucci, R. W. (1968): Ruminant-like digestion of the langur monkey. *Science* **161**, 698–700.

Benson, A. A. & Lee, R. F. (1975): The role of wax in oceanic food chains. *Sci. Am.* **232**, 77–86.

Björnhag, G. (1987): Comparative aspects of digestion in the hindgut of mammals. The colonic separation mechanism (CSM) (a review). *Dtsch. Tierärztl. Wschr.* **94**, 33–36.

Bryant, M. P. (1977): Microbiology of the rumen. In *Dukes' Physiology of Domestic Animals*, 9th ed., ed M. J. Swenson, pp. 287–304. Ithaca: Cornell University Press.

Clemens, E. T., Stevens, C. E. & Southworth, M. (1975): Sites of organic acid production and pattern of digesta movement in the gastrointestinal tract of geese. *J. Nutr.* **105**, 1341–1350.

Cloudsley-Thompson, J. L. (1972): The classification and study of animals by feeding habits. In *Biology of nutrition*, Vol. 18, ed R. N. T-W-Fiennes, pp. 439–470. Elmsford, N. Y: Pergamon Press.

Crompton, A. W. (1980): Biology of the earliest mammals. In *Comparative physiology: primitive mammals*, ed K. Schmidt-Nielsen, L. Bolis, and C. R. Taylor, pp. 1–12. New York: Cambridge University Press.

Crompton, A. W. & Parker, P. (1978): Evolution of the mammalian masticatory apparatus. *Am. Sci.* **66**, 192–201.

Davis, D. D. (1961): Origin of the mammalian feeding mechanism. *Am. Zoologist* **1**, 229–234.

Denis, C., Jeuniaux, C., Gerebtzoff, M. A. & Goffart, M. (1967): La digestion stomacale chez un paresseux: l'unau *Choloepus hoffmanni* Peters. *Ann. Soc. R. Zool. Belg.* **97**, 9–29.

Fänge, R., Lundblad, G., Lind, J. & Slettengren, K. (1979): Chitinolytic enzymes in the digestive system of marine fishes. *Marine Biol.* **53**, 317–321.

Guard, C. L. (1980): The reptilian digestive system: general characteristics. In *Comparative physiology: Primitive mammals*, ed K. Schmidt-Nielsen, L. Bolis and C. R. Taylor, pp. 43–51. Cambridge: Cambridge University Press.

Harder, W. (1975a): *Anatomy of Fishes, Part 1*. Stuttgart: E. Schweizerbart'sche Verlagsbuchhandlung.

Harder, W. (1975b): *Anatomy of Fishes, Part 2*. Stuttgart: E. Schweizerbart'sche Verlagsbuchhandlung.

Haslewood, G. A. D. (1964): The biological significance of chemical differences in bile salts. *Biol. Rev.* **39**, 537–574.

Haslewood, G. A. D. (1967): Bile salt evolution. *J. Lipid Res.* **8**, 535–550.

Hörnicke, H. & Björnhag, G. (1979): Coprophagy and related strategies for digesta utilization. In *Digestive physiology and metabolism in ruminants*, ed Y. Ruckebusch and P. Thivend, pp. 707–730. Westport, Conn: AVI Publishing.

Hume, I. D. (1984): Microbial fermentation in herbivorous marsupials. *BioScience* **34**, 435–440.

Hungate, R. E. (1968): Ruminal fermentation. In *Handbook of physiology*, Sec. 6: *Alimentary canal*, Vol. 5: *Bile, digestion; ruminal physiology*, Sec. 6, ed C. F. Code and W. Heidel, pp. 2725–2745. Washington, D.C: American Physiological Society.

Janis, C. (1976): The evolutionary strategy of the equidae and the origins of rumen and cecal digestion. *Evolution* **30**, 757–774.

Jeuniaux, C. (1962): Digestion de la chitine chez les oiseaux et les mammifères. *Ann. Soc. R. Zool. Belg.* **92**, 27–45.

Kapoor, B. G., Smit, H. & Verighina, I. A. (1975): The alimentary canal and digestion in teleosts. *Adv. Mar. Biol.* **13**, 109–239.

Kay, R. N. B. & Pfeffer, E. (1970): Movements of water and electrolytes into and from the intestine of sheep. In *Physiology of digestion and metabolism in the ruminant*, ed A. T. Phillipson, pp. 390–402. Newcastle upon Tyne: Oriel Press.

Koldovsky, O. (1970): Digestion and absorption during development. In *Physiology of the perinatal period*, ed U. Stave, pp. 379–415. New York: Appleton-Century-Crofts.

Lee, R. F., Hirota, J., Nevenzel, J. C., Sauerheber, R., Lewis, A. & Benson, A. A. (1972): Lipids in the marine environment. *Calif. Mar. Res. Comm., CalCOFI Rep.* **16**, 95–102.

Lönnberg, E. (1902): On some points of relation between the morphological structure of the intestine and the diet of reptiles. *Bih. Svensk Vet. Ak. Handl.* **28**, 1–51.

Luppa, H. (1977): Histology of the digestive tract. In *Biology of the reptilia*, Vol. 6., ed C. E. Gans and T. S. Parsons, pp. 225–314. New York: Academic Press.

McBee, R. H. & West, G. C. (1969): Cecal fermentation in the willow ptarmigan. *Condor* **71**, 54–58.

Moir, R. J., Somers, M. & Waring, H. (1956): Studies on marsupial nutrition. I. Ruminant-like digestion in a herbivorous marsupial *Setonix brachyurus* (Quoy and Gairmard). *Aust. J. Biol. Sci.* **9**, 293–304.

Parsons, T. S. & Cameron, J. E. (1977): Internal relief of the digestive tract. In *Biology of the reptilia*, Vol. 6, ed C. Gans and T. S. Parsons, pp. 159–224. New York: Academic Press.

Phillipson, A. T. (1977): Ruminant digestion. In *Dukes' physiology of domestic animals*, 9th ed., ed M. J. Swenson, pp. 250–286. Ithaca, New York: Cornell University Press.

Powell, D. W. (1987): Intestinal water and electrolyte transport. In *Physiology of the gastrointestinal tract*, 2nd ed., Vol. 2, ed L. R. Johnson, J. Christensen, M. J. Jackson, E. D. Jacobson, and J. H. Walsh, pp. 1267–1306. New York: Raven Press.

Reeder, W. G. (1964): The digestive system. In *Physiology of the amphibia*, Vol. 1, ed J. A. Moore, pp. 99–149. New York: Academic Press.

Skoczylas, R. (1978): Physiology of the digestive tract. In *Biology of the reptilia*, Vol. 8, ed C. G. Gans and K. A. Gans, pp. 589–717. New York: Academic Press.

Smith, H. W. (1943): The evolution of the kidney. In *Lectures on the kidney, Porter Lectures*, Ser. IX. Lawrence, Kansas: University of Kansas Press.

Soergel, K. H. & Hofmann, A. F. (1972): Absorption. In *Pathophysiology: Altered regulatory mechanisms in disease*, ed E. D. Frohlich, pp. 423–453. Philadelphia: J. B. Lippincott.

Sperber, L., Björnhag, G. & Ridderstrale, Y. (1983): Function of proximal colon in lemming and rat. *Swed. J. Agric. Res.* **13**, 243–256.

Stevens, C. E. (1973): Transport across rumen epithelium. In *Transport mechanisms in epithelia*, ed H. H. Ussing and N. A. Thorn, pp. 404–426. New York: Academic Press.

Stevens, C. E. (1977): Comparative physiology of the digestive system. In *Duke's physiology of domestic animals*, ed M. J. Swenson, 9th ed., pp. 216–232. Ithaca, New York: Cornell University Press.

Stevens, C. E. (1988): *Comparative physiology of the vertebrate digestive system.* Cambridge: Cambridge University Press.

Stevens, C. E., Argenzio, R. A. & Clemens, E. T. (1980): Microbial digestion: rumen versus large intestine. In *Digestive physiology and metabolism in ruminants*, ed Y. Ruckebusch and P. Thivend, pp. 685–706. Lancaster, U.K: MTP Press.

Stevens, C. E., Argenzio, R. A. & Roberts, M. C. (1986): Comparative physiology of the mammalian colon and suggestions for animal models of human disorders. *Clin. Gastroenterol.* **15**, 763–786.

Van Soest, P. J. (1982): *Nutritional ecology of the ruminant.* Corvallis, Oregon: O & B Books.

Vonk, H. J. & Western J. R. H. (1984): *Comparative biochemistry and physiology of enzymatic digestion.* New York: Academic Press.

Ziswiler, V. & Farner, D. S. (1972): Digestion and the digestive system. In *Avian biology*, Vol. 2, ed D. S. Farner, J. R. King and K. C. Parkes, pp. 343–430. New York: Academic Press.

* * * * *

Discussion

Dr Widdowson asked *Dr Stevens* to say something about comparative aspects of digestive tract activity during suckling.

Dr Stevens said that the available information was largely limited to laboratory rodents, the domestic pig, and ruminants. The level of digestive enzymes change during the nursing period, but the most pronounced changes are seen following weaning. The development of HCl secretion can also vary, being present at birth in the guinea pig, beginning after a delay of hours in humans, or after days in other species. The large intestine is also not completely developed at the time of birth in mammals.

Sir Kenneth Blaxter mentioned that in the ruminant there was evidence of considerable development of the rumen attendant on the concommitant development of an active flora and he wondered whether the same was true of the large intestine. *Dr Stevens* stated that the microbial population of the hind gut develops fairly quickly but in the pig the capacity of the hind gut to ferment carbohydrate and absorb electrolytes and water continues after the weaning process.

Dr Bassett observed that it was now recognized that gastrointestinal tract function was regulated by a very complex neuroendocrine system and wondered to what extent variations between species in salt and water reabsorption by the hind gut might be related to differences in this regulatory system. *Dr Stevens* replied that this is complicated by the discovery of additional neurosecretory agents and the dual neurosecretory and endocrine effects of some hormones. However Burnstock has provided some excellent reviews on the evolution of the autonomic nervous system, neurosecretory agents and hormones in vertebrates.

Dr Elia also wondered what proportion of protein was indeed absorbed intact in marine fish and neonatal mammals, where it was subsequently dealt with, and what the implications were for the immune system. *Dr Stevens* replied that there appeared to be little information on this, though phagocytosis by midgut mucosa seems to have generally disappeared with the appearance of the brush border in some invertebrates and all vertebrates.

Dr Stevens mentioned the role of bacteria in digestion of endogenous carbohydrates, such as mucus, and of endogenous protein, and stated that this topic would be dealt with later by Professor Van Soest.

Professor Jackson raised the question of retrograde flow, to which *Dr Stevens* replied that examples of retrograde flow could be found in the opossum where the pacemaker is situate at the cloaca, as it is in reptiles and birds, but in most animals the pacemaker is situated more proximally in the colon where its role appears to be that of retaining digesta in the proximal colon and cecum. He also mentioned the studies of Sperber *et al.*, which showed a mechanism in the spiral colon of the lemming that selectively traps bacteria in mucus and transports them back into the cecum.

Professor Stock said that most rodents seemed unable to vomit and asked whether this was a morphological problem, to which *Dr Stevens* replied that the reason was unknown, but the absence of vomiting in rats was associated with highly developed senses of taste and smell which protected them against toxic substances. He went on to refer to the absence of vomiting in horses in which the stomach will often rupture upon extreme distention. They may be protected from toxic substances by their selective grazing and rapid transit of digesta through the stomach and small intestine.

Dr McCracken emphasized the role of diet in the induction of digestive enzymes and this led to a discussion relating to the role of fore-stomach fermentation as seen in ruminants and certain herbivorous species on the detoxification of plant toxins.

Dr Coates pointed out that evidence with experimental animals suggested that although vitamins were synthesized by microbes in the lower gut they were not available to the host without coprophagy. For example germ-free rats do not survive on a vitamin-K-deficient diet, whereas their conventional counterparts thrive. If, however, coprophagy is prevented, the conventional rats also die. This is also true for the B vitamins. She also mentioned that comparisons between germ-free and conventional chicks had shown that the gut microflora have a protein-sparing effect. In New Guinea Highlanders eating a very low protein diet the oral administration of urea labelled with N^{15} resulted in the labelling of lysine in plasma proteins, which could only have come about through the microbial degradation of protein and subsequent absorption of its constituent amino acids. [Tanaka, N., Kubo, K., Shiraki, K., Hoishi, H. & Yoshimura, H. (1980): A pilot study on protein metabolism in Papua New Guinea Highlanders. *J. Nutr. Sci. Vitaminol.* **26**, 247–59.]

Dr Tomkins asked whether there were major structural differences in terms of the mucosa in different species. Morphological variations were extremely interesting but surely the functional problems relate to the nature of the mucosa. *Dr Stevens* replied that in comparing different species there were no differences in the rates of volatile fatty acid absorption per unit surface area but there were differences in the rate of sodium absorption and bicarbonate appearance in the lumen among species, and between the proximal and distal colon of some species. It appears that the proximal colon and caecum retain water and provide the buffer required for microbial activity, whereas the distal colon absorbs sodium and water at much more rapid rates. The distal colon of the horse, for example, absorbs sodium at a rate six times that of the proximal colon. Therefore in thinking of structural and functional aspects, the emphasis must be on the role of the large intestine in the recovery of water and sodium.

Professor Armstrong mentioned that studies had been made in the horse by infusion of ^{35}S into the large intestine. The results of these experiments in Australia had shown that there was no label found in methionine or cystine in the body. This experiment is not in agreement with that quoted by Dr Coates in man. Professor Armstrong also commented on experiments undertaken in his department in which higher fibre levels in the diet of pigs led to increasing levels of butyrate and which appeared to provide the preferred substrate for large intestine metabolism and to stimulate the growth of the epithelium, a phenomenon similar to that noted in the calf. *Dr Stevens* stated that in the horse the butyrate arising from the fermentation may well be the major metabolite, as it is rapidly absorbed and metabolized by the epithelium of the large intestine.

Professor Conning asked about the similarity of strains of bacteria in the hind guts of different species, to which *Dr Stevens* replied that many common bacterial species have been isolated. However, methanogenic bacteria are absent in most species, probably due to the more rapid transit of digesta through the hind gut.

Professor Care asked whether the butyrate in the large intestine increased the rate of blood flow to the epithelium, to which *Dr Stevens* replied that he did not know, but high concentrations of butyrate did produce inflammation of the epithelium, similar to that seen in the rumen.

3

Comparative aspects of the energy exchange

A. J. F. WEBSTER

Introduction

This paper will consider energy exchanges in animals primarily from the standpoint of the nutritionist who is concerned with the one-way flow of chemical energy in food towards work necessary for the maintenance of life, activity, thermoregulation etc, and to synthetic processes of growth, pregnancy and lactation. Nutrient energy supply will generally be described by metabolizable energy (ME), defined as the gross energy of food less that lost as faeces, urine and combustible gases. This is a precise and readily measurable description of the energy absorbed from the gut and available to do work in the body ('physiological fuel'). It does not, of course, describe the chemical nature of the absorbed substrates, eg, the balance between lipogenic 2-C and glucogenic 3-C fragments, and this precludes any more than an empirical description of the partition of ME between heat production (H) and energy retained in body tissues or secreted in milk as protein (RE_p) or fat (RE_f). Nevertheless, most of the important comparative aspects of energy exchange in mammals and birds can still be described perfectly satisfactorily using absolute energy units (watts, kJ/d or MJ/d). Energy exchange is therefore described simply by

$$ME = H \pm (RE_p + RE_f) \qquad (1)$$

The energy content of protein and fat may be assumed as constant at 23.5 kJ/g and 39.0 kJ/g respectively. The elements of food chemistry that define the ME concentration in dry matter (M/D, kJ/g) will be considered only briefly. This paper is therefore principally an analysis of the factors that determine metabolic heat production and the energetic efficiency of processes such as growth and lactation.

Scaling rules for body size

Brody (1945) and Kleiber (1961) produced the first clear description of the allometric relationship between the rate of metabolic processes and body size by relating basal metabolism or fasting heat production (Hmin) in different species of mammal to *metabolic body size*, or $W^{3/4}$. King & Farner (1961) derived essentially the same exponent for birds. The differences between the published exponents (Kleiber = 0.75, Brody = 0.734, King & Farmer = 0.744) is trivial. I accept Kleiber's conclusion that the fractional exponent ¾ conveys all the precision that is necessary, or indeed justified. It follows that physiological rate functions other than Hmin, such as cardiac output, and less obviously, appetite, metabolizable energy (ME,MJ/d) and growth rate (dw/dt,kg/d) also scale across species according to $W^{3/4}$. Several authors (eg Haysson & Lacy, 1985; Heusner, 1982; Thonney *et al.*, 1976) have variously criticized the validity of $W^{3/4}$ as a means to confer proportionality on measurements of rate processes in species differing greatly in body size. However, these reviews are themselves open to criticism on several grounds, most especially failure to account properly for differences in body composition or physiological state (q.v.). At this stage, it can be said with confidence that provided the comparison is made between species, and the animals are in a similar physiological state (eg fasting), then the use of the exponent $W^{3/4}$ to define metabolic body size is, as a first approximation, a satisfactory way to compare energy exchanges independently of body weight.

Taylor (1965) and Ricklefs (1968) examined the time taken to mature in mammals and birds respectively and revealed that maturing interval is a constant function of mature, asymptotic body weight (Wa,kg) raised to an exponent close to $Wa^{1/4}$. Taylor (1965) coined the phrase *metabolic age* (θ metabolic days) to relate maturing time (t, days from conception) to $Wa^{1/4}$. Thus

$$\theta = t.A^{-1/4} \qquad (2)$$

In this paper, two expressions are used to provide size-independent indices of postnatal maturation time; (i) θ_{50} = metabolic age in days from conception/$A^{1/4}$ at 50% maturity (0.5 Wa); (ii) $\theta(25 \text{ to } 75)$ = metabolic time ($t.A^{-1/4}$) to grow from 0.25 to 0.75 Wa. Once again, the concept of metabolic time can be applied to a range of metabolic intervals as widely disparate as blood circulation time, cellular turnover and longevity, although in the latter case the human species is particularly aberrant.

The link between the concepts of metabolic size ($fW^{3/4}$) and metabolic time ($fW^{-1/4}$) should be self-evident.

In any allometric relationship

$$y \alpha x^{b}$$

$$\text{so } y/x \, \alpha \, x^{(b-1)}$$

Suppose y = Hmin or dw/dt, which are known to be proportional to $W^{3/4}$ and $Wa^{3/4}$ respectively, then

$$\text{Metabolic turnover time Hmin}/W \alpha W^{-1/4}$$

$$\text{Maturation time, } dw/dt.Wa^{-1} \alpha Wa^{-1/4}$$

It follows from this that fasting metabolism (Hmin), maintenance requirement for ME (ME_m), growth rate, energy retention, and thus appetite for ME with respect to maintenance (ME/ME_m) all scale, as a first approximation, according to $W^{3/4}$ (Kirkwood & Webster, 1984). This implies that if the concept of metabolic size ($W^{3/4}$) were able to account for all variations between species in ME intake and H, then the efficiency of utilization of ME for maintenance and growth would be identical for all homoeotherms. On evolutionary grounds one might expect this to be reasonably close to the truth. However, the power of these scaling laws lies not in the fact that they appear to make all animals appear the same but that they can reveal the genuine anatomical and physiological basis for differences in energy exchange within and between species. It is these differences that I wish to consider.

Analysis of metabolic heat production

The nutritionist conventionally analyses metabolic heat production according to measurable factors relating to whole-body energy exchange. Usually, these are:

1. *Basal or standard metabolism.* Hmin measured at rest in a thermal environment and a post-absorptive state. This is defined principally by body size so is usually expressed as $MJ/kgW^{3/4}$.
2. *Heat increment of feeding.* HIF describes the increment in H above Hmin due to the work of digestion and metabolism of food, usually expressed as kJH/MJME.
3. *Energy cost of activity.* This describes the energy cost of all activities additional to the minimal activity performed during measurement of Hmin, eg in a calorimeter.
4. *Energy cost of thermoregulation.* This describes the increase necessary to maintain homoeothermy in an animal exposed to cold stress (Monteith & Mount, 1974).

The factorial approach to the prediction of H is very useful for the practical business of predicting ME requirement but it reveals nothing about where and how the heat is produced. To answer these questions, we need to measure H in specific organs and tissues and relate these measurements to the rate of specific processes in metabolism such as protein turnover and ion translocation (eg Na^+/K^+ pumping).

Heat increment of feeding

In all mammals and birds H increases to some extent as a consequence of eating food. The magnitude of HIF (which describes the *inefficiency* of utilization of ME) is determined mainly by the following factors.

(1) The work of ingestion and digestion (including fermentation).
(2) The chemical composition of nutrients absorbed from the gut.
(3) The metabolic fate of absorbed nutrients.

Simple-stomached animals

Table 1 lists some measurements of HIF in adult or near-adult animals retaining energy almost entirely as fat. In mature individuals of simple-stomached species (rat,

Table 1. *Some estimates of the heat increment of feeding (kJH/MJME) in animals retaining energy principally as fat.*

Species	*Diet*	*HIF*	*Reference*
Rat	synthetic	220–260	Barr & McCracken (1984)
			Pullar & Webster (1977)
	cafeteria	700	Rothwell & Stock (1983)
Pig	mixed (principally carbohydrate)	260–320	ARC (1982)
Man	'food'	250	Rosenberg & Durnin (1978)
	alcohol	100	
Sheep	forage	620	Blaxter & Boyne (1978)
	forage + cereal	450	
	intra-gastric infusion	370	Ørskov *et al.* (1979)

pig and man) eating foods with less than 40% of ME as fat, HIF is within the range 200–300 kJ/MJME. In rats, HIF appears to be the same whether animals eat naturally or are force-fed (Barr & McCracken, 1984). The energy costs of fat synthesis in rats from glucose, amino acids and long-chain fatty acids is 190, 400 and 15 kJ/MJ fat (McGilvey, 1970). Thus when men overeat high-fat diets HIF is about 100 kJ (MJME) (Dallosso & James, 1984). In simple-stomached species the act of eating *per se* appears to have a negligible effect on HIF which can therefore be attributed almost entirely to the metabolic costs of metabolizing absorbed nutrients.

During growth, energy is retained as protein (RE_p) and fat (RE_f). Kielanowski (1976) partitioned energy in growing pigs according to equation (3).

$$ME = aW^n + bRE_p + cRE_f \tag{3}$$

The expression of aW^n defines the effect of body weight on ME requirement for maintenance. HIF above maintenance is given by

$$HIF = (b - 1)RE_p + (c - 1)RE_f \tag{4}$$

Kielanowski recognized that the large degree of autocorrelation between the different terms in equation 3 and the smallness of bRE_p with respect to aW^n could seriously distort the prediction of b in particular. Nevertheless, he concluded from a review of the extremely variable published evidence that the mean efficiency of utilization of ME for protein and fat deposition in simple-stomached animals (rat and pig) was 0.45 and 0.75 respectively, corresponding to heat increments of 0.55 and 0.25 when the principal source of dietary energy was carbohydrate.

Pullar & Webster (1977) avoided the autocorrelation implicit in equation 3 by measuring energy exchanges during growth in lean and congenitally obese (fatty) Zucker rats, which show gross differences in the partition of RE between protein and fat at the same size or stage of growth. The values we obtained for HIF were as follows:

$$HIF = 1.25\ RE_p + 0.36\ RE_f \tag{5}$$

which implies efficiencies of utilization of ME of 0.44 for RE_p and 0.74 for RE_f, or HIF values of 560 kJ/MJME for protein deposition and 260 kJ/MJME for fat deposition. Although the difference between HIF for protein and fat depositions is substantial, differences in overall HIF during growth are relatively small. Even the very young rat retains about 60% of energy in the form of fat (although this corresponds to only about 10% of body weight gain). HIF is therefore 430 kJ/MJME in early growth and declines to 260 kJ/MJME at maturity.

These simple rules reliably predict the effect of food intake on H in most simple-stomached species in most circumstances. The one glaring exception to this rule is the very high HIF observed consistently by Rothwell & Stock (1983) in rats seduced to gluttony by a delectable and constantly changing cafeteria diet (Table 1). The very high HIF is associated with a large increase in brown adipose tissue (BAT) which, in response to sympathoadrenal stimulation, produces heat at a rate far in excess of any other tissue in the body (Trayhurn & Nicholls, 1986). Rothwell & Stock describe this phenomenon as dietary-induced thermogenesis which is confusing since, in a strictly semantic sense, the phrase is synonymous with HIF. I prefer to call it *regulatory diet-induced thermogenesis* (RDIT, Webster, 1983).

This is a fascinating mechanism because it appears to offer a partial solution to overeating. It is important however to put it in perspective. Although the evidence of Rothwell & Stock (1983) is consistent and convincing, other workers (Barr & McCracken, 1984, Hervey & Tobin, 1982) have equally consistently failed to elicit RDIT in rats cafeteria- or force-fed. Moreover, it can only be of relevance to those species that possess significant amounts of BAT in adult life. This, in nature, means small mammals of temperate and colder climates with an adult body weight below 3 kg. Synthesis of BAT is normally triggered by acclimation to cold but only occurs if this acclimation is associated with increased food intake, especially iodine-rich diets (Heroux, 1969). It may be that in these small mammals the natural stimulus of cold (or the onset of winter, which is not the same thing) triggers BAT synthesis and overrides normal satiety mechanisms, thereby ensuring that they take in more energy and dissipate more simply as heat without doing effective work. The evolutionary advantages of such a mechanism are obvious for small boreal mammals or species like the brown bat (*Eptesicus fucus*, Hayward & Lyman, 1967) which exhibit daily torpor. It may be that the unusually attractive and confusing nature of the cafeteria diet triggers this adaptive mechanism in the laboratory rat to a degree that is possibly related to the cooling power of the environment.

Ruminants

HIF is considerably greater in ruminants than simple-stomached animals (Table 1) mainly due to the heat of fermentation and the fact that the volatile fatty acids absorbed as a result of fermentation are used less efficiently than monosaccharides (Blaxter, 1967). Table 2 (adapted from Webster, 1980) attempts an analysis of HIF in sheep eating chopped hay or barley pellets. In this example the difference between the two feeds can be attributed mainly to the energy cost of eating and increased thermogenesis within the digestive tract. Effects of varying proportions of 2-C acetate and 3-C propionate on HIF in ruminants have been studied intensively for over 30 years yet the interpretation is still not entirely clear. The most convincing explanation at present is that diets (such as forages) which generate a high C2:C3 ratio of absorbed VFA are utilized for growth and fattening with a low efficiency when there is a shortage

Table 2. *Analysis of the heat increment of feeding (HIF) in sheep fed chopped hay or a barley-based pellet at and above maintenance* (adapted from Webster, 1980).

	Chopped hay	*Barley pellets*
Total HIF (kJH/MJME)	600	520
HIF due to		
eating	22	3
rumination	5	nil
fermentation	80	80
digestive tract	156	112
residual	335	325

of glucogenic substrate to provide reducing equivalents to convert acetate into fatty acid. When acetate is the predominant end-point of carbohydrate fermentation, glucogenic substrate can only come from glucogenic amino acids (MacRae & Lobley, 1982).

Energy cost of maintenance

Strictly speaking, maintenance describes the situation in an adult animal where ME = H, so that it neither gains nor loses energy (hereafter called ME_m). This is determined by size, physiological state and energy costs of activity and thermoregulation where relevant. In growing or lactating animals maintenance becomes an operational description of ME_m or H when energy exchange is adjusted to RE = O by subtraction (or addition) of HIF associated with gains (or losses) of energy as protein and fat.

The terms *standard metabolism* or *fasting metabolism* usually describe H measured under standard conditions, at rest, at thermal neutrality and in the latter case, post-absorptive. Ruminants take at least two days to achieve a post-absorptive state for measurement of fasting metabolism (Hmin) and even then Hmin is affected by prior nutrition (Blaxter, 1967). HIF between fasting and maintenance is larger and slightly more variable in ruminants than simple-stomached species, which implies that ME_m is affected slightly by food quality. However, this effect is small enough to be discounted when making intraspecies comparisons of *standard metabolism*, which corresponds to ME_m at thermal neutrality and when activity is at a minimal level consistent with life. In these circumstances the energy cost of maintenance is determined entirely by size ($W^{3/4}$) and physiological state.

Durnin & Passmore (1967), summarizing short-term measurements of standard metabolism in man, concluded that the main determinant of physiological state was fatness. Thus ME_m (kJ/kg$W^{3/4}$ per d) ranged from 318 at 5% fatness down to 285 at 20% fatness. They also concluded that sex differences in ME_m could be interpreted simply in terms of differences in fat concentration. Other authors have since confirmed this (Cunningham, 1982, Webb, 1981). Most values for ME_m in humans have been based on short-term measurements of respiratory exchange. Only in recent years has a substantial body of data emerged to describe ME_m in man from 24-hr calorimetric measurements similar to those used with high precision for farm animals and with strict control of ME intake.

Table 3. *Metabolizable energy requirement for maintenance (MEm) for different species under 'standard metabolism' conditions expressed per kg body weight (W)$^{3/4}$ and per kg body protein (P)$^{3/4}$.*

	Body wt (kg)	*MEm(MJ/d)* kg$W^{3/4}$	kg$P^{3/4}$	*Reference*
Interspecies mean	—	420	—	Kleiber (1961)
Rat, lean	0.35	425	1550	Pullar & Webster (1977)
fatty	0.35	275	1550	
Pigs, growing	50–100	458	—	ARC (1982)
sows	100	439	—	
Kestrel (*Falco tinnunculus*)	0.24	610	1750	Kirkwood (1981)
Humans	57	376	(1574)	Dauncey (1981)
	71	432	(1882)	van Es *et al.*, (1984)
Sheep, yearling	56	385	1975	Webster (1983)
5-year-old, thin	73	260	1295	*Ibid.*
5-year-old, fat	58	310	1290	*Ibid.*
Cattle, castrate males				
dairy type		585	2305	*Ibid.*
beef type		500	2145	*Ibid.*

Table 3 compares a range of measurements made of ME_m in different species under 'standard metabolism' conditions. The values for the simple-stomached mammals correspond closely to an inter-species mean estimate of 420 kJ/kg$W^{3/4}$ per d based on Kleiber (1961) which provides confirmation, if confirmation were needed, of the correctness of $W^{3/4}$ to account for effects of size, and so permits a first examination of differences attributable to physiological state. Expressing values for ME_m per kg body protein $(P)^{3/4}$ removes all the difference between lean and obese rats and between thin and fat 5-year-old sheep. It also brings the very high value for the extremely lean kestrel (*Falco tinnunculus*) (Kirkwood, 1981) into line with the mammalian species. My own values for ME_m in cattle and sheep (Webster, 1981) are close to preferred values (kJ/kg$W^{3/4}$ per d) for the two species (Agricultural Research Council, 1980). They are included in Table 3 because protein and Hmin were measured in the same individuals. One would expect ME_m to be slightly higher in ruminants than in simple-stomached species because of their higher HIF below maintenance. Sheep however carry relatively large amounts of metabolically inactive mass in the form of fat and wool. The difference between 5-year-old thin and fat sheep disappears when related to $P^{3/4}$. The decline in ME_m between yearling and 5-year-old sheep is of the same order as that observed in man after changes in fat content and muscle mass have been taken into account (Tzankoff & Norris, 1977). In cattle there appears to be a clear between-strain difference in ME_m attributable to selection for beef or dairy production. This has recently been confirmed by Taylor *et al.* (1986) using an approach based on long-term changes in body mass.

Table 3 indicates that differences between animals in ME_m (kJ/kg$^{3/4}$ per d) can be attributed in large part to differences in proportions of metabolically active protein and relatively inactive fat. This rather obvious conclusion provokes the more searching question 'to what extent can differences in ME_m be attributed to differing proportions of the different organs and tissues of the body each having different metabolic rates?' This question is of enormous importance to the science of nutrition since it is a question that needs to be resolved (but seldom is) prior to any hypothesis that differences between

Table 4. *Effects of different feeding regimes on organ size and fasting metabolism (Hmin) in pigs and sheep* (Koong *et al.*, 1982).

	Pig		*Sheep*	
Plane of nutrition	low	high	low	high
Weight (kg)				
whole body (W)	40.7	40.5	32.7	50.0
abdominal viscera (V)	2.07	2.85	1.59	2.78
V/W	0.051	0.070	0.048	0.056
Hmin, $kJ/kg^{3/4}$ per d	280	396	289	382

individuals in standard metabolism can be attributed to RDIT, 'luxus konsumption', 'futile cycles' or any other such departure from the normal energetic efficiency of metabolic processes.

Koong *et al.* (1982) measured Hmin in pigs and sheep having previously kept them on different planes of nutrition and, in consequence, achieved significant differences in the proportion of total body mass made up of metabolically active tissues of the abdomen (gut, liver, kidney, spleen and pancreas). Table 4 summarizes these results and suggests that although the contribution of the (empty) abdominal viscera to total body weight is small (3–7%), their mass is radically affected by prior nutrition. Moreover changes in the relative mass of abdominal viscera are closely linked to changes in Hmin. This is illustrated most clearly by the pigs which were matched for body weight. A 37% increase in weight of abdominal viscera was associated with a 41% increase in Hmin.

Sites of heat production

Most measurements of tissue thermogenesis have been made *in vitro*. Coulson has drawn attention, rather ruthlessly, to the flaw in this approach (Coulson *et al.*, 1977; Coulson & Herbert, 1981). His critique begins, 'modern biochemists usually live in the realms of the very small or the totally disintegrated' and he cites evidence to show that between-species comparisons of *in vitro* measurements of tissue thermogenesis give results that are ludicrously at variance with the concept of metabolic body size ($W^{3/4}$) for comparing metabolic rates *in vivo* between species. In other words, metabolic rates *in vivo* are constrained less by the capacity of enzymes to drive reactions in an ideal medium than by the rate at which the circulation can supply the tissues with substrates and sustain tissue respiration.

The classic approach to the measurement of organ thermogenesis *in vivo* is to measure blood flow and the arterio-venous difference in O_2 concentration. The latter is difficult to measure in small vessels but can, for the purposes of intraspecies comparisons, be assumed to vary to a negligible degree relative to changes in blood flow. It is therefore possible to estimate the contribution of different organs to H, as a first approximation, simply from measurements of regional blood flow, eg using radio-labelled microspheres, after making appropriate corrections for tissues such as the viscera drained by the hepatic portal vein, where a substantial proportion of arterial flow passes not through the capillary bed but through arterio-venous anastomoses.

Foster & Frydman (1978) used this approach to estimate organ thermogenesis in the rat at thermal neutrality and during non-shivering thermogenesis. From their

Table 5. *Distribution of blood flow and estimated O_2 consumption for rats at rest* (adapted from Foster & Frydman, 1978).

	Blood flow	*Heat production*	
	(ml/min)	*(J/min)*	*(% of total)*
Whole rat	89.0	125	—
Muscle (including heart)	18.3	26	20
Brain, skeleton, spinal cord	12.7	18	14
Liver	3.5 + 12.9*	15	12
Gut	12.9	10	8
Skin	10.0	14	11
Kidneys	12.5	18	14
BAT	0.8	1	1

*3.5 from hepatic artery + 12.9 from portal vein.

Table 6. *Fractional distribution of blood flow, protein synthesis and heat production in ruminants* (from Webster, 1980).

		% total	
	Cardiac output	*Protein synthesis*	*Heat production*
Abdominal organs	48	50	40
Muscle	15	20	
Skin	11	17	60
Others	26	13	

data, my estimates of organ thermogenesis at thermal neutrality are given in Table 5 (Webster, 1983). In this example, muscle is contributing only 20% to total H and liver and gut a further 20%. Grande (1980) has reviewed the limited information on organ thermogenesis in resting man. Once again muscle appears to contribute only about 20% of H; the hardest working organs—liver, heart, kidney—about 40%, and brain a further 20%. In ruminants the abdominal organs (gut and liver) contribute about 50% to both total H and total protein synthesis (Table 6, Webster, 1980) at maintenance. A three-fold intake in food consumption of sheep doubles the mass of the rumen and interstitial epithelium and total H in these tissues (Fell & Weekes, 1975; Webster, 1980). Thus changes in organ thermogenesis and resultant changes in ME_m or Hmin (Koong *et al.*, 1982) can probably be attributed simply to the changing mass of tissue involved, without any necessity to invoke fundamental changes in specific metabolic rate per unit mass.

Energy costs of metabolic processes

The alternative approach to the analysis of H is to consider the energy costs of the main physical and chemical processes in metabolism. Baldwin *et al.* (1980) concluded that maintenance thermogenesis was, in the first instance, almost equally divided between functions concerned with cell maintenance, e.g. protein turnover and service

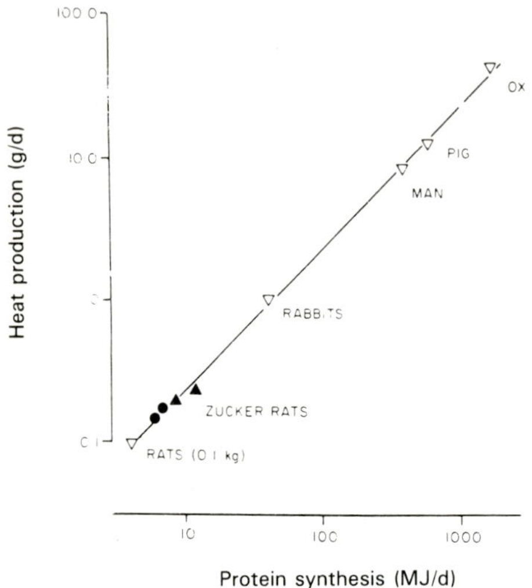

Fig. 1. *The relationship between heat production (MJ/d) and estimated protein synthesis (g/d)* (from Webster, 1983).

functions such as respiration and circulation. Obviously these two functions overlap. The two largest contributors to the cost of cell maintenance are protein turnover and Na^+/K^+ transport, each contributing, very approximately, 20% to total H (Baldwin *et al.*, 1980; Reeds & Fuller, 1983; Milligan & Summers, 1986). I think it a mistake to call these 'futile cycles' as Baldwin does, since they are so obviously vital to normal cellular function.

Figure 1 (from Webster, 1983) illustrates the intraspecies relationship between H and whole-body protein synthesis. Values for protein synthesis (Ps) are taken from various sources reviewed by Reeds & Lobley (1980). Values for H from the same species at the same size and physiological state are those which my colleagues and I obtained when at the Rowett Institute, Aberdeen.

The goodness-of-fit is not entirely surprising for a log-log plot with such wide ranges on both x and y axes. The most interesting feature of Fig. 1 is that the slope of the line is not significantly different from 1.0. In its simplest form therefore the interspecies relationship between H and Ps is

$$H = 20\ \mathrm{kJ/gPs}^{1.0} \tag{6}$$

Since the theoretical energy cost of protein synthesis is approximately 4.5 kJ/g (Reeds & Lobley, 1980), equation 6 tends to confirm the fact that in animals at rest Ps contributes about 20–25% to H. However the closeness of the linear relationship between H and Ps when compared on an intraspecies basis and the closeness of the relationship between H and Ps in organs within a species (Table 6) strongly suggest that differences in resting metabolism both within and between species can, in nearly all cases, be attributed entirely to essential metabolic processes such as protein synthesis and linked functions such as membrane transport mostly within the lean body mass and especially in organs such as the liver and intestinal epithelium which have to process nutrients. The one obvious exception to this rule is non-shivering thermogenesis in BAT in some small animals. This apart, the evidence from a study of comparative energetics is heavily weighted against the existence of 'futile cycles' or other mechanisms such as RDIT which serve no apparent purpose other than to waste energy.

Table 7. *Estimates of the metabolic rates of some free-living mammals and birds* (from Nagy, 1987).

Class	*Typical weight (kg)*	*Field metabolic rate ($kJ/kg^{3/4}$ per d)*	*b in W^b**
Eutherian mammals			
rodents	0.10	620	0.51
herbivores	50	840	0.73
desert eutherians	0.05	660	0.78
Marsupials	10.0	360	0.56
Birds			
passerines	0.05	1590	0.75
desert birds	0.1	600	0.66
sea birds	1.0	1420	0.70

*b is the exponent relating field metabolic rate to W for each class of animals.

Energy cost of activity

For wild animals the costs of activities essential to life and the cost of maintaining homoeothermy elevate the energy cost of maintenance above that measured under conditions of standard metabolism.

Nagy (1987) recently presented estimates of 'field metabolic rate' in a wide range of mammals and birds based on the doubly-labelled water method for measurement of CO_2 production. Some of his conclusions are summarized in Table 7. Assuming an intraspecies mean value of 420 $kJ/kg^{3/4}$ per d for standard metabolism in simple-stomached species (Kleiber, 1961) and 500 $kJ/kg^{3/4}$ per d for ruminants (Webster, 1983), Nagy's data indicate that for most eutherian mammals the additional energy cost of activity necessary for survival in the field increases ME_m by about 50–60% above standard metabolism. Passerine and sea birds, however, appear from Table 7 to work very hard. I shall reconsider the work done by domestic animals at the end of the paper.

In general the allometric regression of H on W yields exponents close to ¾ (Table 7). For rodents and marsupials the exponent is significantly below ¾. This does not imply that these species depart in some profound biochemical way from the intraspecies rule, but simply that the essential energy costs of activity and especially thermoregulation elevate ME_m above standard metabolism to a greater extent in the smaller species within each class.

Energetic efficiency of lactation

There is a great deal of reliable information on energy exchanges during lactation in domestic animals, especially the dairy cow, but very little for wild species.

One can, however, get a reasonably clear picture of the energetic efficiency of lactation from a knowledge of the quantity and composition of milk secreted by different mammals at peak lactation. This is a salutary experience, particularly for breeders of dairy cattle. Table 8 (from Webster, 1987) compares the yields of energy and protein in the milk of typical Friesian and Jersey cattle, the Saanen goat, the sow, a Labrador

Table 8. *Typical yields of nutrients, expressed as energy and protein from some lactating mammals* (from Webster, 1987).

	Friesian cow	*Jersey cow*	*Saanen goat*	*Sow*	*Bitch*	*Woman*
Body weight (kg)	600	400	65	200	26	60
Offspring, number	1	1	1	12	8	1
total weight at birth	45	30	4.5	16	2.0	3.5
Peak milk yield (1/d)	31	21	5	7.5	1.3	1.0
Yield of nutrients/kg$^{3/4}$ per d						
energy (kJ)	745	820	700	770	715	132
protein (g)	8.4	8.7	7.6	8.4	9.4	0.6

bitch, and last (and by every means least) woman. The remarkable thing about the other examples is their similarity. The highly-selected Friesian cow giving 10 000 l per lactation is not only no more efficient at converting ME into milk than the Jersey—merely bigger—she also operates at about the same efficiency as the goat and, if anything, at a slightly lower overall efficiency than the sow or bitch, because HIF (kJH/MJME) associated with milk synthesis is slightly higher in ruminants than in a simple-stomached animal such as the pig (Agricultural Research Council, 1980, 1982). This is not to say that the energetic efficiency of lactation cannot be manipulated by selection—the Friesian dairy cow is undoubtedly more efficient than the Hereford beef cow—but it does reveal the power of the scaling rules in separating real differences in energetic efficiency from the illusion of improvement created (eg) by selecting for increased milk yield and simply achieving larger cows.

Energetic efficiency of growth

The scaling rules assume even greater power when used to evaluate differences in the energetic efficiency of growth. I stated earlier that, as a first approximation, the time taken to mature increases with mature size, $Wa^{1/4}$. Absolute growth rate (dw/dt), H and ME intake all scale according to $W^{3/4}$ (although ME intake may be restricted by food availability or quality). Scaling maturation interval according to $Wa^{1/4}$ and energy exchanges according to $W^{3/4}$ permit an analysis of differences in the energetic efficiency of growth that is independent of size. Table 9, condensed from Kirkwood & Webster (1984), presents values for θ_{50} (metabolic days or $t.A^{-1/4}$) at 50% maturity and $\theta_{(25-75)}$ the time, once again in metabolic days, to progress from 25 to 75% mature weight in a range of mammals and birds. The mouse data reveal that divergent selection for and against liveweight gain sufficient to achieve a two-fold difference in body weight (Falconer, 1973) accelerated maturation by only 2–12%, dependent on the index used. Similarly, selection for growth rate in Merino sheep did not significantly accelerate maturation rate (Butterfield *et al.*, 1983). Conventional selection methods for growth in pigs and beef cattle (usually liveweight gain per day) do appear to have achieved some acceleration in maturation rate, particularly when the data in Kirkwood & Webster (1984) are compared with those in Brody (1945), but the response to selection by man has been relatively small.

Table 9. *Maturation rates of some mammals, precocial and altricial birds* (condensed from Kirkwood & Webster, 1984; for full explanation see text).

	Wa (kg)	*Metabolic age* ($t.A^{1/4}$) *0.5 Wa*	θ (25 to 75)
Mammals			
Mice, small	0.023	112	56
large	0.947	110	49
Pig	320	98	68
Sheep, small	91	130	69
large	117	123	69
Cattle, Hereford	947	98	92
Friesian	1000	117	110
Man	760	1536	1350
Birds: precocial			
quail	0.11	64	25
domestic fowl (broiler)	5.5	60	38
Birds: altricial			
starling	0.07	37	11
kestrel	0.26	55	11

Precocial birds mature approximately twice as fast as mammals, and altricial (nest-fed) birds twice as fast again. It is interesting to speculate on the evolutionary reasons for this. Certainly an altricial bird such as the kestrel is extremely inactive throughout most of development and has little need to use energy for maintenance activity or to grow in such a way as to be capable of a reasonably independent life from the time of hatching. It can therefore accumulate nutrients first and reorganize them later into a perfect flying machine. Maturation rate in humans is extremely slow compared to the other species in Table 9, although Kirkwood (1985) has demonstrated gradual changes in maturation rate within primates from prosimians via the great apes that make man appear less exceptional. The evolutionary advantages of retarding maturation rate in man become clear when one considers that if humans did not depart from the interspecies mean, sons would be as big as their fathers before they reached two years of age!

Figure 2 (from Webster, 1985) illustrates the pattern of energy exchange during growth in two mammals (pig and ox), a precocial bird (quail *Coturnix japonica*), and an altricial bird (kestrel), all scaled by $W^{3/4}$. The curves for pig and ox are typical for mammals (ME-H) thus relative growth rate ($dw/dt.W^{3/4}$) and the energetic efficiency of growth peak at 0.2 Wa but decline rapidly after 0.3 Wa. Precocial birds (eg quail) achieve a greater efficiency not by eating more ($M = 1.2$ MJ/kg$^{3/4}$ per d in both mammals and precocial birds) but by extending the impetus for growth, and thus ME intake, over a longer period of growth. The very high efficiency of the altricial bird (eg kestrel) is achieved by a slightly greater ME intake prolonged until 0.7 Wa and a reduced H until 0.6 Wa, linked to a lower body temperature than in the active adult bird. This body temperature is largely independent of air temperature and appears therefore to reflect an active physiological strategy for maximizing energy retention rather than a passive response to environmental cooling (Kirkwood, 1981).

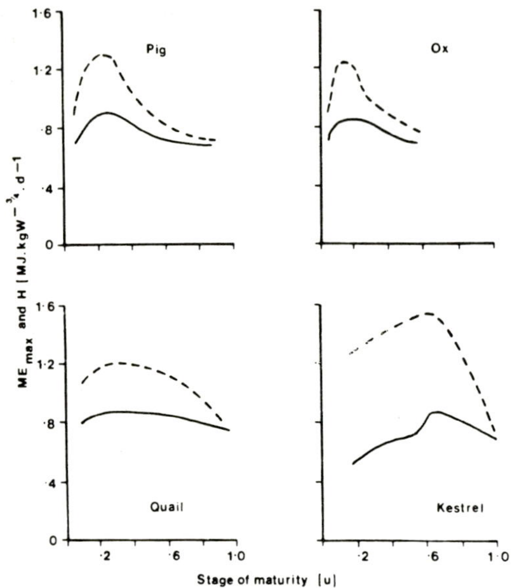

Fig. 2. *Energy exchanges during growth in the pig, ox, Japanese quail and kestrel.* The dotted line indicates *ad lib.* intake of ME, the solid line, H. (from Webster, 1985).

Coda—how hard do animals work?

It may reasonably be assumed that few animals work harder than they need. With the exception of some small mammals and passerine birds, life in the wild is not particularly hard. Man, however, demands harder work from his own species and, particularly, his domesticated animals. Table 10 presents some examples of ME intake and work rate (expressed as H) in man and animals. The daily energy expenditure of a clerk is about 25% greater than that of someone doing absolutely nothing. A UK miner, given the mechanical aids available in 1946, worked about 50% harder than a man at rest, and Czech foresters, the hardest-working group that I have discovered (Wirths, 1957), almost twice as hard (800 kJ/kg$^{3/4}$ per d). The work done by a lactating woman is intermediate between that of the miner and the forester. The work of growth, even in intensively reared pigs and poultry, is no greater than hard manual labour for humans. The hardest worked animal is the high-yielding dairy cow (or goat) required to sustain a work load more than twice maintenance and consume ME at a rate more than three times maintenance. It is no suprise that the major diseases of the high-yielding dairy cow are disorders of digestion and metabolism (Webster, 1987).

It is possible to increase lean tissue growth rate and milk production in farm animals by injecting or implanting exogenous anabolic and/or lactogenic hormones. Speaking strictly in terms of comparative energetics, the use of anabolic steroids to accelerate growth looks like an acceptable way to speed up a process that is not particularly arduous. The use of a lactogenic hormone to increase milk production in the dairy cow becomes less acceptable when her work load is compared with that of the coal miner and frankly irrational when it is appreciated that in most areas of the world and on most cost-effective and healthy roughage-based diets her capacity to sustain lactation is constrained less by the physiological potential of the mammary gland to

Table 10. *Some examples of the effects of activity and the work of growth and lactation on energy exchange in man and animals.*

Species	*Energy exchange ($kJ/kg^{3/4}$ per d)* *ME*	*H*	*Reference*
Man, clerk	520	520	Garry *et al.* (1955)
UK miner (1946)	625	625	*Ibid.*
Czech forester (1950)	800	800	Wirths (1957)
Woman, lactating	830	700	Webster (1987)
Dairy cow (Friesian, 31 l/d)	1800	1000	*Ibid.*
Growing pig (20 kg)	1200	800	Kirkwood & Webster (1984)
Broiler fowl (2 kg)	1000	600	*Ibid.*
Wild, eutherian 'mammal' (300 g)	860	860	Nagy (1987)
Passerine 'bird' (5 kg)	1580	1580	*Ibid.*

produce milk than by the digestive and metabolic capacity of the cow upstream to supply the mammary gland with nutrients.

The comparative approach to nutrition offers a range of fascinating and extremely important insights that could not emerge from the most profound study of the metabolism of a single species. It should confirm, for one, the old adage that all animals are equal—once one has accounted for all the differences. It can protect the fundamental scientist, investigating his own particular mystery of life, from inventing (and investigating at great cost) hypotheses that may explain his own data set but which look extremely unlikely when examined on an intraspecies basis. Finally, it can help the applied animal scientist, working to improve animal productivity, to distinguish between the realistic, the unlikely and the unfair.

References

Agricultural Research Council (1980): *The nutrient requirements of farm livestock No. 2. Ruminants*, 2nd ed. Farnham Royal: Commonwealth Agriculture Bureau.

Agricultural Research Council (1982): *The nutrient requirements of farm livestock No. 3. Pigs*. 2nd ed. London: Agricultural Research Council.

Baldwin, R. L., Smith, N. E., Taylor, J. & Sharp, M. (1980): Manipulating metabolic parameters to improve growth rate and milk secretion. *J. Anim. Sci.* **51**, 1416–1428.

Barr, H. G. & McCracken, K. J. (1984): High efficiency of energy utilization in cafeteria and force-fed rats kept at 29°C. *Br. J. Nutr.* **51**, 379–387.

Blaxter, K. L. (1967): *The energy metabolism of ruminants*, 2nd ed. London: Hutchinson.

Blaxter, K. L. & Boyne, A. W. (1978): The estimation of the nutritive value of feeds as energy sources for ruminants and the derivation of feeding systems. *J. Agric. Sci., Camb.* **90**, 47–68.

Brody, S. (1945): *Bioenergetics and growth*. New York: Reinhold Publs.

Butterfield, R. M., Griffiths, D. A., Thompson, J. M., Zamora, J. & James, A. M. (1983): Changes in body composition relative to weight and maturity in large and small strains of Merino rams. *Anim. Prod.* **36**, 29–37.

Coulson, R. A. & Herbert, J. D. (1981): Relationship between metabolic rate and various physiological and biochemical parameters. A comparison of alligator, man and shrew. *Comp. Biochem. Physiol.* **69**, 1–13.

Coulson, R. A., Hernandez, T. & Herbert, J. D. (1977): Metabolic rate, enzyme kinetics *in vivo*. *Comp. Biochem. Physiol.* **56A**, 251–262.

Cunningham, J. J. (1982): Body composition and resting metabolic rate: the myth of female metabolism. *Am. J. Clin. Nutr.* **35**, 721–726.

Dallosso, H. M. & James, W. P. T. (1984): Whole-body calorimetry studies in adult man. 1. The effect of fat overfeeding on 24-hr energy expenditure. *Br. J. Nutr.* **52**, 49–64.

Dauncey, M. J. (1981): Influence of mild cold on 24 hr energy expenditure, resting metabolism and diet-induced thermogenesis. *Br. J. Nutr.* **45**, 257–267.

Durnin, J. V. G. A. & Passmore, R. (1967): *Energy, work and leisure.* London: Heinemann.

Falconer, D. A. (1973): Repicated selection for body weight in mice. *Genet. Res.* **22**, 291–321.

Fell, B. F. & Weekes, T. E. C. (1975): In *Digestion and metabolism in the ruminant*, eds I. W. McDonald and A. C. E. Warner, pp. 101–118. Armidale, N.S.W., Australia: Univ. New England Publ. Unit.

Foster, D. O. & Frydman, Lorraine M. (1978): Non-shivering thermogenesis in the rat. 2. Measurements of blood flow with microspheres point to brown adipose tissue as the dominant site of calorigenesis induced by noradrenaline. *Can. J. Physiol. Pharmacol.* **56**, 110–122.

Garry, R. C., Passmore, R., Warnock, G. M. & Durnin, J. (1955): *Studies on expenditure of energy and consumption of food by miners and clerks. Fife, Scotland, 1952.* Med. Res. Council Special Report No. 289. London: HMSO.

Grande, F. (1980): Energy expenditure of organs and tissues. In *Assessment of energy metabolism in health and disease*, ed J. M. Kinney, pp. 88–92. Columbus, Ohio: Ross Laboratories.

Haysson, V. & Lacy, R. C. (1985): Basal metabolic rate in mammals: taxonomic differences in the allometry of BMR and body mass. *Comp. Biochem. & Physiol.* **81**, 741–754.

Hayward, J. S. & Lyman, C. P. (1967): Non-shivering thermogenesis during arousal from hibernation and evidence for the contribution of brown fat. In *Mammalian hibernation III*, ed K. C. Fisher, pp. 346–355. New York: American Elsevier.

Heroux, O. (1969): Catecholamines, corticosteroids and thyroid hormones in non-shivering thermogenesis under different environmental conditions. In *Physiology and pathology of adaptation mechanisms*, ed E. Bajusz. Oxford: Pergamon Press.

Hervey, G. R. & Tobin, G. (1982): The part played by variation of energy expenditure in the regulation of energy balance. *Proc. Nutr. Soc.* **41**, 137–154.

Heusner, A. A. (1982): Energy metabolism and body size. 1. Is the 0.75 mass exponent of Kleiber's equation a statistical artefact? *Resp. Physiol.* **48**, 1–12.

Kielanowski, J. (1976): Energy cost of protein deposition. In *Protein metabolism and nutrition*, ed D. J. A. Cole, pp. 207–216. EAAP Publ. No. 165. London: Butterworths.

King, J. R. & Farner, D. S. (1961): Energy metabolism, thermoregulation and body temperature. In *Biology and comparative physiology of birds*, Vol. II, ed A. J. Marshall, pp. 215–288. New York: Academic Press.

Kirkwood, J. K. (1981): Bioenergetics and growth in the kestrel (*Falco tinnunculus*). Ph.D. thesis, University of Bristol.

Kirkwood, J. K. (1985): Patterns of growth in primates. *J. Zool. (Lond, A.)* **205**, 123–136.

Kirkwood, J. K. & Webster, A. J. F. (1984): Energy budget strategies for growth in mammals and birds. *Anim. Prod.* **38**, 147–155.

Kleiber, M. (1961): *The fire of life.* New York: John Wiley.

Koong, L. J., Ferrell, C. L. & Nienaber, J. A. (1982): Effects of plane of nutrition on organ size and fasting heat production in swine and sheep. *Proc. 9th symposium energy metabolism of farm animals*, ed A. Ekern and F. Sundstøl, pp. 245–249. EAAP Publ. 29. Agricultural Institute of Norway.

McGilvey, R. W. (1970): *Biochemistry, a functional approach.* Philadelphia & London: W. B. Saunders.

MacRae, J. R. & Lobley, G. E. (1982): Some factors which influence thermal energy losses during the metabolism of ruminants. *Livestock Prod. Sci.* **9**, 447–456.

Milligan, L. P. & Summers, M. (1986): The biological basis of maintenance and its relevance to assessing responses to nutrients. *Proc. Nutr. Soc.* **45**, 185–193.

Monteith, J. & Mount, L. E. (1974): *Heat loss from animals and man.* London: Butterworths.

Nagy, K. A. (in press): Field metabolic rate and food requirement scaling in mammals and birds. *Ecol. Mono.*

Ørskov, E. R., Grubb, D. A., Smith, J. S., Webster, A. J. F. & Corrigal, W. (1979): Efficiency of utilization of volatile fatty acids for maintenance and energy retention in sheep. *Br. J. Nutr.* **41**, 541–551.

Pullar, J. D. & Webster, A. J. F. (1977): The energy costs of protein and fat deposition in the rat. *Br. J. Nutr.* **37**, 355–363.

Reeds, P. J. & Fuller, M. F. (1983): Nutrient intake and protein turnover. *Proc. Nutr. Soc.* **42**, 463–472.

Reeds, P. J. & Lobley, G. E. (1980): Protein synthesis; are there real species differences? *Proc. Nutr. Soc.* **39**, 43–51.
Reeds, P. J., Wahle, K. W. J. & Haggarty, P. (1982): Energy costs of protein and fatty acid synthesis. *Proc. Nutr. Soc.* **41**, 155–160.
Ricklefs, R. E. (1968): Patterns of growth in birds. *The Ibis*, **110**, 419–451.
Rosenberg, K. & Durnin, J. V. G. A. (1978): The effect of alcohol on resting metabolic rate. *Br. J. Nutr.* **40**, 293–298.
Rothwell, N. J. & Stock, M. J. (1983): Dietary-induced thermogenesis. In *Mammalian thermogenesis*, ed L. Girardier and M. J. Stock, pp. 208–233. London: Chapman & Hall.
Taylor, St. C. S. (1965): A relation between mature weight and the time taken to mature in mammals. *Anim. Prod.* **7**, 203–220.
Taylor, St. C. S., Theissen, R. B. & Murray, J. (1986): Inter-breed relationship of maintenance efficiency to milk yield in cattle. *Anim. Prod.* **43**, 37–62.
Thonney, M. L., Touchberry, R. W., Goodrich, R. D. & Meiske, J. C. (1976): Intraspecies relationships between fasting heat production and body weight: a re-evaluation of $W^{0.75}$. *J. Anim. Sci.* **43**, 697–704.
Trayhurn, P. & Nicholls, D. G. (1986): *Brown adipose tissue*, p. 374. London: Edward Arnold.
Tzankoff, S. P. & Norris, A. H. (1977): Effect of muscle mass decrease on age-related BMR changes. *J. App. Physiol.* **43**, 1001–1006.
Van Es, A. J. H., Vogt, J. E., Niessen, C. H., Veth, J., Rodenburg, L., Teeuwse, V., Dhuyvetter, J., Deurenberg, P., Hautvast, J. G. A. T. & Beek, E. van der (1984) Human energy metabolism below, near and above energy equilibrium. *Br. J. Nutr.* **52**, 429–442.
Webb, P. (1981): Energy expenditure and fat-free mass in men and women. *Am. J. Clin. Nutr.* **34**, 1816–1826.
Webster, A. J. F. (1980): The energy costs of digestion and metabolism in the gut. In *Digestive physiology and metabolism in ruminants*, ed Y. Ruckebusch and P. Thivend, pp. 423–438. Lancaster: MTP Press.
Webster, A. J. F. (1981): The energetic efficiency of metabolism. *Proc. Nutr. Soc.* **40**, 121–128.
Webster, A. J. F. (1983): Energetics of maintenance and growth. In *Mammalian thermogenesis*, ed L. Girardier and M. J. Stock, pp. 178–207. London: Chapman & Hall.
Webster, A. J. F. (1985): Differences in the energetic efficiency of animal growth *J. Anim. Sci.* **61**, Suppl. 2, 92–103.
Webster, A. J. F. (1987): *Understanding the dairy cow*. London: Blackwell Scientific Publications.
Wirths, W. (1957): The cost of human energy in agriculture. *J. Farm Econ.* **39**, 155–161.

* * * * *

Discussion

Dr McCracken commented that in experiments in which he overfed adult rats there was an increase of 50% in body mass, a 37% increase in heat production and metabolic body size but only an 8–10% increase in lean body mass or in viscera weight. This would suggest that the hypothesis put forward by Professor Webster and Dr Koong relating to the role of the viscera might not be correct. *Professor Webster* replied that his data did not include animals with very large amounts of fat and thus skin. In continuing this discussion *Dr McCracken* stated that the main increase in total mass was an increase in adipose tissue, suggesting that the energy costs associated with adipose tissue may be higher than commonly assumed. *Sir Kenneth Blaxter* then asked why the figures for the component costs did not add up to 100%. *Professor Webster* replied that not all tissues were measured, for example peripheral nervous tissue and bone marrow, both of which were likely to have high activity. In this respect *Professor Waterlow* commented that in early measurements of the uptake of labelled amino acids in the rat, summing all the tissues left a discrepancy of 16% and he wondered whether lymphoid tissue could be responsible.

Dr Ingram asked what advantage there might be to having more than one copy of the growth hormone gene in an animal, in terms of the effect on the efficiency of growth. *Professor Webster* replied that the evidence suggested that doubling the size of animals by conventional genetic means has so far had relatively little effect. He re-emphasized the importance of altering the shape of the growth/food relationship.

Dr Speakman commented on the high metabolic rate observed in wild animals and wondered why this was so different from that in the domestic cow, and hence the nature of limitation on energy expenditure for the domesticated ruminant. *Professor Webster* replied that the limitation in forage-consuming animals was that ME intake was constrained by the capacity of the gut and rate of fermentation.

Dr Widdowson commented on the relation between the habitual energy expenditure of man and of animals in the wild, suggesting that man and animals in the wild were really sedentary and spent most of their time sleeping or sitting around, to which *Professor Webster* added the comment that he thought that the differences between people in terms of their maintenance costs were most probably due to differences in time spent on activity.

Dr Stevens asked about the animals such as elephants that eat fairly continuously and *Professor Webster* then commented on the fact that in grazing ruminants it was usual to find some 13 hours out of 24 spent in eating. In these circumstances field metabolic rate was only about 60% above resting metabolism.

Professor Peters commented that movement need not necessarily be expensive. The calculations made by him relating to whales show that the increase in metabolic weight was only a few percent, largely because they were moving in a buoyant medium.

Professor Goldspink commented that gliding flight in birds was associated with 2 times the basal metabolic rate whilst in flapping flight the metabolic rate reached 7 times basal values, which was sometimes maintained. He gave as an example the migrating Arctic tern which travels about 26 000 miles per year. *Professor Webster* thought that more usually the maximal sustainable metabolism during flight was probably four to five times basal metabolic rate.

4
Nitrogen metabolism and protein requirements

P. J. REEDS

Introduction

The study of comparative nutrition serves a number of useful purposes. First and foremost, similarities between species may enable us to identify certain general principles of nutrition as well as the metabolism that underlies nutrient requirements. For example, the amino acids found in proteins and the genetic codes used to direct their incorporation into protein are common to both bacteria and man. In addition, metabolic peculiarities of one species may often enable us to understand the nutritional physiology of others. For example, the relatively low capacity for ornithine synthesis from glutamate in the intestine of the cat and hence the inability of this species to sustain a nutritionally significant rate of net arginine synthesis (Rogers & Morris, 1978; MacDonald *et al.*, 1984) renders the cat extremely sensitive to an arginine-deficient diet. Even a single protein-containing but arginine-deficient meal leads to hyperammonaemia accompanied by neurological disturbances, which not only emphasizes the crucial role of arginine synthesis in ammonia metabolism (see Motil *et al.*, 1981a), but also illustrates the pathological consequences of high systemic levels of ammonia.

Comparative nutritional studies, however, may be of particular importance at the practical level. The use of tractable animal models would be a considerable advantage to the formulation of dietary recommendations for man, especially in the development of a more precise understanding of the subtle interactions between nutrients and their effects on human health. For this reason, this paper is presented within a framework of the protein requirements of mammals and examines the extent to which they differ in this vital area of nutrition.

Table 1. *Components of body nitrogen in the rat and human.* Values in parentheses are %.

	Rat *(g)*	*Man* *(kg)*
Body weight	300	70
Total body N	8.6	2.46
Total body protein N	8.0	2.38
	(93)	(96)
		(g)
Total body nucleic acid N	0.3	4.4
	(3)	(0.2)
Free amino acid N	0.1	6.3
	(1)	(0.2)
Creatine	0.17	31
	(2)	(1.3)

Table 2. *Conversion of amino acids to other nitrogenous compounds.*

Amino acids	*End-products*
Glycine	Creatine
	Purines
	Porphyrins
Methionine	Choline
	Creatine
	Polyamines
Glutamine	Purines
	Pyrimidines
Aspartate	Pyrimidines
Tyrosine	Catecholamines
	Thyroid hormones
Tryptophan	Pyridine nucleotides
	Serotonin
Lysine	Carnitine
Histidine	Histamine

Table 3. *Utilization of glycine for haem and creatine synthesis in man.*

Compound	*Body content (mmol)*	*Glycine/mol*	*Loss/d (mmol)*	*Maximum glycine required (mmol [mg])*
Haem	9.8	4	0.68	2.7 (170)
Creatine	710	1	14	14 (910)

Components of the body nitrogen pool

At the outset, it is important to emphasize that it is incorrect to speak of a 'nitrogen' requirement; the use of this short-hand description has caused a certain confusion in the literature. Organisms, with the exception of the nitrogen-fixing bacteria, appear not to metabolize elemental nitrogen, but rather metabolize nitrogen-containing compounds. Table 1 presents a partial list of some of the nitrogen-containing

Table 4. *Utilization of dietary nucleic acids.*

	Nucleic acid source	*Method*	*Utilization (%)*	*References*
Man	^{15}N nucleic acid	^{15}N excretion	10 for pyrimidines 30 for purines	Golden *et al.* (1982)
	^{15}N nucleic acid	^{15}N excretion	10	Bien *et al.* (1953)
Rat	^{15}N nucleic acid	^{15}N excretion	2	Roll *et al.* (1949)
Mice	^{15}N nucleic acid	^{14}C incorporation	2	Burridge *et al.* (1976)
Sheep	Nucleic acid infusion	Balance	2	Fujihara *et al.* (1987)

components of the body. Even though this list is incomplete, it shows in a quantitative manner that the nitrogen pools of the body are dominated by the body proteins. Furthermore, with the exception of some, but not all, nitrogen-containing vitamins, virtually all the nitrogenous compounds of the body can be and often are derived from amino acids. Table 2 lists some of the pathways of 'nonprotein' routes of amino acid use, some of which could be significant contributors to the requirements for specific amino acids. Glycine, for example, is utilized for the synthesis of purine bases, creatine, haem, and other respiratory pigments. In adult man, the use of glycine for creatine and porphyrin synthesis might amount to 1 g per day (Table 3), and for such a man receiving 0.6 g protein/kg per day the total supply of glycine, including its synthesis *de novo*, is approximately 8 g (Yu *et al.*, 1985). Given the similarities of the pool sizes and turnover rates of creatine and haemoglobin in different species, their contributions to glycine requirement will presumably be similar among mammals.

Relatively little attention has been focused on the study of glycine, glutamine, and aspartate usage for nucleic acid synthesis. Newsholme *et al.* (1985) have emphasized this role for glutamine in rapidly dividing cells. In theory, because of the existence of the salvage pathways of base reutilization, dietary nucleic acids could make a significant contribution to nucleic acid synthesis, but this seems minor. Studies of the utilization of isotopically-labelled dietary nucleic acids in rats (Roll *et al.*, 1949), mice (Burridge *et al.*, 1976) and man (Bien *et al.*, 1953; Golden *et al.*, 1982), and of the excretion of the end-products of purine metabolism in man (Bowering *et al.*, 1970) and sheep (Fujihara *et al.*, 1987), all suggest a virtually complete catabolism of dietary nucleic acids (Table 4). The observations in a ruminant are particularly interesting; up to 10% of 'absorbed nitrogen' in ruminants that are receiving conventional forage diets may be in the form of bacterial nucleic acids (Table 4). Although nucleic acid accretion is a minor component of total nitrogen retention (Table 1), nucleic acid turnover is of greater importance. Recently Sander *et al.* (1986) have calculated the turnover rates of the three main species of RNA, on the basis of the excretion of post-transcriptionally-modified bases. Their results suggest that approximately 100 mg of RNA (0.8% of the nucleic acid pool) is catabolized per day in adult humans. This value compares with a fractional rate of body protein turnover of about 2.5% per day. Furthermore, the turnover rate of nucleic acids parallels the rate of growth and probably protein turnover (Sander *et al.*, 1986). Nevertheless, even if none of the bases so released were reutilized, the use of approximately 30 mg of amino acid N would be required, a low proportion even of the endogenous losses of body nitrogen.

In view of these comments, it seems a reasonable proposition that the nitrogen requirement is not only largely a requirement for amino acids, but is also dominated by the needs of protein accretion and metabolism.

Components of the protein requirement

Four general factors should be considered in a review of the components of the protein requirement: (1) a requirement for 'nonessential' nitrogen from which other nitrogenous compounds, including nonessential amino acids, can be synthesized; (2) a specific pattern of essential amino acids within the protein supply to allow the optimal utilization of dietary protein for productive processes, such as foetal and body growth and lactation; (3) a supply of protein to replace basal losses; and (4) an appropriate balance of protein and energy within the diet, because amino acids are readily used in intermediary metabolism.

Nutritionally, amino acids may be divided into two main groups. The essential (indispensible) amino acids, that by virtue of the pecularities of their carbon skeletons cannot be synthesized by animals, and the nonessential amino acids that can be synthesized given a suitable source of carbon and amino groups. A common series of amino acids appear to be essential for all the animal eukaryotes. In some species, additional amino acids also appear to be essential elements of the diet. We have already alluded to the low rate of net arginine synthesis in cats. The same applies to birds, and perhaps other uricotelic species, which, lacking mitochondrial carbamyl phosphate synthase, are also unable to synthesize arginine (Boorman & Lewis, 1971).

Attention has been focused recently (Laidlaw & Kopple, 1987) on a third group of amino acids that, although synthesized by mammals, are either synthesized only from other essential amino acids (tyrosine and cysteine), or are synthesized from a strictly limited number of nonessential amino acids, or have a limited maximum rate of synthesis. Here again, glycine appears to occupy a special place. Experiments both in rats (Alqvist, 1951; Jackson & Golden, 1980) and man (Jackson & Golden, 1980; Matthews *et al.*, 1981) have shown that glycine neither readily donates nor readily receives amino groups from amino acids other than serine. Given that serine, via its involvement in the synthesis of cystathionine, is closely involved in cysteine synthesis, one can imagine circumstances in which the protein status of an individual could be compromised by limitation in the supply of any two of these three amino acids. Indeed, it has been hypothesized that, because of their limited ability to synthesize glycine, this so-called nonessential amino acid may be the first rate-limiting one for the newborn (Jackson *et al.*, 1981). If so, the low concentration of glycine in milk proteins is difficult to understand. Birds also appear to have a limited ability to synthesize glycine in high net amounts, despite its involvement in uric acid synthesis.

These considerations apart, dietary protein is utilized largely for two purposes: (1) for the deposition of protein within the foetus and the body, in milk and wool and (2) for the replacement of body protein that appears to be lost inevitably via integumental and gastrointestinal losses and by the irrevocable catabolism of amino acids.

One immediate area in which substantial interspecific differences might exist is the pattern of amino acids deposited during growth. When we compare whole body

Table 5. *Contribution of specific proteins to whole body protein in the rat (total body protein = 50 g).*

Proteins	*(g)*
Contractile	11
Ribosomal	1.3
'Extracellular'	3.6
Collagen	3
	(38% of total)

$\frac{\text{Muscle protein}}{\text{body protein}} = 0.5$ and assuming $\frac{\text{contractile protein}}{\text{muscle protein}} = 0.4$.
Average RNA/protein ratio = 1.2 mg/g and protein/RNA in ribosome is 1.6.
Plasma proteins = 10 g/100 ml.
$\frac{\text{Collagen}}{\text{total protein}} = 0.06$.

Table 6. *Gross amino acid composition of muscle protein.*

Amino acid	*Mean of 5 vertebrate species** *(g/16 g N ± 1 s.d.)*	*Man*† *(g/16 g N)*
Leucine	8.1 ± 0.2	7.9
Isoleucine	4.7 ± 0.1	4.8
Valine	5.2 ± 0.1	5.8
Methionine	2.9 ± 0.1	2.9
Phenylalanine	4.4 ± 0.2	4.2
Threonine	4.6 ± 0.1	4.8
Lysine	8.9 ± 0.1	8.6
Tryptophan	1.3 ± 0.1	1.4
Histidine	4.1 ± 0.1	3.4
Nonessential	53 ± 1.6	55

*Rat, pig, cattle, sheep and chickens. †Smith (1980) and Posati (1979); Anderson (1983); Anderson *et al.* (1986).

amino acid compositions (Reeds & Harris, 1981; Smith, 1980), there is little evidence to suggest that the essential amino acids deposited, and hence obligatorily required for growth, are greatly different among mammals. This is perhaps not surprising; as shown in Table 5, a limited number of abundant proteins account for approximately 30% of whole body protein. Although there are important interspecific differences in the details of the primary structures of these proteins, the major elements of their amino acid sequences have been highly conserved. For example, if we compare the average amino acid content of skeletal muscle (Table 6), we can observe few substantial differences. In fact, the variability of the amino acid composition of the protein of a given tissue between species (c.v. 2 to 5%) is much smaller than the variation in the compositions of different tissues within the same species (c.v. 11 to 42%). An important interspecific difference might be the tissue composition of growth. With the exception of the high contribution of skin in small mammals, however, the tissue composition of growth is largely a function of age and not of species. In support of this observation, we know that despite substantial differences in the nutrient densities of different milks (themselves related to the lactational behavior of the species and the postnatal growth rate of the sucklings), and apart from an important but

Table 7. *Calculated and measured compositions of milks of different species.*

Component	*Rat**	*Rabbit*	*Species* *Pig**	*Cattle†*	*Man‡*
Protein g/l	84	136	48	34	14
Amino acids					
Leucine	10.5	10.5	10.8	10.5	10.2
Isoleucine	6.6	6.6	6.6	6.2	5.4
Valine	6.6	6.9	6.5	6.4	5.8
Methionine	3.0	3.0	2.7	2.6	1.4
Phenylalanine	5.4	5.4	5.5	5.4	3.8
Threonine	4.7	4.7	4.8	4.5	4.5
Lysine	8.6	8.6	8.8	7.9	6.6
Tryptophan	1.6	1.6	1.6	ND	2.1
Histidine	2.7	2.7	2.5	2.8	2.4
Nonessential	50.3	50.0	50.2	52.1	58.2

*Based on the distribution of total protein between different components and the amino acid composition of each protein fraction (see Kirchgessner *et al.*, 1967; Davies *et al.*, 1983).
†Amino acid composition from Janas *et al.* (1985).
‡Amino acid composition from Svanberg *et al.* (1977).

Table 8. *Nitrogen excretion under conditions of 'protein-free feeding'.*

Species	*Total N loss (mg/kg$^{0.75}$/d)*	*Reference*
Rat	144	Lin & Huang (1986)
Chicken	152	Marumatsu *et al.* (1986)
Dog	201	Kendal *et al.* (1982)
Sheep	178	See Hovell *et al.* (1983)
Pig	193	Fuller & Crofts (1977)
Man	145	Summary of the literature*
Cattle	175	See Hovell *et al.* (1983)
Cat	381	Miller & Allison (1958)

*Young & Scrimshaw (1968); Calloway & Margen (1971); Huang *et al.* (1972); Nichol & Phillips (1975); Fujita *et al.* (1984).

unexplained difference in the ratio of cysteine to methionine in human milk, the amino acid compositions of different milks appear to be remarkably constant (Table 7). Surprisingly the amino acid composition of milk is quite poorly correlated with the presumed amino acid composition of growth in the preweaning phase.

Nevertheless, the argument persists that the protein requirement of man, when expressed in terms of a dietary allowance to support normal growth and development, is much lower than that of other mammals. The critical phrase is 'normal growth and development', because the rates of growth and development of man are substantially slower than those of all other mammals.

The importance of the replacement of basal losses of body amino acids to the overall protein requirement must be emphasized as the major single component of the lifetime requirement for protein. During the growth phase, the relative requirements for protein deposition and maintenance clearly depend on the relative rate of growth.

Table 9. *Protein-sparing effect of energy under conditions of negative nitrogen balance.*

Species	*Fasting nitrogen loss (mg N/kg$^{0.75}$/d)*	*Protein-free N loss (mg N/kg$^{0.75}$/d)*	*N spared /KJ*	*References*
Sheep	321	220	0.23	Asplund *et al.* (1986)
Cattle	272	189	0.18	Summary of literature
Man	239	145	0.19	See Reeds & Garlick (1984)
Pig	220	175	0.22	Fuller & Crofts (1977)
Rat	218	124	0.22	Lin & Huang (1986) Schemmel *et al.* (1983)

The maintenance component of the protein requirement for growth accounts for about 22% of the total in the rat and 90% of the total in man.

One approach to the quantification of the basal or maintenance component of the dietary protein requirement has been to investigate the rate of body nitrogen loss (by both the fecal and urinary routes) in individuals receiving no protein in their diets. Table 8 shows data from a number of species; differences emerge, with the dog, and not suprisingly the domestic cat, losing more nitrogen than average, and man, and suprisingly the rat, losing somewhat less than average.

As we point out above, this basal nitrogen loss consists predominantly of two components. The first is the loss of amino acids and other nitrogenous components by catabolism. On the basis of urinary nitrogen loss, this accounts for approximately 60% of the total and is principally derived from skeletal muscle (Uezu *et al.*, 1983). Unfortunately, the basis of this continual loss of amino acids by irrevocable catabolism is still unclear. At the simplest level it is rare for enzyme activities to disappear entirely and the preservation of some amino acid catabolic capacity will allow the organism to avoid the deleterious consequences of a sudden increase in protein intake following a period of protein-free feeding. Even after prolonged ingestion of protein-free diets, humans retain the ability to increase amino acid catabolism rapidly when protein is reintroduced into the diet (Clugston & Garlick, 1982).

In addition, other metabolic pathways such as choline, creatine and haem synthesis that use amino acids are sustained at a low rate even when no protein is supplied in the diet. When no protein is supplied in the diet, the loss of an essential amino acid into some other pathway will automatically restrict the degree to which the other amino acids can be reincorporated. The catabolism of the 'excess' amino acids must then occur if an amino acid imbalance is to be avoided. For example the provision of methionine alone will significantly spare the loss of body protein in animals receiving protein-free diets (see for example, Yoshida & Moritoki, 1974; Maramatsu *et al.*, 1986) and the provision of choline in the diet will spare methionine catabolism (Benenvenga, 1984). In this respect the cycling of urea nitrogen into the rumen may confer an adaptive advantage to ruminants receiving very low protein diets, for a proportion of this nitrogen will be reabsorbed as protein following its fixation by rumen microbes.

Amino acid carbon may also play an important role in intermediary metabolism and dietary energy will spare body nitrogen loss even when no protein is supplied in the diet (Table 9). Essentially the same quantity of nitrogen is spared in animals and man so that differences in the relationships between energy supply and protein deposition do not appear to explain the apparently low rate of basal nitrogen loss in man. Perhaps we should seek an answer within the dynamics of protein metabolism.

Body protein metabolism

Protein digestion, absorption and visceral metabolism

During the foregoing discussion, we have qualified our use of the term 'requirement' with the adjective 'obligatory'. A problem arises when the obligatory or minimal requirement is converted into a dietary allowance, because the ultimate utilization of the amino acids of the diet involves a number of processes within the body, and potential reductions in amino acid availability occur within each process.

The true digestibility of dietary proteins remains an unresolved area of investigation. Faecal nitrogen (which in general accounts for 30 to 40% of total basal N loss) represents a complex mixture of dietary protein and endogenous secretions that escaped digestion, together with the proteins and nucleic acids which have been synthesized by the colonic flora from the exogenous and endogenous components of the luminal contents. Although apparent N digestibility can give a general picture of the net availability of dietary proteins, it is of limited use in assessing the availability of any one amino acid. Furthermore, faecal nitrogen losses are increased in the presence of abundant supplies of undigestible carbohydrates and are generally higher in ruminant than in nonruminant species. The extent to which these losses represent protein of direct dietary origin, and hence are a function of digestibility, and the extent to which endogenous losses (a component of the protein requirement) contribute are often known with little certainty.

A further point of potential loss, and hence of potential variation in the efficiency of dietary protein utilization, is the 'first-pass' metabolism of amino acids at the early stages of their assimilation. Although the accretion and secretion of protein by the gastrointestinal tract is part of nitrogen retention, if the pattern of amino acids that leave the gut is different from that provided in the diet, it may no longer be appropriate for the efficient deposition of protein elsewhere in the body. As more comparisons have been made of amino acid losses from the gut lumen and appearances in the hepatic portal circulation, a significant difference has emerged in these two measures of protein digestion. Typically smaller quantities of amino acids appear in the portal circulation that disappear from the lumen of the small intestine (Tagari & Bergman, 1978; Low, 1980; Rerat *et al.*, 1980; Darcy & Rerat, 1983) and the hepatic portal appearance bears only a loose relationship to the composition of dietary protein. This phenomenon is common to both ruminant and nonruminant species and may represent metabolism by the cells of the gastrointestinal tract, metabolism in this case being taken to mean catabolism. This interpretation, however, may not be entirely correct. The contents of the intestine contain components derived from the diet and components secreted into the gut by the host animal. Amino acids utilized to produce these secretions have to be supplied from one of two sources: those from the lumen and those presented to the gut in the mesenteric arterial circulation. If these amino acids are derived in large part from the blood, they are removed from the mesenteric artery and replaced in the hepatic portal vein with a mixture of amino acids derived both

Table 10. *Comparison of apparent losses of essential amino acids during absorption with the amino acid composition of ileal digesta of pigs and sheep receiving protein-free diets.* Data from Low (1980); Rerat *et al.* (1979); Darcy & Rerat (1983); Tagari & Bergman (1978).

Amino acid	*Pig*	*Sheep*	*Composition of ileal digesta*
	Composition of amino acid loss (% of total)		
Lysine	10.7	12.6	11.4
Histidine	3.4	4.7	6.2
Threonine	18.9	15.5	18.4
Valine	18.4	17.9	16.9
Isoleucine	15.1	13.6	13.6
Leucine	21.5	21.6	19.8
Methionine	4.2	4.5	3.1
Phenylalanine	9.7	8.9	10.5

from the dietary protein and from the digestion of the secreted proteins themselves. Support for the idea that the anomalies in essential amino acid absorption result from this phenomenon is provided by the results in Table 10. Tagari & Bergman (1978) have presented data on the quantites of essential amino acids lost from the small intestine that fail to appear in the hepatic portal blood of sheep; estimates in the pig can be derived from results summarized by Low (1980) and Darcy & Rerat (1983). Low (1980) has also presented information on the amino acid composition of the ileal contents of pigs that were receiving protein-free diets. From these data, we can calculate the apparent composition (with respect to essential amino acids) of the endogenous proteins. As shown by the results in Table 10, a close similarity exists between the compositions of the amino acid mixture that apparently fails to appear in the hepatic portal blood and that of the endogenous secretions. The patterns appear similar in both sheep and pigs. These findings suggest that at least a portion of the apparent inefficiency of the absorption of these essential amino acids may result from a failure to account completely for the essential amino acids that are removed from the arterial circulation to supply the needs for secretory and constitutive protein production in the gut.

Nevertheless, these comments apply only to the essential amino acids. Strong evidence suggests that major changes occur in the mixture of nonessential amino acids that cross the gut wall. There is a substantial interconversion involving net metabolism of glutamine, glutamate and aspartate, with an output of alanine and ammonia. Furthermore, these transformations occur with both lumenal (Bergman & Pell, 1986) and systemic (Wahren *et al.*, 1976; Windmueller & Spaeth, 1978; Heitman & Bergman, 1980) amino acids and continue in the postabsorptive state (Table 11). Thus a metabolic cycle exists whereby glutamine and alanine, which are released from skeletal muscle even in the fed state in sheep (Heitman & Berman, 1980), rats (Lund, 1982), and man (Wahren *et al*, 1976), pass to the viscera where they are metabolized by the gut, the liver and the kidney (see Tables 11 and 12). In these respects, there seem few fundamental differences in the metabolism of these amino acids in the mammalian species for which we have information.

Apparent metabolic differences do exist, however, in other areas of amino acid metabolism, especially between nonruminants (as exemplified by man and the dog)

Table 11. *Splanchnic exchange of amino acids in fasted and fed man and sheep.* From Wahren *et al.* (1976); Heitman & Bergman (1980).

	Splanchnic exchange µmol/min			
	Fasted		Fed	
Amino acid	*Man*	*Sheep*	*Man*	*Sheep*
Aspartate	37	27	0	17
Glutamine	68	60	105	61
Alanine	97	64	83	16
Glycine	26	51	– 14	28
Leucine	– 7‡	10†	– 80	– 6
Isoleucine	– 7	7	– 40	– 3
Valine	– 18	13	– 64	– 7
Phenylalanine	14	16	– 4	– 4

†Positive values = utilization; ‡Negative values = output.

Table 12. *Limb exchange of amino acids in fasted and fed man and sheep.* From Wahren *et al.* (1976); Heitman & Bergman (1980).

	Hind limb exchange µmol/min			
	Fasted		Fed	
	Man	*Sheep*	*Man*	*Sheep*
Aspartate	18	ND	8	ND
Glutamine	– 40	– 28	– 50	– 18
Alanine	– 30	– 30	– 30	– 17
Glycine	– 6	– 31	4	– 14
Leucine	5†	– 9‡	23	3
Isoleucine	3	– 5	11	2
Valine	9	– 9	24	8
Phenylalanine	– 2	– 8	7	3

†Positive values = utilization; ‡Negative values = output.

Table 13. *Leucine oxidation either by the whole body or by a limb in sheep, cattle, dogs, and man in fed and fasted states.*

	Leucine oxidation (% of leucine turnover)				
	Whole body		Limb metabolism		
Species	*Fed*	*Fasted*	*Fed*	*Fasted*	*Reference*
Sheep	15.0	21.0	8	15.7	Pell *et al.* (1986)
Cattle	9.0	11.9	ND	ND	Lobley *et al.* (1987)
Man	20.6	13.2	30.7	4.8	Cheng *et al.* (1987)
Dog	19.6	13.3	ND	ND	Nissen & Haymond (1986)

and ruminants (as exemplified by the sheep). Measurements of leucine oxidation in sheep, cattle, man, and dog (Table 13) show that when expressed as a proportion of leucine flux, a short fast reduces leucine oxidation in the nonruminants and increases its oxidation in the ruminants. This difference is even more apparent when leucine metabolism in peripheral tissues is considered; ie, in the fed state, the limb tissues of man catabolize about 30% of the total leucine uptake while the sheep oxidizes only 8%. The position was reversed in fasted individuals. This description should not be interpreted to imply that a reduction does not occur in total leucine oxidation in the fasted state in both man and the sheep, but the results do imply that leucine (as opposed to α-keto isocaproic acid) catabolism between the musculature and the viscera is quite different. Further support is provided by measurements that show a significant splanchnic output of branched-chain amino acids in fasted man (Wahren *et al.*, 1976) but a significant uptake in fasted sheep (Heitman & Bergamn, 1980; Pell *et al.*, 1986) (Tables 11, 12). However, the differences in the response to fasting in ruminant and non-ruminant species shown in Table 13 may be misleading; the length of the fast was significantly different in the ruminants (4–5 days) and in the nonruminants (12 to 24 hours). When rats were fasted for 2 (Sketcher *et al.*, 1974) or 4 days (Meikle & Klein, 1971), the proportion of leucine flux that passed into leucine oxidation also rose. These results are supported by a recent study in man (Nair *et al.*, 1987).

Amino acid losses also occur in the liver and significant changes in the amino acid pattern occur between the hepatic portal vein and the hepatic vein. Unfortunately the results of studies of hepatic exchange of amino acids have been largely confined to adult animals in which amino acid intakes are low and in which all amino acids are eventually catabolized. However, this point of loss may be of particular importance to the high protein requirements of cats (and perhaps of other carnivores), because of evidence to suggest that this species lacks the ability to effect substantial changes in either hepatic protein catabolism (Silva & Mercer, 1986) or amino acid catabolism (Rogers & Morris, 1978) in relation to hepatic amino acid supply.

Protein turnover

The premise that animals continue to degrade and resynthesize body proteins even under conditions of severe protein-loss is now well-established. Thus, the ultimate utilization of dietary protein represents a balance between the incorporation of amino acids into protein and irrevocable amino acid catabolism. Nevertheless, it is important to recognize that protein turnover itself does not necessarily result in a net loss of amino acids from the body protein.

Although this last comment is qualitatively true, important quantitative and mechanistic questions remain. For example, there is no certainty whether amino acid catabolism is largely dominated by the need to remove amino acids that are not incorporated into protein, and is hence set by the overall balance between protein synthesis and degradation, or whether specific pathways of amino acid use exert a direct controlling influence, interacting with protein turnover, and thus with overall protein balance. Under some circumstances, such as in the severely protein-depleted state, this consideration may be important.

Nevertheless, some quantitative questions with regard to protein turnover must be examined. The first of these relates simply to the magnitude of the protein turnover (see Young, 1987). Tables 14 and 15 provide a summary of data obtained in mature and immature individuals studied in a state close to nitrogen equilibrium. Two points emerge: first, that the immature animals clearly synthesize more protein per $kg^{0.75}$ than mature individuals; and second, that in both comparisons, body protein synthesis in man is significantly lower than in nonhuman species. Although these points suggest

Table 14. *Whole body protein turnover in adults.*

Species	*Whole body protein turnover (g protein/kg$^{0.75}$/d)*	*References*
Rat	15.4	Goldspink & Kelly (1984)
Rabbit	14.6	Lobley, G. E. *et al.* (unpublished)
Dog	16.5	Nissen & Haymond (1986)
Sheep	14.0	Pell *et al.* (1986)
Cattle	14.5	Reeds *et al.* (1981)
Man	11.9	Reeds & Garlick (1984)
	.	Hoffer *et al.* (1985)

Table 15. *Whole body protein turnover in immature mammals restricted to energy equilibrium.*

Species	*Whole body protein turnover (g protein/kg$^{0.75}$/d)*	*Reference*
Rat	17.5	Reeds *et al.* (1982)
Pig	18.9	Reeds *et al.* (1980)
Cattle	19.6	Lobley *et al.* (1987)
Man	13.5	Golden *et al.* (1977)
	10.5	Jackson *et al.* (1983)

Table 16. *Increments in protein synthesis per unit increment in protein deposition in immature mammals.*

Species	*Increase in protein synthesis / Increase in protein deposition*	*% Mature weight*	*Reference*
Rat	1.20	11	Reeds *et al.* (1982)
Pig	2.17	16	Reeds *et al.* (1980)
Man	1.36	10	Golden *et al.* (1977)
Sheep	2.38	41	Davis *et al.* (1981)
Cattle	4.16	80	Lobley *et al.* (1987)

that protein metabolism in man is maintained more efficiently and the results in Table 16 suggest that growth is also achieved more effectively, the interpretation may be incorrect. Lobley *et al.* (1987) have pointed out that a major influence on the relationship between protein turnover and growth appears to be the developmental age of the subject. When humans and rats are compared at the same proportion of mature body weight, they appear remarkably similar.

However, a further and important point emerges from the data in Table 14. The subjects reported by Golden *et al.* (1977) were infants recovering from malnutrition who may have adapted to their condition, so that the relationship between protein turnover and nitrogen loss (ie, the balance between protein synthesis and amino acid catabolism) was altered in a manner that conserved body protein. Indeed, Golden went on to show that malnourished children required significantly less dietary protein to maintain their body protein stores than when they had recovered from malnutrition. Similar results have been obtained in protein-depleted immature sheep (Hovell *et al.*, 1987). These findings also apply to adults; in a recent study in young men, Young *et al.* (1987) have shown that a period of low leucine intake induces an accommodation

Table 17. *Protein turnover and amino acid recycling in rats, chicks and humans fed 'protein-free' diets.*

Species	*Protein turnover* (*g protein/kg$^{0.75}$/d*)	*Protein loss*	*Recycled* (*%*)	*Reference*
Rat	8.06	0.83	90	Garlick *et al.* (1975)
				Uezu *et al.* (1985)
Chick	7.8	1.16	85	Marumatsu *et al.* (1986)
Man	9.20	0.94	90	Motil *et al.* (1981b)
	9.03	1.16	87	Garlick *et al.* (1980)

associated with a reduction in protein turnover that enables the individual to conserve this amino acid. Interestingly, if we compare protein turnover rates and nitrogen losses in different species which have received protein-free diets for a considerable time (Table 17), we find that essentially the same process of conservation occurs in man, the rat, and the chick.

The findings of these investigators have an important bearing on the theme of this paper. In Table 9, two species, the rat and man, have an apparent low rate of basal nitrogen loss. The measurements were reported after a prolonged period of ingestion of a protein-free diet (3 weeks in both cases). It could be argued that, had a sufficiently long period been allowed to elapse, the other monogastric animals may well have given similar results, with the possible exception of the cat. This may be of great importance to an understanding of the needs of any species, for it can be argued that because of metabolic adaptation, basal protein loss is an inappropriate measure of maintenance protein requirements.

Nevertheless, the fact that man is capable of surviving, if not prospering while ingesting a wide variety of diets, demonstrates his considerable metabolic adaptive capabilities. The mechanistic basis for this ability is still poorly understood and is discussed elsewhere (Young, 1987). Certainly it is an important area for future research.

It is proposed that few fundamental protein metabolic differences exist between man and other mammals. However, humans stand alone in their slow rate of normal growth and their habitual low voluntary intakes of the major nutrients. Perhaps when we study normal man, we are studying a mammal that has adapted to a life-time of intakes that are remarkably close to those required for protein and energy maintenance.

Acknowledgement—The author is extremely grateful to Professor V. R. Young for his helpful comments and stimulating discussions concerning this paper.

References

Alqvist, S. E. G. (1951): Metabolic relationships among amino acids studied with isotopic nitrogen. *Acta Medica Scand.* **5**, 1046–1064.

Anderson, B. A. (1983): *Composition of pork products.* Agricultural Handbook 8–10, Washington DC: United States Department of Agriculture.

Anderson, B. A., Lauderdale, J. L. & Hoke, I. M. (1986): *Composition of beef products.* Washington DC: United States Department of Agriculture.

Asplund, J. M., Orskov, E. R., Hovell, F. D. deB. & MacLeod, N. A. (1986): The effect of infusion of glucose, lipids or acetate on fasting nitrogen excretion and blood metabolites in sheep. *Br. J. Nutr.* **54**, 189–195.

Benevenga, N. J. (1984): Evidence for alternative pathways of methionine catabolism. *Adv. Nutr. Res.* **6**, 1–18.

Bergman, E. N. & Pell, J. M. (1986): Interorgan movement of amino acids. In *Proceedings of the XIII International Congress of Nutrition*, eds T. G. Taylor and N. K. Jenkins, pp. 370–374. London: John Libbey.

Bien, E. J., Yu, T. T., Benedict, J. D., Gutman, A. B. & Steffen, D. (1953): The relationship of dietary nitrogen consumption to the rate of uric acid synthesis in normal and gouty man. *J. Clin. Invest.* **32**, 778–780.

Boorman, K. N. & Lewis, D. (1971): Protein metabolism. In *Physiology and biochemistry of the domestic fowl*, eds D. J. Bell and B. M. Freeman, pp. 339–372. London: Academic Press.

Bowering, J., Calloway, D. H., Margen, S. & Kaufman, N. A. (1970): Dietary protein level and uric acid metabolism in normal man. *J. Nutr.* **100**, 249–261.

Burridge, P. W., Woods, R. A. & Henderson, J. F. (1976): Utilization of dietary nucleic acid purines for nucleotide and nucleic acid synthesis. *Can. J. Biochem.* **54**, 500–506.

Calloway, D. H. & Margen, S. (1971): Variation in endogenous nitrogen excretion and dietary nitrogen utilization as determinants of human protein requirements. *J. Nutr.* **101**, 205–216.

Cheng, K. N., Pacy, P. J., Dworzak, F., Ford, G. C. & Halliday, D. (1987): Influence of fasting on leucine and muscle protein metabolism across the human forearm determined using L-[^{13}C, ^{15}N]-leucine as the tracer. *Clin. Sci.* **73**, 241–246.

Clugston, G. A. & Garlick, P. J. (1982): The response of whole-body protein turnover to feeding in obese subjects given a protein-free low energy diet for three weeks. *Hum. Nutr: Clin. Nutr.* **36C**, 391–397.

Darcy, B. & Rerat, A. (1983): Protein digestion and absorption of the hydrolysis products in the small intestine of the pig. In *Protein metabolism and nutrition*, ed M. Arnal, M. Pion and D. Bonnin, pp. 233–244. Paris: I.N.R.A.

Davies, D. T., Holt, C. & Christie, W. W. (1983): The composition of milk. In *Biochemistry of lactation*, ed T. B. Mepham, pp. 71–120. Amsterdam: Elsevier.

Davis, S. R., Barry, T. N. & Hughson, G. A. (1981): Protein synthesis in tissues of growing lambs. *Br. J. Nutr.* **46**, 409–419.

Fujihara, T., Orskov, E. R., Reeds, P. J. & Kyle, D. J. (1987): The effect of protein infusion on urinary excretion of purine derivatives in ruminants nourished by intragastric infusion. *J. Agric. Sci.* (Camb.). **109**, 7–12.

Fujita, Y., Okuda, T., Rikimaru, T., Ichikawa, M., Miyatami, S., Kajiwara, N. M., Yamaguchi, Y., Oi, Y., Koishi, H., Alpers, M. P. & Heywood, P. F. (1984): Endogenous nitrogen excretion in male highlanders of Papua, New Guinea. *J. Nutr.* **114**, 1997–2002.

Fuller, M. F., & Crofts, R. M. J. (1977): The protein sparing effect of carbohydrate. *Br. J. Nutr.* **38**, 479–488.

Garlick, P. J., Clugston, G. A. & Waterlow, J. C. (1980): Influence of low-energy diets on whole-body protein turnover in obese subjects. *Am. J. Physiol.* **238**, E235–E244.

Garlick, P. J., Millward, D. J., James, W. P. T. & Waterlow, J. C. (1975): The effect of protein deprivation and starvation on the rate of protein synthesis in tissues of the rat. *Biochim. Biophys. Acta* **414**, 71–84.

Golden, M. H. N., Waterlow, J. C. & Picou, D. (1977): Protein turnover, synthesis and breakdown before and after recovery from protein energy malnutrition. *Clin. Sci.* **53**, 473–477.

Golden, M. H. N., Waterlow, J. C. & Picou, D. (1982): Metabolism of ^{15}N-nucleic acids in children. In *Nitrogen metabolism in man*, eds J. C. Waterlow and J. M. L. Stephen, pp. 269–274. London: Applied Science Publishers.

Goldspink, D. F. & Kelly, F. J. (1984): Protein turnover in the whole body, liver and kidney of the rat from the foetus to senility. *Biochem. J.* **217**, 507–516.

Heitman, R. N. & Bergman, E. N. (1980): Integration of amino acid metabolism in sheep. Effects of fasting and acidosis. *Am. J. Physiol.* **239**, E248–E254.

Hoffer, L. J., Yang, R. D., Matthews, D. E., Bistrian, B. R., Bier, D. M. & Young, V. R. (1985): Effects of meal consumption on whole body leucine and alanine kinetics in young adult men. *Br. J. Nutr.* **53**, 31–38.

Hovell, F. D. deB., Orskov, E. R., Grubb, D. A. & MacLeod, N. A. (1983): Basal urinary nitrogen excretion and growth response to supplemental protein by lambs close to energy equilibrium. *Br. J. Nutr.* **50**, 173–182.

Hovell, F. D. deB., Orskov, E. R., Kyle, D. J. & MacLeod, N. A. (1987): Undernutrition in sheep. Nitrogen repletion by N-depleted sheep. *Br. J. Nutr.* **57**, 77–88.

Huang, P. C., Chong, H. E. & Rand, W. M. (1972): Obligatory urinary and fecal nitrogen losses in young Chinese men. *J. Nutr.* **102**, 1605–1614.

Jackson, A. A., Byfield, R., Jahoor, F., Royes, J. & Soutter, L. (1983): Whole body protein turnover and nitrogen balance in young children at intakes of protein and energy in the region of maintenance. *Hum. Nutr: Clin. Nutr.* **37C**, 433–466.

Jackson, A. A. & Golden, M. H. N. (1980): ^{15}N-glycine metabolism in normal man: metabolic a-amino nitrogen pool. *Clin. Sci.* **58**, 517–522.

Jackson, A. A., Shaw, J. C. L., Barber, A. & Golden, M. H. N. (1981): Nitrogen metabolism in pre-term infants fed human donor breast milk: the possible essentiality of glycine. *Pediatr. Res.* **15**, 1454–1461.

Janas, L. M., Picciano, M. F. & Hatch, T. F. (1985): Indices of protein metabolism in term infants fed human milk, whey predominant formula or cow's milk formula. *Pediatrics* **75**, 775–784.

Kendal, P. T., Blaza, S. E. & Holme, D. W. (1982): Assessment of endogenous nitrogen output in adult dogs of contrasting size using a protein-free diet. *J. Nutr.* **112**, 1281–1286.

Kirchgessner, M., Frisecke, H. & Koch, G. (1967): *Nutrition and the composition of milk*. Philadelphia: J. B. Lippincott.

Laidlaw, S. A. & Kopple, J. D. (1987): Newer concepts of the indispensible amino acids. *Am. J. Clin. Nutr.* **46**, 593–605.

Lin, C. P. & Huang, P.-C. (1986): Comparison of control diets containing various protein levels for determining Net Protein Utilization in rats. *J. Nutr.* **116**, 216–222.

Lobley, G. E., Connell, A. & Buchan, V. (1987): Effect of food intake on protein and energy metabolism in finishing beef steers. *Br. J. Nutr.* **57**, 457–465.

Low, A. G. (1980): Nutrient absorption in the pig. *J. Sci. Fd. Agric.* **31**, 1087–1130.

Lund, P. (1982): Metabolism of glutamine, glutamate and aspartate. In *Nitrogen metabolism in man*, eds J. C. Waterlow and J. M. L. Stephen, pp. 155–168, London: Applied Science Publishers.

MacDonald, M. L., Rogers, Q. L. & Morris, J. G. (1984): Nutrition of the Domestic Cat. *Ann. Rev. Nutr.* **4**, 521–562.

Maramatsu, T., Kato, M., Tasaki, I. & Okamura, J. (1986): Enhanced whole-body protein synthesis by methionine and arginine supplementation in protein-starved chicks. *Br. J. Nutr.* **55**, 635–641.

Matthews, D. E., Conway, J. E., Young, V. R. & Bier, D. M. (1981): Glycine nitrogen metabolism in man. *Metabolism* **30**, 886–893.

Meikle, A. W. & Klein, G. J. (1972): Effects of fasting and fasting-refeeding on conversion of leucine to CO_2 and lipids in rats. *Am. J. Physiol.* **222**, 1246–1250.

Miller, S. A. & Allison, J. B. (1958): The dietary nitrogen requirements of the cat. *J. Nutr.* **64**, 493–501.

Motil, K. J., Harmon, W. E. & Grupe, W. E. (1981a): Complications of essential amino acid hyperalimentation in children with acute renal failure. *J. Parent. Enteral Nutr.* **4**, 32–35.

Motil, K. J., Matthews, D. E., Bier, D. M., Burke, J. F., Munro, H. N. & Young, V. R. (1981b): Whole body leucine and lysine metabolism: response to dietary protein intake in young men. *Am. J. Physiol.* **240**, E712–E721.

Nair, K. S., Woolf, P. D., Welle, S. L. & Matthews, D. E. (1987): Leucine, glucose and energy metabolism after 3 days of fasting in healthy human subjects. *Am. J. Clin. Nutr.* **45**, 557–562.

Newsholme, E. A., Crabtree, B. & Ardawi, M. S. M. (1985): Glutamine metabolism in lymphocytes: its biochemical, physiological and clinical importance. *Quart. J. Exp. Physiol.* **70**, 473–489.

Nichol, B. M. & Phillips, P. G. (1975): Endogenous nitrogen excretion and utilization of dietary protein. *Br. J. Nutr.* **35**, 181–188.

Nissen, S. & Haymond, M. W. (1986): Changes in leucine kinetics during meal absorption: effects of dietary leucine availability. *Am. J. Physiol.* **250**, E695–E701.

Pell, J. M., Caldarone, E. M. & Bergman, E. N. (1986): Leucine and a-keto iso caproate metabolism and interconversions in fed and fasted sheep. *Metabolism* **35**, 1005–1006.

Posati, L. P. (1979): *Composition of poultry products*. Agricultural Handbook 8-5, Washington DC: United States Department of Agriculture.

Reeds, P. J., Cadenhead, A., Fuller, M. F., Lobley, G. E. & McDonald, J. D. (1980): Protein turnover in growing pigs. Effects of age and food intake. *Br. J. Nutr.* **43**, 445–455.

Reeds, P. J. & Garlick, P. J. (1984): Nutrition and protein turnover in man. *Adv. Nutr. Res.* **6**, 93–138.

Reeds, P. J., Haggarty, P., Wahle, K. W. J. & Fletcher, J. M. (1982): Tissue and whole body protein synthesis in immature Zucker rats and their relationship to protein deposition. *Biochem. J.* **204**, 393–398.

Reeds, P. J. & Harris, C. I. (1982): Protein turnover in animals: Man in his context. In *Nitrogen metabolism in man*, eds J. C. Waterlow and J. M. L. Stephen, pp. 391–408. London: Applied Science Publishers.

Reeds, P. J., Orskov, E. R. & MacLeod, N. A. (1981): Whole body protein synthesis in cattle sustained by infusion of volatile fatty acids and casein. *Proc. Nutr. Soc.* **40**, 50A.

Rerat, A., Vaissade, P. & Vangelade, P. (1979): Absorption kinetics of amino acids and reducing sugars during digestion of barley and wheat meals in the pig. *Ann. Biol. Anim. Biochim. Biophys.* **19**, 739–747.

Rogers, Q. R. & Morris, J. G. (1978): Why does the cat require a high protein diet? In *Nutrition of the dog and the cat*, ed R. S. Anderson, pp. 521–532. Oxford: Pergamon Press.

Roll, P. M., Brown, G. B., Di Carlo, F. G. & Schultz, A. S. (1949): Utilization of ^{15}N-glycine for purine synthesis. *J. Biol. Chem.* **180**, 329–340.

Sander, D., Topp, H., Heller-Schorch, G., Wieland, J. & Schorch, G. (1986): Ribonucleic acid turnover in man: RNA catabolites in urine as a measure for the metabolism of each of the three major species of RNA. *Clin. Sci.* **71**, 367–374.

Schemmel, R. A., Stone, M., Warren, M. J. & Stoddart, K. A. (1983): Nitrogen and protein losses in rats during weight reduction with a high-protein, very low energy diet or fasting. *J. Nutr.* **113**, 727–734.

Silva, S. V. P. S. & Mercer, J. R. (1986): Protein degradation in cat liver cells. *Biochem. J.* **240**, 843–846.

Sketcher, R., Fern, E. & James, W. P. T. (1974): The adaptation in muscle oxidation of leucine to dietary protein and energy intake. *Br. J. Nutr.* **31**, 333–342.

Smith, R. H. (1980): Comparative Amino Acid Requirements. *Proc. Nutr. Soc.* **39**, 71–77.

Svanberg, V., Gebre-Medhin, M., Lindqvist, B. & Olsson, M. (1977): Breast-milk composition in Ethiopian and Swedish mothers. *Am. J. Clin. Nutr.* **30**, 499–507.

Tagari, H. & Bergman, E. N. (1978): Intestinal disappearance and portal appearance of amino acids in sheep. *J. Nutr.* **98**, 790–803.

Uezu, N., Yamamoto, S., Rikimaru, T., Kishi, K. & Inoue, G. (1985): Contributions of individual body tissues of nitrogen excretion in adult rats fed protein-deficient diets. *J. Nutr.* **113**, 105–114.

Wahren, J., Felig, P. & Hagenfeldt, L. (1976): Effect of protein digestion on splanchnic and leg metabolism in normal man and in patients with Diabetes Mellitus. *J. Clin. Invest.* **57**, 987–999.

Windmueller, H. G. & Spaeth, A. E. (1978): Identification of ketone bodies and glutamine as major respiratory fuels *in vivo* for post-absorptive rat small intestine. *J. Biol. Chem.* **253**, 69–76.

Young, V. R. (1987): Kinetics of human amino acid metabolism: nutritional implications and some lessons. *Am. J. Clin. Nutr.* **46**, 709–725.

Young, V. R., Gucalp, C., Rand, W. M., Matthews, D. E. & Bier, D. M. (1987): Leucine kinetics during three weeks at submaintenance-to-maintenance intakes of leucine in men: adaptation and accommodation. *Hum. Nutr: Clin. Nutr.* **41C**, 1–18.

Young, V. R. & Scrimshaw, N. S. (1968): Endogenous nitrogen metabolism and plasma free amino acids in young adults given a 'protein-free' diet. *Br. J. Nutr.* **22**, 9–20.

Yoshida, A. & Moritoli, K. (1974): Nitrogen sparing action of methionine and threonine in rats receiving a protein-free diet. *Nutr. Rep. Int.* **9**, 159–168.

Yu, M., Yang, R. D., Matthews, D. E., Burke, J. F., Bier, D. M. & Young, V. R. (1985): Quantitative aspects of glycine and alanine nitrogen metabolism in young men: effect of level of nitrogen and dispensible amino acid intake. *J. Nutr.* **115**, 339–410.

* * * * *

Discussion

Dr Widdowson recalled that when she had looked at the amino acid composition of the human fetus and of breast milk, she had realized that milk could not supply the amounts of glycine that the fetus had been obtaining from the maternal supply and concluded that the baby must be able to synthesize considerable amounts. *Dr Reeds* commented that the same is true of sheep, for experiments by Robinson showed a similar large requirement for glycine. He showed that the sources of this were indeed rather limited and that it probably mostly came from serine.

Dr Elia commenting on the table dealing with the splanchnic exchange, stated that there was perhaps room for confusion since some of the experiments quoted related to the ingestion of a meal containing protein only rather than a mixed meal. *Dr Reeds* agreed, but pointed out that the difference was still present and was as marked in fasted as in fed animals.

Dr Fuller commented that although the concentrations of sulphur amino acids appear to be relatively low in the milk-to-tissue comparison, other essential amino acids were present in relative excess.

Professor Jackson commented with respect to glycine that in tissue culture there is a need for very large amounts of glycine. In this respect he mentioned that Professor Vernon Young had shown that on low protein diets *de novo* synthesis of glycine by man may not always be sufficient to meet requirements. *Dr Reeds* replied that it seemed important to look at complete amino acid balances in approaching many of these problems and went on to point out that glutamine and glycine together are required in considerable amounts by rapidly developing cells. This had certainly been shown with respect to oxidative changes, but from the point of view of nucleic acid metabolism much more needed to be done. *Professor Armstrong* commented on comparative aspects of allowances for protein in ruminants and pointed out that there was a considerable component of nitrogen turnover related to events in the digestive tract itself involving protozoa and bacteria. He also pointed out that protein had a role in appetite regulation.

In relation to the latter *Professor Forbes* stated that appetite was certainly reduced in ruminants when rate of digestion in the rumen was limited by nitrogen deficiency; diets deficient in protein or with imbalanced amino acids also depress intake in all species, possibly by reducing metabolic rate.

Dr Millward commented on the efficiency quotients of net body gain in protein over synthesis, and wondered whether the comparisons made in Table 16 were really comparable since the human data related to catch-up growth in children, which may well be more efficient than normal growth. *Dr Reeds* stated that whilst all these results related to the consequences of increases in the amount of diet, he nevertheless accepted that this was a valid criticism.

Professor James then asked how far these ratios depended on the nature of the growth process in relation to particular tissues. *Dr Reeds* stated that they might very well and Professor James continued by saying that the potential of tissues to modify synthesis following nutritional insult could perhaps be very great.

Dr Reeds then commented that where there were experimental differences it was extremely difficult in some instances to attribute errors to them but it did appear that the differences largely reflect differences in experimental protocols in design and that an underlying coherence appeared to be present.

Professor Waterlow then asked whether the recycling of some essential amino-acids, eg lysine, was more efficient than others, to which *Dr Reeds* replied that there was insufficient evidence. *Dr Millward* pointed out that the problem is largely one of measurement. He said however that he was very uneasy about the recycling (Table 17) particularly in so far as the data related to a ratio calculated from a small value—nitrogen excretion, with a much larger one, nitrogen turnover. The ratio is relatively insensitive to changes in the magnitude of nitrogen loss. *Dr Reeds* said that all the measurements had been made over long periods on low protein diets and the conditions under which the measurements were made were very similar; clearly more work needed to be done. The interesting point was that all three species came down to the same rate of protein turnover and essentially the same efficiency of recycling.

5

Comparative aspects of nutrient metabolism: lipid metabolism

M. I. GURR

Introduction

Lipids perform two major functions in the animal body: as structural components of membranes and as an efficient means of storing energy. There are major chemical differences between the structural and storage lipids and their fatty acids and there are also significant differences between the lipids that predominate in plants and in animals. These differences are important when considering the composition of the dietary lipids of carnivores, herbivores and omnivores, since the quantity and nature of dietary lipids influence the subsequent pathways of metabolism and the structure, composition and function of the animal's tissues and organs.

Major differences in lipid digestion occur between ruminants, other herbivores and carnivorous or omnivorous simple stomached animals. In ruminants, lipids are digested mainly by the bacteria in the rumen giving rise to free fatty acids and glycerol. Most simple stomached animals break down lipids in the duodenum with the aid of a pancreatic lipase, the main products being monoacylglycerols and free fatty acids. In many species the newborn begins lipid digestion in the stomach making use of a lingual or gastric lipase. In large herbivores such as the horse, the large intestine is a major digestive organ, bacterial fermentation giving rise to very short chain fatty acids which are absorbed in the lower gut and metabolized to lipids in the liver.

Despite these differences in digestion, the mechanism of absorption of long chain fatty acids seems to be quite similar in most species. After absorption, the basic principles of the transport of lipids in the blood as lipoproteins, their assimilation by tissues and the anabolic and catabolic biochemical pathways of lipid metabolism are similar in most species, although there are many differences in detail. For a general

Comparative Nutrition, ed K. Blaxter & I. Macdonald. ©John Libbey 1988.

review, the reader is referred to Gurr & James (1980). This paper will concentrate on two aspects: lipid storage and the metabolism of the unsaturated fatty acids.

Lipid storage

Most animal species store their lipid reserves in adipose tissue, but fish are notable exceptions since they store them in the liver (eg cod, sharks) or in the flesh (eg mackerel, herring) (Opstvedt, 1984). In all the fish species that we are accustomed to eat, the stored lipids are mainly triacylglycerols (Opstvedt, 1984), but some fish, such as the orange roughy, use wax esters as a storage form (Buisson, 1983). There are two forms of adipose tissue, designated 'brown' and 'white'. Brown adipose tissue is not involved in lipid storage: it has a specialized function in generating heat for the maintenance of body temperature, especially in the newborn of some species (eg man, rat, guinea pig, but not, apparently, the pig) and in species that hibernate (Hull & Hardman, 1970; Cannon & Nedergaard, 1985). It will not be further discussed here; the reader is referred to these excellent reviews that take a comparative approach.

White adipose tissue: species similarities

White adipose tissue is the major organ for storing lipids as energy reserves and the primary stored lipids are triacylglycerols in all species. The mature adipocyte is characterized by a single globule of fat that occupies the centre of the cell forcing the nucleus and cytoplasm, with its various organelles to the periphery of the cell. Circulating plasma lipoproteins, that are primary carriers of triacylglycerols, become entrapped in the capillaries supplying the adipose tissue by interaction with the enzyme lipoprotein lipase. This enzyme, whose activity is stimulated by insulin, catalyses the hydrolysis of the lipids to free fatty acids, which are taken into the cell. There they are esterified back into triacylglycerols, primarily via the glycerol phosphate pathway. Adipocytes can also synthesize fatty acids and glycerol phosphate from glucose as precursors for the storage lipid. Fatty acids are mobilized from the fat stores when the body requires oxidative substrates. This is accomplished by lipolysis catalysed by a lipase that is repressed by insulin but stimulated by the catecholamines. For a general background see Gurr & James (1980) and for more detail, Vernon & Clegg (1985). A principle that is common to most species is the accumulation of maternal fat depots during early pregnancy and their subsequent mobilization in late gestation. Such fat mobilization leads to hyperlipidaemia of pregnancy and its extent depends on the litter size and maternal nutritional status (Battaglia & Meschia, 1986).

White adipose tissue: species differences

A. Tissue development. As long ago as the 1870s (eg see Flemming, 1871) it was postulated that adipocytes had their origins in connective tissue and since then, numerous authors have provided supporting evidence (eg see Leat & Cox, 1980). Nevertheless, other data do not support this concept since, although fibroblasts are distributed throughout the body, some areas of the body never contain adipocytes (eg see Hausman, 1985). Flemming (1871) had already noted that adipose tissue cells first appeared near

Table 1. *Adipose tissue in the new-born.*

Species	*Placental permeability to free fatty acids*	*Fat at birth g/100 g*	*Fat cell diameter μm*
Man	+ + + +	16.1	50–80
Guinea pig	+ + + +	10.1	130
Rabbit	+ + +	5.8	35
Lamb	+ +	3.3	
Calf	+ +	2.8	
Foal	+ +	2.6	
Cat	+	1.8	
Rat	+	1.1	10
Pig	+	1.1	20

blood vessels and not randomly in the connective tissue. These observations suggest that some local, as yet unknown, humoral factors are responsible for modifying fibrous connective tissue into immature adipose tissue (Hausman, 1985). This author has suggested that the extensive distribution of adipose tissue in the fetus is related to the downgrowth of epithelium into underlying connective tissue, based on observations of adipocyte development at sites where developing hair follicles and mammary gland ducts invade connective tissue in the fetal pig and rat respectively (Hausman & Martin, 1982; Hausman, 1982). Preadipose tissue, which contains primitive fat cells characterized by numerous small lipid globules, similar in appearance to brown adipocytes (multilocular cells), can be found in the fetus of most species. Its development into mature tissue, characterized by unilocular cells, may occur in the fetus or postnatally depending on the species.

Man and guinea pig are species which have a high proportion of their body weight as fat at birth, mainly in the white adipose tissue; in contrast, pigs, cats and rats are born with little or no adipose tissue, while ruminants and rabbits have an intermediate amount (Table 1). In man, development of fat cells begins mainly in the last third of gestation and at birth the average size of the cells is relatively large (Table 1). The guinea pig is similar and provides a good model for man in regard to fat cell development (Kirtland *et al.*, 1976). Despite the lack of fat at birth in pig and lamb, preadipocytes can be observed in fetal pig at 70 days gestation (Desnoyers & Vodovar, 1974) and in the fetal lamb at 60 days (Wensvoort, 1967).

The origins of fetal fat and the reasons for the extensive prenatal accumulation of fat in some species and the almost entirely postnatal accumulation in others are subjects of some controversy. The fetus is totally dependent on the placental transfer of substrates from the mother's circulation. At least four sources can be envisaged for the fetal accumulation of lipid: glucose transferred from maternal to fetal circulation; free fatty acids transferred across the placenta; maternal circulating lipoproteins, and substrates provided by the mother but synthesized into lipid in the placenta.

Most authors seem to agree that glucose is a major source of energy for the fetus (eg see Heim, 1983; Kimura & Warshaw, 1983). The fetuses of most species possess the enzymic activities for conversion of glucose into fatty acids and in any case glucose is necessary for the provision of the glycerol moiety of triacylglycerols via glycerol

Table 2. Amounts of lipid in the milks of different species.

Species	*Lipid in milk (g/100 g)*	*Species*	*Lipid in milk (g/100 g)*
Horse	2	Brown bear	10
Cow	4	Elephant	15
Guinea pig	4	Sperm whale	16
Human	5	Rabbit	18
Sheep	8	Polar bear	32
Pig	9	Fur seal	53
Rat	10	Harp seal	58

phosphate (Martin *et al.*, 1985). Animals are incapable of synthesizing all their lipid requirements. The fetus needs an external source of the essential fatty acids as discussed later.

The dominance of glucose as a source of fatty acids has been questioned (Szabo & Szabo, 1974). There are large differences between species in the rates of placental transfer of free fatty acids and these seem to correlate well with the observed accumulation of fat *in utero*. Thus the placentas of man, guinea pig and rabbit are relatively permeable to free fatty acids and these are species that develop white adipose tissue *in utero*, while those of sheep, cat and rat are relatively impermeable and their fetuses accumulate very little fat (Szabo & Szabo, 1974; Battaglia & Meschia, 1986) (Table 1). The high permeability of guinea pig placenta is demonstrated by studies in which pregnant guinea pigs were fed diets whose differing fatty acid compositions were faithfully reflected in the composition of the adipose tissue of the newborn animals (Pavey *et al.*, 1976). The guinea pig was chosen as a model for man, since Widdowson *et al.* (1975) had obtained evidence that the fat depots of Dutch babies at birth contained a higher concentration of linoleic acid than those of British babies and supposed that this might be related to differences in fatty acid composition of the mothers' diets.

The concentrations of all lipoprotein classes increase in the maternal circulation during pregnancy, a process that is mediated by the sex hormones (Knopp *et al.*, 1986). These authors have demonstrated the presence of lipoprotein lipase in rat and human placenta. This is consistent with the hypothesis that during the hyperlipidaemia of pregnancy, release of fatty acids by the placental lipoprotein lipase could generate substrates for synthesis of lipids by the fetus, but does not explain the extreme differences between these two species in the extent of fat accumulation by the fetus in late gestation. The transfer of intact lipoproteins by a receptor mediated pathway has not been demonstrated but cannot be ruled out (Battaglia & Meschia, 1986; Knopp *et al.*, 1986).

Immediately after birth, the newborn animal relies entirely on mother's milk as a source of its lipids. In the milks of most species, fat provides the major source of energy, although there are tremendous variations between species (Table 2). The way in which the fat depots of the neonate develop during suckling and thereafter depends on a number of interacting factors: the plane of nutrition and the physiological demands on the animal for lipid mobilization and energy expenditure.

More interesting are the differences between species in the relative distribution of adipose tissue between body sites. Subcutaneous adipose tissue is the major storage site in pig, sheep and man; in cattle the intramuscular site is most important while in the rabbit, perirenal fat is the largest site (Leat and Cos, 1980). In cats and many other carnivores the primary site of fat deposition is in the abdomen (Pond, 1984).

B. Fatty acid composition of the fat stores. In simple stomached animals, the fatty acid composition of the fat stores is influenced markedly by the fatty acid composition of the diet. This is seen at the very earliest age. In Dutch babies who received infant formulas in which the fat component was derived from a vegetable oil, the proportion of linoleic in the adipose tissue increased to around 4% of fatty acids in the first year of life. This contrasted with British babies fed formulas based on cow's milk fat: their adipose tissue contained only 1–2% linoleic acid in the same period (Widdowson *et al.*, 1975).

Recently, there has been much interest in the composition of adipose tissue in relation to mortality and morbidity from cardiovascular disease. A lower content of linoleic acid has been found in the adipose tissue of men living in Edinburgh (where cardiovascular disease incidence is relatively high) compared with those in Stockholm where it is lower. It was also lower in Scottish men prone to coronary heart disease compared with those without the disease (Wood *et al.*, 1987). It is unlikely that the metabolism of this fatty acid in adipose tissue is directly related to the disease but it is probable that compositional differences reflect at least one difference in habitual dietary intake between the two populations. Katan *et al.* (1986) have further developed the technique of fatty acid analysis of human adipose tissue biopsy samples as a tool in epidemiological studies to indicate long term fatty acid intakes of individuals, since there is a very high correlation between dietary linoleic acid intake and its content in adipose tissue. Estimates by dietary survey methods are subject to large random errors. The same authors have also used this method to assess intake of *trans* fatty acids, for which there is also a high correlation between dietary intake and adipose tissue composition (British Nutrition Foundation, 1987). This relationship does not hold true for all dietary fatty acids. For example, adipose tissue concentrations of α-linolenic acid and arachidonic acid are generally lower than would be predicted from the amounts present in the diet. This is true even for those species in which these fatty acids contribute a considerable proportion of the total dietary fatty acids (herbivores and carnivores respectively). This probably arises because of discrimination against certain fatty acid structures by the enzymes that incorporate fatty acids into triacylglycerols; these acids are preferentially esterified in membrane phospholipids. It is possible, however, to elevate the proportion of linolenic acid in the backfat of pigs by feeding inordinately large amounts of linseed oil for a long period (Anderson *et al.*, 1972).

The fat depots of laboratory rodents (eg see Kirtland and Gurr, 1978; Pavey *et al.*, 1976) and of species commercially reared for human food, such as pigs and hens (Wood, 1984; Fisher, 1984) respond in a similar manner to the composition of the dietary fat. Ruminants, however, present a completely different picture. Although traditionally consuming diets relatively low in fat, the composition of the dietary fatty acids is highly unsaturated, with α-linolenic acid predominating. During passage through the rumen, the double bonds of these fatty acids are extensively hydrogenated so that the concentrations of polyunsaturated fatty acids are drastically reduced and those of monounsaturated fatty acids and of stearic acid are significantly increased before absorption. During hydrogenation, isomerization of the double bonds occurs so that ruminant fat depots (and milk fats) are significantly enriched in saturated acids and in monounsaturated acids with *trans* double bonds and isomers in which the double bonds are shifted along the chain from the normal 9,10 position. In consequence, the fatty acid composition of adipose tissue of ruminants reared normally is relatively insensitive to diet. Deposition of polyunsaturated fatty acids can be encouraged by feeding the animals diets in which the fatty acids have been 'protected' against hydrogenation in the rumen. This has been accomplished, for example, by treating sunflower seeds with formaldehyde which crosslinks the seed protein and renders the unsaturated fatty acids unavailable to rumen microorganisms. When the food enters the abomasum, the cross-links are broken in the acid environment and the fatty acids pass into the duodenum where lipid digestion and absorption take place in the same way as in non-ruminants. Smaller changes in ruminant fat depot composition can be induced by supplementing the feed with fat without taking any special measures to 'protect' the fat (Palmqvist, 1984). High inclusions of fat inhibit the activities of the rumen microorganisms allowing more unsaturated acids to be absorbed.

The fatty acid composition of the fat stores can differ significantly between different sites of deposition in the body in several different species. Thus Brook (1971) observed a greater degree of unsaturation in the subcutaneous adipose tissue of the lower leg of children than in other subcutaneous sites, while Pittet *et al.* (1979) and Kokatnur *et al.* (1979) have demonstrated considerable site differences in adult humans, both lean and obese. Even in ruminants, where fat stores are relatively insensitive to changes in composition induced by diet, there are significant differences in fatty acid composition according to site of deposition (Wood, 1984).

Finally, the composition of the lipid stores of fish, which are in the flesh or the liver rather than adipose tissue, are quite different from those of any other type of animal. They are characterized by large concentrations of highly unsaturated C20 and C22 fatty acids which are elaborated from simpler precursors present in the phytoplankton that constitute the fishes' diet. These fatty acids are largely of the n-3 family, in marked contrast with the absence of n-3 fatty acids in the adipose tissue of mammals (Opstvedt, 1984).

C. Turnover of fatty acids in adipose tissue

Adipose tissue has evolved to respond to acute changes in the influx and efflux of lipids according to pressures resulting from the intake of dietary lipids and the demands for energy respectively. Underlying these acute changes are subtle, continuous, minute to minute modifications of lipid composition in the fat stores catalysed by concerted action of the enzymes of esterification and lipolysis. In regard to this 'turnover' of lipids, adipose tissue is no different from most other body tissues and its dynamic nature was first demonstrated in the 1930s by the classic experiments of Schoenheimer & Rittenberg (1937). Since that time, however, there have been surprisingly few studies on adipose tissue turnover and none to my knowledge that have taken a comparative approach, either between species or, within a species, between different ages, sites of deposition, or comparing different fatty acids. The number of individual fatty acids that have been studied is limited.

Table 3. *Turnover times of storage fats.*

Species	*Depot*	*Fatty acid*	*Label*	*Half-life (days)*	*References*
Rat	carcass	all	^{14}C-acetate	16–20	Stein & Stein 1962
Rat	adipose	22:1	feed 22:1	18–31	Wagner *et al.*, 1958a
Rat	adipose	18:3	feed 18:3	46–76	Wagner *et al.*, 1961
Rat	adipose	18:2	feed 18:2	60–77	Wagner *et al.*, 1958b
Rat	adipose	all	$^{3}H_2O$	70–80	Thompson & Ballou 1956
Rat	adipose	16:0	^{14}C-16:0	163	Stein & Stein 1962
Rat	adipose	18:2	^{14}C-18:2	187	Stein & Stein 1962
Pig	structural	18:3	feed 18:3	47	Anderson *et al.*, 1972
Pig	muscle TAG	18:3	feed 18:3	175	Anderson *et al.*, 1972
Pig	adipose	18:3	feed 18:3	300	Anderson *et al.*, 1972
Man	adipose	18:2	feed 18:2	350–750	Hirsch *et al.*, 1960

Hirsch *et al.* (1960), Dole (1965) and Fleischmann *et al.* (1968) measured changes in fatty acid composition in adipose tissue of human beings who had previously ingested high levels of dietary polyunsaturated fatty acids and estimated the half-lives to be between 350 and 700 days. Stein & Stein (1962) used a technique for incorporating radiolabelled fatty acids directly into epididymal fat pads of rats and estimated the half lives of palmitic and linoleic acids to be 163 and 187 days respectively. These are considerably longer than half-lives determined in this species using other labelling techniques and other fatty acids (Table 3) (Wagner *et al.*, 1958a,b; 1961; Thompson & Ballou, 1956).

The half-life of linolenic acid in pig adipose tissue of 300 days (Anderson *et al.*, 1972) is similar to that reported for linoleic acid in man by Hirsch *et al.* (1960). Palmitic acid labelled with ^{14}C had a half life of 180 days in pig adipose tissue (Cunningham, 1968).

It is clear from the work of Anderson *et al.* (1972) that fatty acids turned over much more rapidly in the intramuscular storage lipid ($t_{1/2}$ = 175 days) and in the structural fat of muscle ($t_{1/2}$ = 47 days). These data are consistent with earlier data from rats and mice in which total carcass lipid was measured, rather than adipose tissue itself, giving a range of half lives between 6 and 40 days (see Stein & Stein, 1962).

An important concept with regard to lipid dynamics in adipose tissue is that of separate compartments of lipids with different turnover rates. Zinder *et al.* (1973) prelabelled isolated adipocytes with radioactive fatty acids or glucose and then transferred them to a medium containing serum albumin and adrenalin. The specific activity of the fatty acids released during the first 15 minutes exceeded that of the bulk glycerides by a factor greater than 10 and then dropped rapidly. The results are consistent with a model in which the adipocyte contains a bulk pool of triacylglycerols which is relatively inert and a separate 'active' pool containing the latest glycerides to be formed. In the presence of adrenalin the 'active' glycerides mix with the bulk pool, equilibration being complete after one hour; in contrast, the half-time of mixing in the absence of adrenalin is 3.5 hours. Whether the compartmentation is physical, in the sense that the triacylglycerols occupy separate regions of the cell, or chemical, in that particular molecular species are metabolically more active than others has not been resolved.

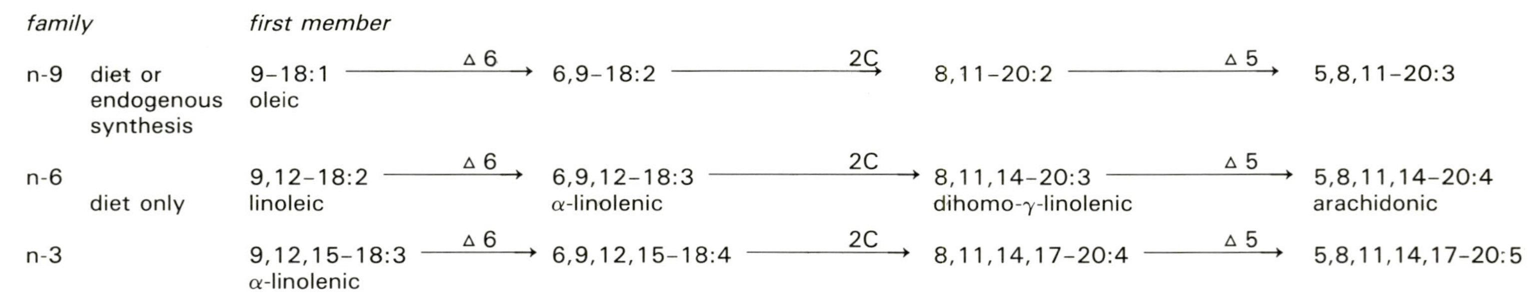

Footnote

The shorthand nomenclature is as follows: the number before the colon indicates the number of carbon atoms in the fatty chain; the number after the colon shows the number of double bonds; the sequence of numbers before the hyphen indicates the positions of the double bonds from the carboxyl carbon which is numbered as carbon-1. All double bonds are in the cisgeometrical configuration. Note that desaturations and chain elongations proceed alternately and that the double bonds are always separated by a methylene (CH_2) group. Thus α-linolenic acid (all-cis-9,12,15–18:3) is:-

$$CH_3.CH_2.CH=CH.CH_2.CH=CH.CH_2.CH=CH(CH_2)_4COOH$$

15 12 9 1

Fatty acids are also grouped in families named by numbering from the methyl end of the chain to the last double bond in the sequence. Thus α-linolenic acid in the above example belongs to the 'n-3' family (sometimes written ω3) while linoleic and oleic acids belong to the n-6 and n-9 families respectively. Because human tissues do not possess the desaturases that insert double bonds in positions 12 or 15, the fatty acids of these different families cannot be interconverted and the parent acids of the n-3 and n-6 family must be obtained from the diet (essential fatty acids). Normally, sufficient linoleic acid is present in the diet for the n-6 pathway to be predominant. When there is little linoleic acid in the diet the n-9 pathway from oleic acid is the major pathway. The end-product 5,8,11–20:3 accumulates. The ratio 5,8,11–20:3/5,8,11,14–20:4 (triene/tetraene ratio) is used as a biochemical index of essential fatty acid deficiency, values above 0.4 being taken arbitrarily as indicative of deficiency.

Fig. 1. *Metabolism of the n-3, n-6 and n-9 series of unsaturated fatty acids.*

In summary, the turnover rate of fatty acids in the bulk pool of triacylglycerols in adipose tissue in most species examined is surprisingly slow, although the cells may have a smaller, rapidly turning over, compartment. The available data do not allow rigorous comparisons between species because of possible age and tissue site differences and because widely different techniques have been used. The subject requires more rigorous investigation.

Unsaturated fatty acid metabolism

All animals are equipped to synthesize lipids from carbohydrates. Whether lipid synthesis occurs at a high rate depends to a large extent on the amount of fat in the diet. Most laboratory rodents, agriculturally important species and many wild animals eat diets in which carbohydrates provide the major source of energy, and lipid synthesis is extensive. The main differences between species are the organs within the body that make the biggest contribution to lipid synthesis. In pigs, guinea-pigs and ruminants, the adipose tissue predominates; in poultry, the liver is the major site, and in rodents both the liver and adipose tissue make an important contribution (Vernon, 1980). In Western man, whose diet generally contains a high proportion of fat, the enzymes of fatty acid synthesis are probably 'switched off' and the needs for storage and structural lipids are satisfied from dietary intake.

The end-products of fatty acid synthesis in animal tissues are the saturated fatty acids. In addition, virtually all tissues contain enzymes (desaturases) that insert a double bond into saturated fatty acids, normally at position 9. Enzymes are also present that insert further double bonds into unsaturated fatty acids to produce polyunsaturated fatty acids (Fig. 1).

Essential fatty acids

No animal species is able to synthesize its entire requirement for lipids. In the course of evolution, animals lost the ability to make the enzymes that insert double bonds at positions 12 and 15. Double bonds in these positions are present in linoleic and α-linolenic acids which are synthesized in plants. Yet these fatty acids and higher polyunsaturated fatty acids derived from them (see Fig. 1) are essential to life, and therefore they must be supplied in the diet (Holman, 1970a,b). Different species have requirements for different types and amounts of essential fatty acids.

As far as we know, linoleic acid (*cis, cis*-9, 12-octadecadienoic acid) is essential for every animal species at a dietary level of approximately 1% of energy (Holman, 1970b). There is less certainty about α-linolenic acid. Fish, where lipid metabolism is geared to processing a high dietary intake of n-3 fatty acids, seem to have a definite and high requirement (2.7% of energy) for fatty acids of this family (Castell *et al.*, 1972). At the other end of the scale, Leat *et al.* (1983) found that α-linolenic acid could not replace linoleic acid in the diet of the rat with regard to the maintenance of testicular function. The testicular lipids of most species consist mainly of phospholipids esterified with a high proportion of n-3 long chain polyenoic acids, whereas those of the rat are dominated by the n-6 long chain polyenoic acids. The brains of most species, however, including the rat, are characterized by a high proportion of the n-3 fatty acids and we can infer that, since these acids cannot be synthesized in the body, there is some dietary requirement for them, however small.

Capuchin monkeys maintained on a diet containing adequate linoleic acid but little or no α-linolenic acid, suffered symptoms closely resembling those of classical essential fatty acid deficiency as described by Holman (1970a). These were cured by the addition of linseed oil (which contains appreciable amounts of linolenic acid) to the diet (Fiennes *et al.*, 1973). In man, the essentiality of α-linolenic acid remained in doubt until Holman *et al.* (1982) described the case of a girl who displayed neurological symptoms 4–5 months after being on total parenteral nutrition in which the fat component was a safflower oil emulsion containing mainly linoleic acid and only a minute amount of α-linolenic acid. When safflower oil was replaced by soyabean oil containing much more linolenic acid, the neurological symptoms disappeared. More recently, Bjerve *et al.* (1987) provided evidence for linolenic acid deficiency in elderly patients fed by gastric tube. It seems quite certain that only very small amounts of this nutrient are needed in human diets (Zöllner, 1986).

Cats are unusual among mammals in that neither linoleic nor α-linolenic acid alone is sufficient to protect against the effects of fatty acid deficiency: these animals require arachidonic acid (all-*cis*-5,8,11,14-eicosatetraenoic acid, see Fig. 1) in their diets because they lack the ability to insert double bonds in positions 6 and 8 as well as 12 and 15 (Rivers *et al.*, 1975, 1976).

The detailed effects of essential fatty acid deficiency vary from species to species but the general pattern is very similar. The first signs are generally dermatosis and reduced water permeability through the skin. Growth and reproductive ability are impaired and there are diverse changes in lipid metabolism, including cholesterol accumulation in many tissues, changes in the fatty acid composition of most tissues, and increased triacylglycerol biosynthesis and release by the liver (Holman, 1970a). Essential fatty acids are required (1) to maintain the structural and functional integrity of biological membranes and (2) to provide precursors for a diverse range of metabolites, now generally categorized as 'eicosanoids', with potent biological effects at extremely low concentrations (Lands, 1979; Needleman *et al.*, 1986). Eicosanoids include the prostaglandins, prostacyclins, thromboxanes, and leukotrienes and are so called because their main precursors are the polyunsaturated fatty acids with chain lengths of 20 carbon atoms — the eicosenoic acids. There is considerable debate about the extent to which these two functions of essential fatty acids are interrelated.

Formation of long chain polyunsaturated fatty acids

Although the principal essential fatty acids required in the diet are linoleic and α-linolenic, the functional requirements are to a considerable degree only satisfied by the longer chain and more highly unsaturated metabolites. Animal tissues metabolize these precursors by the introduction of further double bonds catalysed by enzymes termed desaturases, and the long chain polyunsaturated end-products are built up by a sequence of alternate desaturations and 2-carbon chain elongations (Fig. 1). These processes give rise to several families of polyunsaturated fatty acids that are not interconvertible in animal tissues. If the diet lacks the essential fatty acids that are the precursors for these biochemical pathways, the major precursor will be oleic acid (either from the diet or endogenous synthesis) which will give rise to a sequence of polyunsaturated fatty acids of the n-9 family which cannot substitute functionally for the n-6 or n-3 series. Holman has used the ratio of the concentrations of 20:3 (n-9)/20:4 (n-6) in tissues as an index of essential fatty acid status, values over 0.4 being arbitrarily designated as indicating essential fatty acid deficiency. This index is remarkably similar for all species examined (Holman 1970a,b).

Our knowledge of the activities of the various desaturases in different species is derived from two main sources: (1) incubations with radio-labelled fatty acids *in vitro* and (2) incorporation of labelled fatty acids into tissue lipids *in vivo*. A third method, which involves making inferences from the fatty acid composition of different tissues, is fraught with difficulty because of the many interacting pathways of lipid metabolism. *In vitro* methods have adequately demonstrated the high activity of the Δ 6-desaturase in rat tissues (Brenner, 1982) and its absence from the tissues of carnivorous fish (Owen *et al.*, 1975). This enzyme has been studied more than other desaturases (apart from the Δ 9-enzyme) since it is regarded as the rate-limiting step on the desaturation-elongation pathway illustrated in Fig. 1 (Hassam, 1984). Claims that it has low activity in human liver (Hassam, 1984) should be treated critically since De Gomez Dumm & Brenner (1975), who published the original work, were at pains to point out that the patients from whom the biopsy samples were taken at operation were elderly and had been fasting: both factors known to reduce the activity of this enzyme. The effects of anaesthesia and premedication are unknown. This illustrates the difficulties of relating *in vitro* activities to physiological activities, especially in human subjects from whom the collection of 'normal' samples is quite unusual.

Radioactive labelling *in vivo* can give a more accurate picture of the true physiological activity of pathways, though not such detailed information on individual enzymic steps. While it is useful for studies with small laboratory animals, the sheer size of many species prohibits the extensive use of radioactivity, although the absence of Δ 6 and Δ 8-desaturation in lions has been shown by this means (Rivers *et al.*, 1976). Moreover, ethical and practical considerations severely restrict its use in man. Substantial advances in mass spectrometry, however, now open up the potential for the more extensive use of stable isotopes for studying lipid metabolism in man. As an example, El Boustani *et al.* (1986) have demonstrated Δ 5-desaturase activity in human plasma using deuterium-labelled dihomo-γ-linolenic acid and observing its conversion into arachidonic acid.

Fetal accumulation of polyunsaturated fatty acids

This detailed knowledge of metabolic pathways has been obtained largely from studies of mature animals. A crucial question in developmental biology is how essential fatty acids are acquired and metabolized in early life, since the cellular components for which they are required are being laid down from the very earliest point in fetal development. There are several sources from which the fetus can obtain the essential fatty acids it needs for its membranes: precursor and product EFA obtained directly from maternal plasma, transferred across the placenta and taken up and used directly by fetal tissues; precursor EFA taken up by the placenta and converted into product EFA in the placenta before transfer to fetal tissues, and precursor EFA transferred across the placenta and converted into product EFA in fetal tissues.

Here the term 'precursor EFA' refers to linoleic and α-linolenic acids in species other than obligate carnivores, while 'product EFA' are their long chain polyunsaturated fatty acid metabolites.

As discussed earlier, the placenta of most mammals is permeable to free fatty acids, although there are large differences between species in rates of transfer (Table 1). In rabbit and man there appear to be no significant differences in rates of transfer between essential and non-essential fatty acids (reviewed by Kuhn & Crawford, 1986). In contrast, linoleic acid traverses the guinea pig placenta with greater facility than palmitic, while the reverse is true in sheep (reviewed by Noble, 1979).

A common finding that has to be explained is a higher concentration of arachidonic acid in fetal than in maternal plasma (Noble, 1979). The relative importance of placental synthesis of 'product EFA' compared with transfer from maternal plasma is still to be resolved. The rat appears to rely more on maternal transfer than on placental synthesis (see Zimmerman *et al.*, 1979). These authors demonstrated that isolated human placenta is capable of synthesizing arachidonic acid from linoleic acid supplied by the mother and concluded that the human fetus is not dependent on a maternal supply of arachidonic acid: the placenta could be a major source. In contrast, Kuhn & Crawford (1986) decided that the ability of a perfused human placenta to desaturate and elongate linoleic acid was quite limited. They concluded that arachidonic acid is selectively incorporated and 'trapped' into phospholipids in placenta for export to the fetal circulation. Crawford has used the term 'biomagnification' for a process in which the proportion of product EFA increases in phospholipids, progressing from maternal blood to cord blood, fetal liver and fetal brain. This sequence is best demonstrated in guinea pigs (Crawford *et al.*, 1976).

The study of fetal conservation of EFA in ruminants is extremely rewarding since the availability of EFA to the mother is limited by rumen hydrogenation. The triene/tetraene ratio in fetal lamb tissues is about 1.6, a value that in simple-stomached animals would be associated with extensive signs of EFA deficiency (Noble *et al.*, 1972). By 10 days after birth, the ratio has fallen to 0.4, and by 30 days, to 0.1. These values are well within the 'normal' range despite the extremely low concentration of linoleic acid in ewe's milk (0.5% of energy). Ruminants are therefore able to conserve EFA with supreme efficiency. Sheep placenta transfers linoleic acid at a relatively slow rate but has a very high Δ 6-desaturase activity by comparison with non-ruminants (Shand and Noble, 1979; Noble 1979) which probably provides the major source of arachidonic acid for the fetus. In addition, the resulting arachidonic acid is concentrated into the phosphoglycerides whereas the linoleic acid precursor is in higher concentration in the triacylglycerols. This 'molecular compartmentation' has the effect of conserving arachidonic acid and directing it into membranes.

Brain lipids

A large proportion of the 'product EFA' synthesized or accumulated during the perinatal period is destined for the growth of the brain, 50% of which may consist of the long chain polyunsaturated fatty acids 20:4 (n-6), 22:4 (n-6), 22:5 (n-6) and 22:6 (n-3) (Crawford *et al.*, 1976). As with adipose tissue, there are large species differences in the time at which birth occurs in relation to the extent of brain development. Peak brain development occurs in guinea pigs in fetal life; in the rat, postnatally; while in man and pig it reaches a peak in late gestation and continues after birth. Clandinin *et al.* (1981) suggested that transfer from placenta is the major source of long chain polyunsaturated fatty acids for the human fetus but recognized the experimental difficulties of demonstrating this in man. Purvis *et al.* (1982) have studied the accumulation of brain lipids in pigs and argued for a remarkable similarity to man. Long chain derivatives of linoleic acid (n-6 family) increase from mid-gestation to term whereas little linoleic acid itself accumulates until birth, when the concentration increases three-fold while product EFA remain constant. Moreover, by labelling with 1-^{14}C linoleic acid *in vivo*, Purvis *et al.* (1983) demonstrated that linoleic acid was metabolized to long chain polyunsaturated fatty acids by piglet brain and liver throughout the perinatal period. The contribution of the liver was many-fold greater than the brain at all stages. Whether this mechanism can supply all the needs of the nervous system without the need for maternal transfer is still to be resolved.

An outstanding feature of the composition of brain phospholipids is its remarkable consistency irrespective of species and diet (Crawford *et al.* 1976). The concentrations of the precursor EFA are extremely low (18:2, n-6, 0.1–1.5%; and 18:3, n-3, 0.1–1.0%) while arachidonic (20:4, n-6) and docosahexaenoic (22:6, n-3) acids predominate at 8–17% and 13–29% respectively in all species. This contrasts with the liver lipids where there is much greater variation between species. The precursor EFA are present in much greater concentrations than in brain and there are major differences in the product EFA. For example, 22:5 is the major n-3 fatty acid in the liver lipids of ruminants and other herbivores while 22:6 predominates in the carnivores and omnivores (Crawford *et al.*, 1976). Fatty acids of the n-6 family usually predominate in liver phosphoglycerides, even when the overwhelming dietary intake is in favour of n-3 fatty acids. Thus zebra and dolphin, both species that have great excess of n-3 fatty acids in the diet (n-6/n-3 = 1:3 and 1:30 respectively) attain ratios of about 8:1 and 1.1:1 respectively in liver phosphoglycerides (Williams & Crawford, 1986).

Our understanding of the significance of these species and tissue differences in EFA metabolism in the perinatal period is rudimentary. Eicosanoids, which are metabolites of the long chain polyunsaturated fatty acids, are known to play important roles in pregnancy and in the mechanism of parturition in all mammalian species that have been studied (Mitchell, 1986). A discussion of the further metabolism of 'product EFA' into eicosanoids is beyond the scope of this review and the state of knowledge in this field hardly allows a comparative approach to be adopted. It is clearly a burgeoning area in which we are likely to see exciting developments in the near future.

Conclusion

There are many reasons for adopting a comparative approach, but one of them is certainly to learn more about general biological principles so that we can gain a better understanding of lipid metabolism, and perhaps more importantly, of aberrations in lipid metabolism in our own species. It is important to distinguish general principles from special characteristics pertaining to a limited set of species. For example, it is possible that we have been led astray by observations of the contribution of brown adipose tissue to the thermogenic response to overfeeding in rodents, and that it may not be a phenomenon having enormous significance for man. The study of the developmental biology of white adipose tissue, however, should give us important clues about factors that may initiate new cell division in this tissue.

As far as one can judge from the published literature, the concept of a two compartment model for the fat store in the adipocyte, in which there are pools with slow and fast turnover times, is general for most species. We know little about this compartmentation, but with the attention that is now being given to the measurement of adipose tissue fatty acid composition as an epidemiological tool it is important to learn how the compartmentation is achieved and what is its significance for fat storage. We are fortunate that adipose tissue fatty acids can be studied in man with relatively simple biopsy techniques and the use of stable isotopes provides a further powerful tool for metabolic studies. Thus comparisons between species can proceed in parallel over a period of time.

Detailed temporal studies of human brain lipids are more problematical and highlight the need for a good animal model. The pig, which is inadequate as a model for the temporal aspects of adipose tissue development, is useful as a model for brain lipid accretion. These studies are important since the increasing expertise in sustaining life in premature infants has bequeathed us the problem of how to feed them to achieve 'normal' development. These children may be born well before brain development has reached its peak. It is crucial therefore, that the lipids in the infant feed are able to contribute to the brain growth that would have occurred in the fetus. Any long-chain essential fatty acids that the fetus could not elaborate for itself and had to be supplied by the mother or the placenta will now have to be contributed by the milk. Greater knowledge of the relative roles of mother, placenta and the fetus or new-born's own tissues in supplying long chain polyunsaturated fatty acids and of the quantitative requirements for these nutrients is therefore needed. There cannot be a better illustration of the value of the comparative approach to the study of lipid metabolism.

References

Anderson, D. B., Kauffman, R. G. & Benevenga, N. J. (1972): Estimate of fatty acid turnover in porcine adipose tissue. *Lipids* **7**, 488–489.

Battaglia, F. C. & Meschia, G. (1986): *An introduction to fetal physiology*. New York: Academic Press.

Bjerve, K. S., Lovold-Mostad, I., & Thoresen, L. (1987): Alpha-linolenic acid deficiency in patients on long term gastric tube feeding: estimation of linolenic and long chain unsaturated n-3 fatty acid requirement in man. *Am. J. Clin. Nutr.* **45**, 66–77.

Brenner, R. R. (1982): Nutritional and hormonal factors influencing desaturation of essential fatty acids. *Prog. Lipid Res.* **20**, 41–47.

British Nutrition Foundation (1987): *Report of the task force on trans fatty acids*. London: BNF.

Brook, C. G. D. (1971): Composition of adipose tissue from deep and subcutaneous sites. *Br. J. Nutr.* **25**, 377–380.

Buisson, D. H. (1983): The future of fish oils in New Zealand. *Proc. Int. Conf. Oils, Fats and Waxes*, eds S. G. Brooker, A. Renwick, S. F. Hamon and L. Eyres, pp. 29–34. Auckland: Duromark.

Canon, B. & Nedergaard, J. (1985): Brown adipose tissue: molecular mechanisms controlling activity and thermogenesis. In *New perspectives in adipose tissue: structure, function and development*, eds A. Cryer and R. L. R. Van, pp. 233–270. London: Butterworth.

Castell, J. D., Sinnhuber, R. O., Wales, J. H. & Lee, D. J. (1972): Essential fatty acids in the diet of the rainbow trout (*Salmo gairdneri*): Growth, feed conversion, and some gross deficiency symptoms. *J. Nutr.* **102**, 77–86.

Clandinin, M. T., Chappell, J. E., Leong, S. E., Heim, T., Swyer, P. R. & Chance, G. W. (1981): Intrauterine fatty acid accretion rates in human brain: implications for fatty acid requirements. *Early Hum. Devel.* **4**, 121–129.

Crawford, M. A., Casperd, N. M. & Sinclair, A. J. (1976): The long chain metabolites of linoleic and linolenic acids in liver and brain in herbivores and carnivores. *Comp. Biochem. Physiol.* **54B**, 395–401.
Crawford, M. A., Hassam, A. G., Williams, G. & Whitehouse, W. L. (1976): Essential fatty acids and fetal brain growth. *Lancet* **1**, 452–453.
Cunningham, H. M. (1968): Effect of caffeine on nitrogen retention, carcass composition, fat mobilization and the oxidation of C^{14}-labelled body fat in pigs. *J. Anim. Sci.* **27**, 424–430.
De Gomez Dumm, I. N. T. & Brenner, R. R. (1975): Oxidative desaturation of α-linolenic, linoleic and stearic acids by human liver microsomes. *Lipids* **10**, 315–317.
Desnoyers, F. & Vodovar, N. (1974): Apparition, origine et evolution des tissues adipeux epididymaire et pericardiaque du foetus de porc. *Ann. Biol. Anim. Biochim. Biophys.* **14**, 769–780.
Dole, V. P. (1965): Energy storage. In *Handbook of physiology, 5. Adipose tissue*, pp. 13–18. Washington DC: American Physiological Society.
El Boustani, S., Descomps, B., Monnier, L., Warnant, J., Mendy, F. & Crastes de Paulet, A. (1986): *In vivo* conversion of dihomogamma-linolenic acid into arachidonic acid in man. *Prog. Lipid Res.* **25**, 67–71.
Fiennes, R. N. T. W., Sinclair, A. J. & Crawford, M. A. (1973): Essential fatty acid studies in primates: linolenic acid requirements of capuchins. *J. Med. Prim.* **2**, 155–169.
Fisher, C. (1984): Fat deposition in broilers. In *Fats in animal nutrition*, ed J. Wiseman, pp. 437–470. London: Butterworth.
Fleischman, A. I., Hayton, T., Bierenbaum, M. L. & Watson, P. (1968): The effect of a polyunsaturated diet upon adipose tissue fatty acids in young coronary males: a five-year cohort study. *Lipids* **3**, 147–150.
Flemming, W. (1871): Observations on adipose tissue. *Arch. Mikrosk. Anat.* **7**, 32–56.
Gurr, M. I. & James, A. T. (1980): *Lipid biochemistry: an introduction*. London: Chapman & Hall.
Hassam, A. G. (1984): The role of evening primrose oil in nutrition and disease. In *The role of fats in human nutrition*, eds F. B. Padley and J. Podmore, pp. 84–100. London: Ellis Horwood/Society of Chemical Industry.
Hausman, G. J. (1982): Adipocyte development in subcutaneous adipose tissues of the young rat. *Acta Anat.* **112**, 185–196.
Hausman, G. J. (1985): The comparative anatomy of adipose tissue. In *New perspectives in adipose tissue: structure, function and development*, eds A. Cryer and R. L. R. Van, pp. 1–21. London: Butterworth.
Hausman, G. J. & Martin, R. J. (1982): The development of adipocytes located around hair follicles in the fetal pig. *J. Anim. Sci.* **54**, 1286–1296.
Heim, T. (1983): Energy and lipid requirements of the fetus and the preterm infant. *J. Pediatr. Gastroenterol. & Nutrition* **2**, (Suppl. 1) S16–41.
Hirsch, J., Farquar, J. W., Ahrens, E. H., Peterson, M. L., & Stoffel, W. (1960): *Am. J. Clin. Nutr.* **8**, 499–511.
Holman, R. T. (1970a): Essential fatty acid deficiency. *Prog. Chem. Fats Other Lipids.* **9**, 275–348.
Holman, R. T. (1970b): Biological activities and requirements for polyunsaturated fatty acids. *Prog. Chem. Fats Other Lipids* **9**, 607–682.
Holman, R. T., Johnson, S. B. & Hatch, T. F. (1982): A case of human linolenic acid deficiency involving neurological abnormalities. *Am. J. Clin. Nutr.* **35**, 617–623.
Hull, D. & Hardman, M. J. (1970): Brown adipose tissue in newborn mammals. In *Brown adipose tissue*, ed O. Lindberg, pp. 97–115. New York: Elsevier.
Katan, M. B., Van Staveren, W. A., Deurenberg, P., Barendse-van Leeuwen, J., Germing-Nouwen, C., Soffers, A., Berkel, J. & Beynen, A. C. (1986): Linoleic and *trans*-unsaturated fatty acid content of adipose tissue biopsies as objective indicators of the dietary habits of individuals. *Prog. Lipid Res.* **25**, 193–195.
Kimura, R. E. & Warshaw, J. B. (1983): Metabolic adaptations of the fetus and newborn. *J. Pediatr. Gastroenterol. Nutr.* **2**, (Suppl. 1) S12–15.
Kirtland, J. & Gurr, M. I. (1978): The effect of different dietary fats on fat cell size and number in rat epididymal fat pad. *Br. J. Nutr.* **39**, 19–26.
Kirtland, J., Gurr, M. I. & Widdowson, E. M. (1976): Body lipids of guinea-pigs exposed to different dietary fats from mid-gestation to three months of age. I. The cellularity of adipose tissue. *Nutr. Metabol.* **20**, 338–350.
Knopp, R. H., Warth, M. R., Charles, D., Childs, M., Li, J. R., Mabuchi, H. & Van Allen, M. I. (1986): Lipoprotein metabolism in pregnancy, fat transport to the fetus and the effects of diabetes. *Biol. Neonate* **50**, 297–317.

Kokatnur, M. G., Oalmann, M. C., Johnson, W. D., Malcolm, G. T. & Strong, J. P. (1979): Fatty acid composition of human adipose tissue from two anatomical sites in a biracial community. *Am. J. Clin. Nutr.* **32**, 2198–2205.

Kuhn, D. C. & Crawford, M. A. (1986): Placental essential fatty acid transport and prostaglandin synthesis. *Prog. Lipid Res.* **25**, 345–353.

Lands, W. E. M. (1979): The biosynthesis and metabolism of prostaglandins. *Ann. Rev. Physiol.* **41**, 633–652.

Leat, W. M. F. & Cox, R. W. (1980): Fundamental aspects of adipose tissue growth. In *Growth in animals*, ed T. L. J. Lawrence, pp. 137–174. London: Butterworth.

Leat, W. M. F., Northrop, C. A., Harrison, F. A. and Cox, R. W. (1983): Effect of dietary linoleic and linolenic acids on testicular development in the rat. *Quart. J. Exp. Path.* **68**, 221–231.

Martin, M. J., Kasser, T. R., Ramsay, T. G. & Hausman, G. J. (1985): Regulation of adipose tissue development *in utero*. In *New Perspectives in Adipose Tissue*, eds A. Cryer and R. L. R. Van, pp. 303–317. London: Butterworth.

Mitchell, M. D. (1986): Pathways of arachidonic acid metabolism with specific application to the fetus and mother. *Seminars in Perinatology* **10**, 242–254.

Needleman, P., Turk, J., Jakschik, B. A., Morrison, A. R. & Lefkowith, J. B. (1986): Arachidonic acid metabolism. *Ann. Rev. Biochem.* **55**, 69–102.

Noble, R. C. (1979): Lipid metabolism in the neonatal ruminant. *Prog. Lipid Res.* **18**, 179–216.

Noble, R. C., Steele, W. & Moore, J. H. (1972): Metabolism of linoleic acid by the young lamb. *Br. J. Nutr.* **27**, 503–508.

Opstvedt, J. (1984): Fish Fats. In *Fats in animal nutrition*, ed J. Wiseman, pp. 53–82. London: Butterworth.

Owen, J. M., Adron, J. W., Middleton, L. & Cowey, C. B. (1975): Elongation and desaturation of dietary fatty acids in turbot (*Scophthalmus maximus*) and rainbow trout (*Salmo gairdneri*). *Lipids* **10**, 528–531.

Palmqvist, D. L. (1984): Use of fats in diets for lactating dairy cows. In *Fats in animal nutrition*, ed. J. Wiseman, pp. 357–381. London: Butterworth.

Pavey, D., Robinson, M. P. & Widdowson, E. M. (1976): Body lipids of guinea pigs exposed to different dietary fats from mid-gestation to three months of age. II. The fatty acid composition of the lipids of liver, plasma, adipose tissue, muscle and red cell membranes at birth. *Nutr. Metabol.* **20**, 351–363.

Pittet, P. G., Halliday, D. & Bateman, P. E. (1979): Site differences in the fatty acid composition of subcutaneous adipose tissue of obese women. *Br. J. Nutr.* **42**, 57–61.

Pond, C. M. (1984): Physiological and ecological importance of energy storage in the evolution of lactation: evidence for a common pattern of anatomical organization of adipose tissue in mammals. *Symp. Zool. Soc. Lond.* **51**, 1–32.

Purvis, J. M., Clandinin, M. T. & Hacker, R. R. (1982): Fatty acid accretion during perinatal brain growth in the pig. A model for fatty acid accretion in human brain. *Comp. Biochem. Physiol.* **72B**, 195–199.

Purvis, J. M., Clandinin, M. T. & Hacker, R. R. (1983): Chain elongation-desaturation of linoleic acid during the development of the pig. Implications for the supply of polyenoic fatty acids to the developing brain. *Comp. Biochem. Physiol.* **75B**, 199–204.

Rivers, J. P. W., Hassam, A. G., Crawford, M. A. & Brambell, M. R. (1976): The inability of the lion (*Panthera leo*) to desaturate linoleic acid. *FEBS Lett.* **67**, 269–270.

Rivers, J. P. W., Sinclair, A. J. & Crawford, M. A. (1975): Inability of the cat to desaturate essential fatty acids. *Nature (Lond.)* **258**, 171–173.

Schoenheimer, R. & Rittenberg, D. (1937): Deuterium as an indicator in the study of intermediary metabolism. IV. Synthesis and destruction of fatty acids in the organism. *J. Biol. Chem.* **114**, 381–396.

Shand, J. H. & Noble, R. C. (1979): Δ9- and Δ6-desaturase activities of ovine placenta and their role in the supply of fatty acids to the fetus. *Biol. Neonate.* **36**, 298–304.

Stein, Y. & Stein, O. (1962): The incorporation and disappearance of fatty acids in rat epididymal fat pad studied by the *in vivo* incubation technique. *Biochim. Biophys. Acta* **60**, 58–71.

Szabo, A. J. & Szabo, O. (1974): Placental free fatty acid transfer and fetal adipose tissue development: an explanation of fetal adiposity in infants of diabetic mothers. *Lancet* **2**, 498–499.

Thompson, R. C. & Ballou, J. E. (1956): Studies of metabolic turnover with tritium as a tracer. V. The predominantly non-dynamic state of body constituents in the rat. *J. Biol. Chem.* **223**, 795–809.

Vernon, R. G. (1980): Lipid metabolism in the adipose tissue of ruminant animals. *Prog. Lipid Res.* **19**, 23–106.

Vernon, R. G. & Clegg, R. A. (1985): The metabolism of white adipose tissue *in vivo* and *in vitro*. In *New perspectives in adipose tissue structure, function and development*, eds A. Cryer and R. L. R. Van, pp. 65–86. London: Butterworths.
Wagner, H., Seelig, E. & Bernhard, K. (1958a): Verteilung und Halbwertszeit der erucasaure nach Rapsolgaben an Ratten. *Z. Physiol. Chemie, Hoppe-Seylers* **312**, 104–110.
Wagner, H., Seelig, E. & Bernhard, K. (1958b): Der Verweilzeit der Linolsaure im Organismus der Ratte. *Z. Physiol. Chemie Hoppe-Seylers* **313**, 235–243.
Wagner, H., Wagner, O. & Bernhard, K. (1961): Untersuchungen uber das Verhalten der Linolensaure im Tierkorper. *Z. Physiol. Chemie Hoppe-Seylers* **323**, 105–110.
Wensvoort, P. (1967): The development of adipose tissue in sheep foetus. *Path. Vet.* **4**, 69–78.
Widdowson, E. M., Dauncey, M. J., Gairdner, J. M. T., Jonxis, J. H. P. & Pelikan-Filipkova, M. (1975): Body fat of British and Dutch infants. *Br. Med J.* **1**, 653–655.
Williams, G. & Crawford, M. A. (1986): Lessons from the fatty acid component in structural lipids from marine and land mammals. *Prog. Lipid Res.* **25**, 421–423.
Wood, D. A., Riemersma, R. A., Butler, S., Thomson, M., Macintyre, C., Elton, R. A. & Oliver, M. F. (1987): Linoleic and eicosapentaenoic acids in adipose tissue and platelets and risk of coronary heart disease. *Lancet* **1**, 177–183.
Wood, J. D. (1984): Fat deposition and the quality of fat tissue in meat animals. In *Fats in animal nutrition*, ed J. Wiseman, pp. 407–435. London: Butterworths.
Zimmerman, T., Winkler, L., Moller, U., Schubert, H. & Goetze, E. (1979): Synthesis of arachidonic acid in human placenta *in vitro*. *Biol. Neonate* **35**, 209–212.
Zinder, O., Eisenberg, E. & Shapiro, B. (1973): Compartmentation of glycerides in adipose tissue cells. 1. The mechanism of free fatty acid release. *J. Biol. Chem.* **248**, 7673–7676.
Zöllner, N. (1986): Dietary linolenic acid in man: an overview. *Prog. Lipid Res.* **25**, 177–180.

* * * * *

Discussion

Professor Beynen said he thought that the information on the turnover of fatty acids was perhaps slightly misleading since in the growing animal there was a considerable component related to accretion of fatty acids and net synthesis from carbohydrate. In humans conversion of carbohydrates into fatty acids is probably negligible. *Professor Gurr* agreed with this and said that he had failed to find other suitable information.

Dr Thurnham asked where the trans-9,11 linoleic acid is deposited in the body, to which *Professor Gurr* replied that his reference to this isomer had been in connection with its formation during ruminal hydrogenation. During this process very little of this isomer remains in ruminant fat. Admittedly traces of the trans-diene can be isolated from milk but these are very minor indeed. *Dr Thurnham* pointed out that this particular isomer represented the largest component of the conjugated dienes in the plasma of man and wondered whether *Professor Gurr* could confirm that this could not be of dietary origin; which *Professor Gurr* did.

Dr Fuller asked whether anything was known about the physiological control of species differences in fat distribution. *Professor Gurr* was not inclined to speculate on this.

Professor Waterlow commented on the strange selective loss of fat seen in malnourished children, in whom the fat content of the lower limbs appears to be better preserved. He thought, and *Professor Gurr* agreed, that perhaps differences in blood flow were responsible.

Dr Dauncey asked what was known about the effects of diet, not on the storage lipids, but on the structural ones, and what were the functional consequences of any changes.

Professor Gurr said that the brain lipids were not very much affected whereas the red cell membranes and membranes of other tissues could be modified by diet. Differences in the rates of lysis of the red cells suggested that membrane structure had changed following change in fatty acid composition of the diet and certainly adenyl cyclase activity could be changed by altering the fatty acid composition of the membrane.

Dr Sanders commented on the n-3/n-6 unsaturation in relation to membrane fatty acid composition and wondered whether Professor Gurr had not been somewhat conservative in his view that the changes were relatively small. Large changes in the balance between n-3 and n-6 fatty acids can be induced by diet and in some cases these were accompanied by functional changes. For example, changes in the electroretinogram patterns of experimental animals and changes in erythrocyte deformability have been noted when n-3 fatty acids replace n-6 fatty acids. *Professor Gurr* agreed that there were large differences between the species in regard to the proportion of n-3 and n-6 fatty acids in membranes which could be related to differences in diet, but said that he would not necessarily conclude from this that dietary changes within a species must be associated with functional changes.

6

Vitamin C (ascorbic acid): antioxidant functions of vitamin C in disease in man and animals

DAVID I. THURNHAM

Introduction

Vitamin C was isolated a little over 50 years ago (Szent-Gyorgyi, 1963; Waugh & King, 1932) although its deficiency disease, scurvy, is one of the oldest diseases known to mankind (Counsell & Hornig, 1981). Many of the manifestations of scurvy can be attributed to a failure of collagen synthesis, especially in skin and bone, which lead to a weakening and failure of repair processes in the extracellular matrix. At the biochemical level, this is due to the reduced activity of two mixed function oxidases, prolyl and lysyl hydroxylase, which hydroxylate the corresponding amino acid residues in nascent collagen to ensure normal triple-helix formation and fibrillogenesis (Bates, 1981). Much of our understanding of the role of ascorbate in this process and in other aspects of metabolism has come from experiments on guinea pigs which, like man, are dependent on an exogenous supply of vitamin C. However, most species of animals can synthesize ascorbic acid (Chatterjee *et al.*, 1975). They synthesize the vitamin from D-glucose via the D-glucouronic acid pathway of metabolism present in the microsomes (Isherwood *et al.*, 1954; Chatterjee *et al.*, 1975). It appears that in evolutionary ascent, the enzyme system for synthesis of vitamin C was originally in the kidney where it is found in amphibians, reptiles, the chicken and pigeon. It then passed to the liver where it is found in most avian and mammalian species, but finally disappeared altogether in man, primates, bats, guinea pigs and the red-vented bulbul (Chatterjee *et al.*, 1975; Binney *et al.*, 1976).

The dependence of man on an exogenous source of vitamin C for his metabolism means that there must be a specific minimum requirement for the vitamin to maintain health. The Sheffield studies in the UK (Bartley *et al.*, 1953) and the later ones of Baker *et al.* (1969) established that 10 mg per day would prevent clinical signs of vitamin C deficiency. There is very little dispute that 10 mg per day is the minimum requirement for man but the various national recommendations as to the daily allowance to cover the needs of most of the population reflect a considerable diversity of opinion as to man's true needs to maintain health as opposed to preventing scurvy. RDAs range from our own of 30 mg (DHSS, 1979), 60 mg in the USA (Food & Nutrition Board, 1979), and 120 mg in some Eastern block countries to the recommendations of Irvin Stone and Linus Pauling (1970) of 10 g per day to suppress or avert infection.

It is not my intention to discuss recommended daily allowances in this chapter, for such issues will only be resolved by a better understanding of the functions of vitamin C; neither will I attempt to cover the enormous amount that has been written on the vitamin. The reader should consult the two symposia of the New York Academy of Sciences (1961, 1975) as well as more recent publications (Counsell & Hornig, 1981; Sieb & Tolbert, 1982). The objective of this symposium is to examine how far observations made with other species of animals have relevance to the newer problems which are being encountered in the nutrition of man. But looking at the problems surrounding vitamin C rather as an onlooker, I am struck by the fact that the problems are not new and the question that constantly recurs is 'What is needed to maintain or attain optimal health?' Animal studies have shown that vitamin C is involved in cholesterol metabolism and heart disease (Ginter, 1977), in cancer and in drug metabolism (Zannoni *et al.*, 1977). Likewise many epidemiological studies have shown inverse relationships between vitamin C status and ischaemic heart disease and cancer (Gey, 1986; Gey *et al.*, 1987). Numerous studies have shown that blood ascorbate concentrations are lower in smokers than in non-smokers (Pelletier, 1977) and in a variety of other situations. Do lower ascorbate values reported in patients with diabetes (Newill *et al.*, 1984), rheumatoid arthritis (Sahud & Cohen, 1971; Thurnham *et al.*, 1987a), schizophrenia (Suboticanec *et al.*, 1986) etc simply mean that there is less vitamin C in their diets or do they represent increased requirement for vitamin C? If they represent increased requirement, do they represent normal functions of vitamin C which are exaggerated in some people?

The antioxidant defence system

I have been involved in measuring and interpreting vitamin status for many years and this interest has evolved into studying ways of assessing the importance of nutrition in maintaining health against oxidant stress. The antioxidant properties of ascorbate have been known since the discovery of the vitamin but its role in the antioxidant defences of the body is an area of expanding interest, since this function may be of relevance to many of the benefits of ascorbate which are in dispute.

Vitamin C is a water-soluble vitamin with pronounced redox properties (Bielski, 1982). Ascorbate undergoes a reversible, 2-step oxidation/reduction process with a free radical intermediate to dehydroascorbate. While ascorbate is a relatively reactive reductant, its free radical is relatively non-reactive. This means that the free radical can act as a chain terminator. Its relative stability will stop a chain of lipid peroxidation, and give it time to move away from the site of oxidation and be reduced, for example, by the pentose phosphate system (Lachant & Tanaka, 1986). In addition, the ascorbate free radical can disproportionate: two radicals can react together to form one molecule

Table 1. *Nutrients with a role in antioxidant metabolism.*

Nutrient	*Biological role*
Selenium	Cofactor for glutathione peroxidase
Zinc and copper	Cofactor for superoxide dismutase
Tocopherol, Carotenoids, Retinol	Radical scavengers in the lipid phase
Ascorbate	Radical scavenger in the aqueous phase
Riboflavin	Coenzyme for glutathione reductase

Table 2. *Ways of expressing serum antioxidant potential.*

[Ascorbate]* × [Cholesterol standardized tocopherol] × [Selenium] × [Beta-carotene] (Gey, 1986)

[Ascorbate × 1.7**] + [Tocopherol × 2] + [Urate × 1.3] + [Sulphydryl × 0.33] (Wayner *et al.*, 1987)

*Plasma concentrations for all nutrients in μmol/l.
**Stoichiometric factors derived using the TRAP assay and representing the efficiency, or capacity of the individual antioxidants for trapping peroxyl radicals.

of ascorbate and one of dehydroascorbate. The presence of dehydroascorbate in tissues is not desirable and if injected into animals it affects insulin secretion by the pancreas and induces diabetes. Hence in both animals and plants there are enzymes for converting dehydroascorbate and the ascorbate free radical back to ascorbate (dehydroascorbate reductase, using reduced glutathione, and the semidehydroascorbate reductase, utilizing NADH [Halliwell & Gutteridge, 1985]).

Ascorbate is just one of several antioxidants with nutritional importance (Table 1) and there is a rapidly expanding body of evidence to suggest that they interact. We looked round for ways of assessing the nutritional status of the antioxidant vitamins which measured the collective response to an oxidant stress but can also measure the components individually. Gey (1986) describes an index of antioxidant status based on the arbitrary multiplication of plasma antioxidants which were correlated with ischaemic heart disease in a cross-cultural study in four countries. His formula is based on the plasma concentrations of vitamins C and E, selenium and beta-carotene (Table 2) but disregards the antioxidant urate which in molar terms is greater than all these put together. We have investigated an alternative approach based on a method of specifically measuring radical-trapping properties of serum which I will describe later in the chapter.

The antioxidant hypothesis suggests that all tissues are under constant attack from oxygen free radicals. Poly-unsaturated fatty acids (PUFA) are easily oxidized and their presence in tissue membranes is universal throughout the animal and plant kingdoms. However, tissues in the living body do not normally oxidize and the concept that PUFA were under constant oxidative attack was overlooked until it was found that an enzyme capable of metabolizing superoxide, viz superoxide dismutase, was widely distributed in all oxidative tissues (see McCord & Fridovich, 1977).

Endogenous oxygen radicals are produced in considerable quantities in normal metabolism, eg flavoproteins (such as xanthine oxidase) and P-450 cytochromes (Paine, 1978), as well as in the normal immune processes, when the phagocytic action of macrophages is facilitated by the cytotoxic action of reactive oxygen species (ROS) in the respiratory burst (Baboir *et al.*, 1973). Such oxygen species include superoxide ($O_2^{\cdot}$), perhydroxyl radicals ($HO_2^{\cdot}$), hydroxyl radicals ($HO^{\cdot}$) and singlet oxygen ($^1O_2$). An increase in endogenous ROS has been implicated with ischaemia, inflammatory and degenerative diseases, hyperbaric oxygen, ionizing radiation (Halliwell & Gutteridge, 1985), kwashiorkor (Golden & Ramdath, 1987) etc. Exogenous radicals or radical precursors are ozone, nitrous oxide, various carcinogens and mitogens, chemotherapeutic drugs, halogenated compounds and other xenobiotics.

Free radicals carry an unpaired electron and are usually highly reactive. PUFA molecules are very vulnerable but any organic molecule, eg protein or DNA, can be attacked. Following the initial contact between the free radical and a PUFA molecule, hydrogen is abstracted and an alkyl free radical is formed ($L^{\cdot}$). This unsaturated molecule undergoes isomerization to form a conjugated diene and under aerobic conditions rapidly reacts with oxygen to form a peroxyl free radical ($LOO^{\cdot}$). The most likely targets of attack by the peroxyl radical are adjoining PUFA molecules to form a new alkyl radical and the formation of a lipid hydroperoxide (LOOH). The new alkyl radical goes on to propagate a new cycle of lipid peroxidation, while the hydroperoxide can also be broken down and generate an alkoxyl radical ($LO^{\cdot}$) to propagate the chain reaction. Lipid hydroperoxides however are metastable and, in contrast to fast reacting free radicals, can diffuse away from the site of formation and thus spread the damage (Halliwell & Gutteridge, 1985).

The consequence of lipid peroxidation is to alter tissue structure and cause tissue damage. Alterations to DNA, protein structures, enzymes, nucleotides, etc may initiate pathological changes in the cell, while damage to membranes or extracellular macromolecules may influence permeability. Pathological changes in cell structure will also propagate lipid peroxidation because tissues depend on organized structural compartments to resist oxidative damage (Dormandy 1978; 1983). Many metal cations are potent catalysts of lipid peroxidation and are normally tightly bound to protein to prevent these effects. Ferrous iron is a particularly powerful initiator of lipid peroxidation since it will catalyse the breakdown of hydrogen peroxide or lipid hydroperoxides with the formation of hydroxyl radicals by the Haber Weiss reaction. The latter are particularly reactive and have very powerful oxidizing capability (see Halliwell & Gutteridge, 1985).

Protection against lipid peroxidation

Protection against lipid peroxidation exists in three forms, viz (i) structural integrity, (ii) enzyme systems which prevent initiation, and (iii) radical quenchers to scavenge radicals and terminate chains of lipid peroxidation (Wayner *et al.*, 1985; 1987). Mention has already been made of the importance of cell structure to minimize initiation of lipid peroxidation by compartmentalizing cell components. Compartmentalization, however, does not entirely prevent ROS being formed, so the second level of defence is to detoxify the ROS and prevent them initiating lipid peroxidation. This includes superoxide dismutase, which converts superoxide to hydrogen peroxide; selenium-dependent glutathione peroxidase for the reduction of lipid hydroperoxides to the corresponding alcohols; catalase to remove hydrogen peroxide; caeruloplasmin to convert ferrous iron to the ferric form; and glutathione-S-transferase, which is important for removing a variety of foreign compounds as mercapturic acids. Finally the radical quenchers, which include the vitamins C and E, carotenoids, urate, glutathione and sulphydryl groups in proteins, are needed to break chains of peroxidation when lipid peroxidation takes place. Glutathione and carotenoids are probably only important within the cell: glutathione since it does not pass through the cell membrane, and carotenoids since they only act efficiently as scavengers at lower oxygen tensions (Burton & Ingold, 1984). Within the extracellular fluids therefore there are four main radical-scavenging antioxidants.

Vitamin C as a radical scavenger

In this chapter I am focusing my attention on vitamin C but it is more likely that antioxidants act collectively in the face of oxidant stress. Tappel (1962) was the first to suggest that there may be an antioxidant chain and, more recently, Packer *et al.* (1979) showed that ascorbate could regenerate tocopherol from the tocopheryl radical *in vitro*. Other workers have suggested that glutathione may regenerate ascorbate from dehydroascorbate, and recent studies of Wayner *et al.* (1987) suggest that, on exposure to a continuous supply of peroxyl radicals, antioxidants in serum disappear in the sequence sulphydryl, urate and finally tocopherol. Ascorbate could not be measured. Vanderpas & Vertongen (1985) obtained similar results with neonatal red blood cells exposed to increasing concentrations of hydrogen peroxide. As haemolysis took place, glutathione was the first to disappear and tocopherol the last.

Tocopherol is localized within lipid structures in the cell, where work in rats has suggested that one molecule protects 220 molecules of PUFA (Fukuzawa *et al.*, 1982). In serum, tocopherol is localized in the low density lipoproteins where most serum cholesterol is also found, and we have noticed a similar ratio of tocopherol to cholesterol in the serum of normal populations which we have studied (Thurnham *et al.*, 1986). Tocopherol can only exert this protective function if the relatively long-lived tocopheryl free radical can be regenerated *in situ* and ascorbate, being water-soluble, is ideally placed to support tocopherol in this role. The protective role of ascorbate in tissues, however, is often obscured by the techniques used to investigate lipid peroxidation, since the addition of ascorbate to tissue preparations is a very good way of generating free radicals to stimulate lipid peroxidation. Any tissue preparation will contain some free iron and the addition of ascorbate maintains this iron in the ferrous form, which then acts as a potent catalyst of lipid peroxidation, as mentioned earlier. Tappel (1980) describes experiments with vitamin-E-deficient rats injected with 0.8 LD_{50} methyl ethyl ketone peroxide. The treatment raised breath pentane production 60 times above basal levels but supplementing the deficient rats with vitamin C (750 mg/kg per day for 3 days) caused a further doubling of pentane output. The pro-oxidant action of ascorbate was probably acting by maintaining iron in the ferrous form and exaggerating the toxic effect of the peroxide to accelerate lipid peroxidation in the vitamin-E-deficient tissue. Such studies may indicate potential difficulties in giving supplementary vitamin C to animals that synthesize their own. However, it is more likely that the anti-oxidant system is delicately balanced and that too little vitamin E in the experiments of Tappel or too much iron as found in patients with iron-overload can adversly affect the utilization of ascorbate. It is reported that the administration of vitamin C to patients with iron overload has sometimes provoked severe reactions (Halliwell & Gutteridge, 1985).

Measuring radical trapping properties in serum

In man and animals, the occurrence of lipid peroxidation can only be measured indirectly and the majority of the assays available measure products of peroxidized lipid, eg malonyldialdehyde (MDA), ethane and pentane. However, radical quenching antioxidants are consumed to stop lipid peroxidation, and following the recent introduction of a method to measure total peroxyl-radical-trapping activity (TRAP) in serum (Wayner *et al.*, 1985; 1987), we investigated three situations where there is evidence of increased oxidant stress, viz rheumatoid arthritis, alcohol abuse and malaria, for evidence of effects of the stress on serum antioxidants.

TRAP is measured by exposing a serum/linoleic acid mixture to a constant source of free radicals generated from a thermolabile azo compound known as ABAP (2,2′-azo-bis-2-amidinopropane hydrochloride, Polysciences, Warrington, PA). ABAP reacts with lipid in the medium, generating chains of lipid peroxidation which consume oxygen. Antioxidants in the serum prematurely break these chains and the delay in the onset of maximum oxygen consumption is measured and compared with the delay produced following the addition of a known amount of a water-soluble vitamin E analogue, Trolox (6-HO-2,5,7,8-tetramethylchroman-2-carboxylic acid, Hoffman-La-Roche, Nutley, NJ). TRAP is expressed as μmol peroxyl radicals trapped per litre serum.

We measured TRAP in serum from 20 patients (17 women and 3 men) with classical rheumatoid arthritis and 20 healthy hospital workers matched by age and sex (Fig. 1). TRAP values in the rheumatoid patients were significantly lower than those in the control subjects and ascorbate and sulphydryl concentrations were lower in the patients (Thurnham *et al.*, 1987). There was also another important difference between the relationships of the individual antioxidants and TRAP in the two groups. In the control group, tocopherol was the only antioxidant significantly related to TRAP ($P<0.001$) and it explained 51% of the variance. However in the patients, only urate explained a significant proportion of the variance (58%, $P<0.001$). Furthermore, in both the other patient groups which we have subsequently examined (alcoholics and malaria patients; unpublished observations), urate has been the main determinant of TRAP.

The technique also enables one to determine the trapping efficiency of the individual antioxidants by adding known concentrations of them to a serum sample and comparing the increase in trapping response with that obtained by the Trolox standard in the same run (Wayner *et al.*, 1985). The factors obtained can then be used to compute theoretical TRAP values for the individual and total antioxidant capacity of the serum. In rheumatoid patients we have reported that there is approximately a 50 μmol/l discrepancy between theoretical and actual TRAP values (Thurnham *et al.*, 1987). However these differences can be greater depending on the stoichiometric factors used (Koottathep & Thurnham, unpublished data). We have suggested that the lower experimental TRAP values in rheumatoid patients may be partly due to ascorbate being present in the form of DHA, as reported by Lunec & Blake (1985). We have

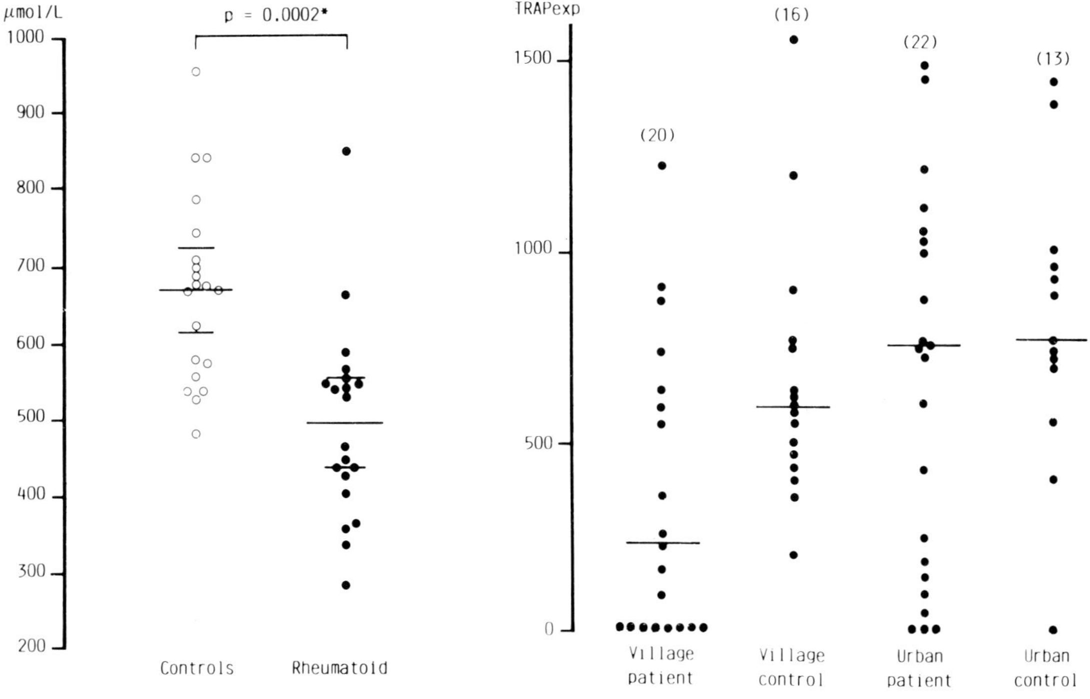

Fig. 1(above, left). *Peroxyl-radical trapping capacity (TRAP) in 20 patients with rheumatoid arthritis and 20 age- and sex-matched control subjects.* Bars show means and SDs. (From Thurnham *et al.*, 1987).
Fig. 2(above, right). *TRAP measurements on serum from patients with malaria from village and urban Thai communities and matched control subjects.* Bars show median values.

also shown that caeruloplasmin, which is increased in rheumatoid arthritis, may play a role in the oxidation of ascorbate because of its ascorbate oxidase activity (Thurnham *et al.*, 1987a). The importance of this observation in serum, however, is open to question since it has been suggested that ascorbate is protected by the copper- or iron-binding capacity of urate (Lam *et al.*, 1984; Sevanian *et al.*, 1985), of which there is a 10-fold molar excess in these patients.

Experimentally-determined TRAP values were lower than calculated TRAP in the rheumatoid patients (Thurnham *et al.*, 1987) and patients abusing alcohol (unpublished) but the discrepancies were very much greater in the patients with malaria. The results shown in Fig. 2 were obtained by my colleague Dr Singkamani from Thailand, who spent several weeks in my laboratory recently. In all cases, calculated TRAP values were greater than 400 μmol/l but were experimentally undetectable in many of the malaria patients. The one control with an undetectable TRAP result may have sickle cell anaemia since he had very high red cell aspartate aminotransferase activity, a feature we reported in such patients previously (Adelekan *et al.*, 1987), but this needs to be confirmed. It is suggested that peroxidative changes may be important in the pathogenesis of sickle cell disease and Lachant & Tanaka (1986) recently recommended that clinical trials should be undertaken to examine

Table 3. *Variables associated with experimentally-determined peroxyl radical trapping properties of serum from patients with malaria.*

Variable	*n*	*Correlation coefficient*	*P*<	*Variance explained (%)**	*P*<
Retinol	42	0.490	0.001	12	n.s.
Ascorbate	22	0.358	0.1	21	0.05
Urate	41	0.381	0.01	35	0.01
Caeruloplasmin	42	– 0.281	0.1	14	n.s.
Malonyldialdehyde: cholesterol ratio	38	– 0.372	0.02	13	n.s.
Combined*	19			54	

*The combined effect of all variables to explain the variance in TRAP was examined for 19 malaria-infected patients in whom all data were available.

the efficacy of vitamin C in the treatment of this disease since they found beneficial effects *in vitro* from ascorbate in protecting red cell from such patients against haemolysis.

Various measurements were made on these samples and some of the factors associated with the TRAP values are shown in Table 3. The ascorbate measurements were made on trichloracetic acid extracts prepared at the time of collection and may have some bearing on the TRAP measurements shown in Fig. 2 which were obtained after storage at – 70°C approximately 5 to 7 weeks later. TRAP measurements on control blood are stable for at least 12 weeks (Thurnham *et al.*, 1987) but ascorbate, measured at the time of the TRAP analysis in some of the Thai samples, was very low to negligible and further analysis was discontinued as sample volume was limited. We have previously shown however that in some malaria samples from Nigeria (Thurnham *et al.*, 1988) the lack of ascorbate itself does not prevent the measurement of TRAP, although it may reduce it. TRAP measurements were inversely associated with MDA or the MDA: cholesterol ratios (Table 2) which is supportive evidence for lipid peroxidation being associated with the low TRAP values. Vitamin E was significantly lower in the patients but at the present time we do not know why approximately 40% of the malaria samples have no apparent radical-trapping activity in spite of there being as much urate and protein sulphydryl in patient serum as in the controls.

The technique has produced some very interesting results and may tell us something about cooperative interaction between serum antioxidants. In the TRAP assay, serum is very dilute and in almost all the patient groups we have studied, urate explains most of the variance in the TRAP results. In molar terms urate is the antioxidant present in highest concentrations with the exception of protein sulphydryl but the latter has only poor trapping efficiency. On a mass action effect therefore, urate might be expected to explain most of the variance in TRAP results since urate would intercept chains of peroxidation more frequently in the dilute solution than tocopherol or ascorbate which each represent less than 10% of the radical scavenging properties. Why then should tocopherol explain most of the variance in TRAP in the control subjects in the rheumatoid study? One possibility which arises from studies in rat microsomes is that there may be protein coupling factors which assist the transfer of electrons from water-soluble reductants. Haenen & Bast (1983) describe a heat-sensitive factor which is necessary to enable GSH to prevent lipid peroxidation in rat microsomes. This substance was destroyed by lipid peroxidation and was absent in microsomal preparations prepared from vitamin-E-deficient rats. In studies in human serum, other workers have also suggested that proteins in serum lipoprotein may be necessary to couple aqueous phase reductants to tocopherol in order to exert the necessary antioxidant activity to prevent lipid peroxidation (Vidlakova *et al.*, 1972).

Vitamin C and malaria parasites

I cannot compare these results on TRAP with any similar work in animals since measurements of this kind have not yet been made. However there are some interesting studies on ascorbate metabolism in experimental malaria which are complementary to our own in man. I shall describe some of these to end this chapter as they are a useful illustration of the role of comparative studies in elucidating human problems.

The interaction of riboflavin, tocopherol and ascorbate with rodent and simian malaria is very interesting, for deficiencies of all three of these antioxidant vitamins suppress parasite multiplication: riboflavin in rats and ducks, tocopherol in mice, and ascorbate in monkeys (Kaikai & Thurnham, 1983; Etkin & Eaton, 1975; McKee & Geiman, 1946). My entry into this area of research was through experiments to show that riboflavin status was important for red cell integrity. Riboflavin is a coenzyme for glutathione reductase, the enzyme needed to maintain glutathione in the reduced form, and energy for this reaction is supplied by the hexose monophosphate shunt. Glucose-6-phosphate dehydrogenase is an integral part of this shunt and it has been recognized for some time that the protection against malaria which is conferred by G-6-PD deficiency is associated with an inability to supply sufficient GSH to maintain red cell integrity and allow normal parasite maturation.

Etkin & Eaten recognized in 1975 that malaria parasites created an oxidant stress within the red cell and that the infection superimposed on vitamin-E-deficient mice resulted in excessive haemolysis. However more interest has developed in this area following the recognition that intra-erythrocytic parasites can be damaged by ROS produced by phagocytic cells (Allison & Clark, 1977; Clark & Hunt, 1983). These studies were done in animals where the parasite load is very high; however, similar results have now been reported for human *falciparum* malaria (Descamps-Latscha *et al.*, 1987). It is also suggested that ROS could be responsible for the severe tissue damage observed in both animal (Clark & Hunt, 1983) and human malaria (Descamp-Latscha *et al.*, 1987). Nutritional factors could influence these effects (Thurnham, 1986) and Australian workers have recently reported changes in ascorbate metabolism in murine malaria suggestive of an adaptive response to the infection (Stocker *et al.*, 1986a; 1986b).

Plasmodium vinckei-infected red blood cells contain levels of ascorbic acid that are more than double those of red blood cells isolated from uninfected mice (Stocker *et al.*, 1986c). Associated with this, ascorbate was taken up readily *in vitro* by infected red cells but not by control cells, and the conversion of dehydroascorbate to ascorbate by infected lysates was higher than that in control lysates (Stocker *et al.*, 1986a). It is also interesting to note that the latter effect was abolished if the lysate was dialysed first, a procedure which removes GSH. It seems highly likely that these changes in the red cell are induced by the parasite and not the host since the duration of the malaria infection was too short to have affected red cell synthesis. It has also been shown that there is an obligatory requirement for ascorbate in the *in vitro* cultivation of *P. vivax* (Brockelman *et al.*, 1987). All this suggests that the parasite is trying to protect itself from ROS and that nutritional status may be an important determinant of human malaria pathology as has been shown in animals.

Conclusions

The use of different animal models to study the antioxidant (radical-scavenging) properties of vitamin C provides some unique opportunities that are not available for other antioxidant nutrients. The rhesus monkey or guinea-pig can be used to study the effects of vitamin C deficiency and mimic the human situation. In contrast, rodent or murine species provide models to examine the effects of host-infection interactions on vitamin C metabolism, since these species can synthesise vitamin C.

These aspects are examined in relation to malaria where in man there is evidence that total radical trapping properties of serum are markedly reduced by the presence of the parasite, and in the rhesus monkey a deficiency of vitamin C is reported to depress parasite growth. The parasites' apparent need for vitamin C is illustrated in murine malaria, where it appears to manipulate vitamin C resources in erythrocytes for its own protection. Furthermore, the *in vitro* cultivation of human *P. vivax* parasites is reported to need exogenous vitamin C to achieve normal multiplication.

There is growing evidence that antioxidants interact, possibly as a chain. It is therefore important to study vitamin C not in isolation but as one component of an integrated system. Different methods of measuring total antioxidant potential are considered and the use of one such method is described in patients with rheumatoid arthritis where preliminary results suggest that disease may disturb interaction between antioxidant nutrients.

Acknowledgements—The author is grateful for continued support by the Department of Health & Social Security, U.K. and for some assistance from British Council in the studies on malaria.

References

Adelekan, D. A., Adekunle, A. D. & Thurnham, D. I. (1987): Dependence of pyridoxine metabolism on riboflavin status in sickle cell patients. *Am. J. Clin. Nutr.* **46**, 86–90.

Allison, A. C. & Clark, I. A. (1977): Specific and non-specific immunity to haemoprotozoa. *Am. J. Trop. Med. Hyg.* **26**, 216–222.

Baboir, M. B. (1973): Oxygen dependent microbial killing of phagocytes. *New Engl. J. Med.* **298**, 659–680.

Baker, E. M., Hodges, R. E., Hood, J., Sauberlich, H. E. & March, S. C. (1969): Metabolism of ascorbic-1-^{14}C acid in experimental human scurvy. *Am. J. Clin. Nutr.* **22**, 549–558.

Bartley, W., Krebs, H. A. & O'Brien, J. (1953): Vitamin C requirements of human adults. In *Medical Research Council special report series, no 280.* London: H.M.S.O.

Bates, C. J. (1981): The function and metabolism of vitamin C in man. In *Vitamin C (ascorbic acid),* ed J. N. Counsell and D. H. Hornig, pp. 1–22. London: Applied Science Publishers.

Bielski, B. H. (1982): Chemistry of ascorbic acid radicals. In *Ascorbic acid, chemistry, metabolism and uses,* ed P. A. Seib and B. M. Tolbert, Adv. Chem. Ser. 200, pp. 81–100. Washington: American Chemical Society.

Binney, E. C., Jeness, R. & Ayuz, K. M. (1976): Inability of bats to synthesize L-ascorbic acid. *Nature* **260**, 626–628.

Brockelman, C. R., Tan-ariya, P. & Menabandhu, C. (1987): The influence of magnesium ion and ascorbic acid on the erythrocytic schizogony of *Plasmodium vivax*. *Parasitol. Res.* **73**, 107–112.

Burns, J. J., editor (1961): In *Vitamin C. Ann. N.Y. Acad. Sci.* **92**, 1–332.

Burton, G. W. & Ingold, K. U. (1984): β-Carotene: an unusual type of lipid antioxidant. *Science* **224**, 569–573.

Chatterjee, I. B., Majumder, A. K., Nandi, B. K. & Subramanian, N. (1975): Synthesis and some major functions of vitamin C in animals. In *Second conference on vitamin C*, ed C. G. King & J. J. Burns. *Ann. N. Y. Acad. Sci.* **258**, 24–47.

Clark, I. A. & Hunt, N. H. (1983): Evidence for reactive oxygen intermediates causing hemolysis and parasite death in malaria. *Inf. Immunol.* **39**, 1–6.

Counsell, J. N. & Hornig, D. H., editors (1981): In *Vitamin C (Ascorbic Acid)*. London: Applied Science Publishers.

Descamps-Latscha, B., Lunel-Fabiani, F., Kara-Binis, A. & Druilhe, P. (1987): Generation of reactive oxygen species in whole blood from patients with acute falciparum malaria. *Parasite Immunol.* **9**, 275–279.

D.H.S.S. (1979): Recommended daily amounts of food energy and nutrients for groups of people in the United Kingdom. London: HMSO.

Dormandy, T. L. (1978): Free-radical oxidation and antioxidants. *Lancet* **1**, 647–650.

Dormandy, T. L. (1983): An approach to free radicals. *Lancet* **2**, 1010–1014.

Etkin, N. L. & Eaton, J. W. (1975): Malaria-induced erythrocyte oxidant sensitivity. In *Erythrocyte structure and function*, ed G. J. Brewer, pp. 219–232. New York: A. A. Liss.

Food & Nutrition Board, (1979): Recommended daily allowances. Washington: US Government Printing Office.

Fukuzawa, K., Tokumura, A., Ouchi, S. & Tsukatani, H. (1982): Antioxidant activities of tocopherols on Fe^{2+}-ascorbate-induced lipid peroxidation in lecithin liposomes. *Lipids* **17**, 511–513.

Gey, K. F. (1986): On the antioxidant hypothesis with regard to arteriosclerosis. *Biblthca Nutr. Dieta* **37**, 53–91.

Gey, K. F., Brubacher, G. B. & Stahelin, H. B. (1987): Plasma levels of antioxidant vitamins in relation to ischemic heart disease and cancer. *Am. J. Clin. Nutr.* **45**, 1368–1377.

Ginter, E. (1977): Vitamin C and cholesterol. In *Re-evaluation of vitamin C*, ed A. Hanck and G. Ritzel, pp. 53–66. Vienna: Verlag Hans Huber.

Golden, M. H. N. & Ramdath, D. (1987): Free radicals in the pathogenesis of kwashiorkor. *Proc. Nutr. Soc.* **46**, 53–68.

Haenen, G. R. M. M. & Bast, A. (1983): Protection against lipid peroxidation by a microsomal glutathione-dependent labile factor. *FEBS Lett.* **159**, 24–28.

Halliwell, B. & Gutteridge, J. M. C., editors (1985): In *Free radicals in biology and medicine*. Oxford: Clarendon Press.

Isherwood, F. A., Chen, Y. T. & Mapson, L. W. (1954): Synthesis of L-ascorbic acid in plants and animals. *Biochem. J.* **56**, 1–15.

Kaikai, P. & Thurnham, D. I. (1983): The influence of riboflavin deficiency on *Plasmodium berghei* infection in rats. *Trans. R. Soc. Trop. Med. Hyg.* **77**, 680–686.

King, C. G. & Burns, J. J., editors (1975): In *Second Conference on vitamin C. Ann. N. Y. Acad. Sci.* **258**, 1–552.

Lachant, N. A. & Tanaka, K. R. (1986): Antioxidants in sickle cell disease: the *in vitro* effects of ascorbic acid. *Am. J. Med. Sci.* **292**, 3–10.

Lam, K. W., Fong, D., Lee, A. & Liu, K. M. D. (1984): Inhibition of ascorbate oxidation by urate. *J. Inorg. Biochem.* **22**, 241–248.

Lunec, J. & Blake, D. R. (1985): Determination of dehydroascorbate and ascorbate in the serum and synovial fluid of patients with rheumatoid arthritis. *Free Rad. Res. Comm.* **1**, 31–39.

McCord, J. M. & Fridovich, I. (1977): Superoxide dismutase: a history. In *Superoxide and superoxide dismutases*, ed A. Michelson, J. M. McCord and I. Fridovich, pp. 1–11. New York: Academic Press.

McKee, R. W. & Geiman, Q. M. (1946): Studies on malarial parasites. V. Effects of ascorbic acid on malaria (*Plasmodium knowlesi*) in monkeys. *Proc. Soc. Exptl Biol. Med.* **63**, 313–315.

Newill, A., Habibzadeh, N., Bishop, N. & Schorah, C. J. (1984): Plasma levels of vitamin C components in normal and diabetic subjects. *Ann. Clin. Biochem.* **21**, 488–490.

Packer, J. E., Slater, T. F. & Willson, R. L. (1979): Direct observations of a free-radical interaction between vitamin E and vitamin C. *Nature* **278**, 737–738.

Paine, A. J. (1978): Excited states of oxygen in biology: Involvement in cytochrome P450 oxidations as well as in the induction of the P450 system by many diverse compounds. *Biochem. Parmacol.* **27**, 1805–1813.
Pauling, L. (1970): In *Vitamin C and the common cold.* London: Academic Press.
Pelletier, O. (1977): Vitamin C and tobacco. In *Re-evaluation of vitamin C*, ed A. Hanck and G. Ritzel, pp. 147–169. Vienna: Verlag Hans Huber.
Sahud, M. A. & Cohen, R. J. (1971): Effect of aspirin ingestion on ascorbic acid levels in rheumatoid arthritis. *Lancet* **1**, 937–938.
Seib, P. A. & Tolbert, B. M., editors (1982): In *Ascorbic acid, chemistry, metabolism and uses*. Adv. Chem. Ser. 200. Washington: American Chemical Society.
Sevanian, A., Davies, K. J. A. & Hochstein, P. (1985): Conservation of vitamin C by uric acid in blood. *J. Free Rad. Biol. Med.* **1**, 117–124.
Stocker, R., Weidemann, M. J. & Hunt, N. H. (1986a): Possible mechanisms for the increased ascorbic acid content of *Plasmodium vinckei*-infected mouse erythrocytes. *Biochim. Biophys. Acta* **881**, 391–397.
Stocker, R., Hunt, N. H., Weidemann, M. J. & Clark, I. A. (1986b): Changes in the endogenous antioxidant levels of plasma and erythrocytes during *Plasmodium vinckei* malaria. *Proc. Nutr. Soc.* **45**, 70A.
Stocker, R., Hunt, N. H., Buffinton, G. D., Weidemann, M. J., Lewis-Hughes, P. H. & Clark, I. A. (1986c): Oxidative stress and protective mechanisms in erythrocytes in relation to *Plasmodium vinckei* load. *Proc. Natl. Acad. Sci. USA* **82**, 348–551.
Suboticanec, K., Folnegovic-Smalc, V., Turcin, R., Mestrovic, B. & Buzina, R. (1986): Plasma levels and urinary vitamin C excretion in schizophrenic patients. *Hum. Nutr: Clin. Nutr.* **40C**, 421–428.
Szent-Gyorgyi, A. (1963): Lost in the twentieth century. *Ann. Rev. Biochem.* **32**, 1–15.
Tappel, A. L. (1962): Vitamin E as the biological lipid antioxidant. *Vitamins & Hormones* **20**, 493–510.
Tappel, A. L. (1980): Vitamin E and selenium protection from *in vivo* lipid peroxidation. In *Micronutrient interactions: vitamins, minerals and hazardous elements. Ann. N. Y. Acad. Sci.* **355**, 18–31.
Thurnham, D. I. (1986): Nutrient deficiencies and malaria: a curse or a blessing? In *Proceedings of XIII International Congress of Nutrition*, ed T. G. Taylor and N. K. Jenkins, pp. 129–131. London: John Libbey.
Thurnham, D. I., Davies, J. A., Crump, B. J., Situnayake, R. D. & Davis, M. (1986): The use of different lipids to express serum tocopherol:lipid ratios for the measurement of vitamin E status. *Ann. Clin. Biochem.* **23**, 514–520.
Thurnham, D. I., Situnayake, R. D., Koottathep, S., McConkey, B. & Davis, M. (1987): Antioxidant status measured by the TRAP assay in rheumatoid arthritis. In *Free Radicals, oxidant stress and drug action*, pp. 169–192. London: Richelieu Press.
Thurnham, D. I., Koottathep, S. & Adelekan, D. A. (1988): Chain-breaking antioxidants in the blood of malaria-infected children. In *Free radicals: recent developments in lipid chemistry, experimental pathology and medicine*. London: Richelieu Press. (In the press).
Vanderpas, J. & Vertongen, F. (1985): Erythrocyte vitamin E is oxidized at a lower peroxide concentration in neonates than in adults. *Blood* **66**, 1272–1277.
Vidlakova, M., Erazimova, J., Norki, J. & Placer, Z. (1972): Relationship of serum antioxidative activity to tocopherol and serum inhibitor of lipid peroxidation. *Clin. Chim. Acta* **36**, 61–66.
Waugh, W. A. & King, C. G. (1932): The chemical nature of vitamin C. *J. Biol. Chem.* **97**, 325–331.
Wayner, D. D. M., Burton, G. W., Ingold, K. & Locke, S. (1985): Quantitative measurement of total peroxyl radical-trapping antioxidant capability of human blood plasma by controlled peroxidation. *FEBS Lett.* **187**, 33–37.
Wayner, D. D. M., Burton, G. W., Ingold, K., Barclay, L. R. C. & Locke, S. J. (1987): The relative contributions of vitamin E, urate, ascorbate and proteins to the total radical-trapping antioxidant activity of human blood plasma. *Biochim. Biophys. Acta* **924**, 408–419.
Zannoni, V. G., Smith, C. R. & Rikans, L. E. (1977): Drug metabolism and ascorbic acid. In *Re-evaluation of vitamin C*, ed A. Hanck and G. Ritzel, pp. 99–125. Vienna: Verlag Hans Huber.

* * * * *

Discussion

Dr Widdowson said that the history of vitamin C showed up comparative nutrition in a very elegant way. She quoted Claude Bernard as saying that in research the choice of animal is very important and she gave an example of guinea pigs which were chosen for work on beri beri and by accident produced ascorbic acid deficiency. She recommended the recent book by K. Carpenter on the History of Vitamins.

Professor Gurr made the point that there were considerable amounts of polyunsaturated fatty acids in the body and so protective factors against oxidation were important. He wondered whether urate could act like ascorbic acid in this respect. *Thurnham* replied that urate tended to be present in high concentrations in those species which were not able to synthesize vitamin C and also made the point that urate may well protect vitamin C from oxidation by metal ions, particularly copper [Lam *et al.* (1984)].

Dr Grimble referred to the patients with rheumatoid arthritis and wondered whether there was any correlation between ascorbic acid levels and urate. Thurnham replied that no correlation was found in any of the groups examined.

Dr Eastwood wondered whether oxalic acid which is a reducing agent had a role to play in the body similar to that of ascorbic acid. *Thurnham* said that he knew of no specific role, though there were many substances which could act as radical quenchers but may not be of any physiological importance.

Professor Waterlow wondered whether the role of ascorbic acid in collagen synthesis and its function as a free radicle scavenger were related, and *Thurnham* replied that they might be.

Dr Coates noted the fact that birds produce large quantities of urates and also synthesize ascorbic acid and she wondered where this fitted in with the scheme that Thurnham had in mind, to which he replied that he knew of no work in this area.

Professor Jackson commented that TRAP was measuring extra-cellular radical-quenching activity whereas pathological peroxidation would tend to start intra-cellularly. *Thurnham* made the point that, while this was true, he believed that the extra-cellular antioxidants were in contact with intracellular antioxidants. *In vivo*, membranes are permeable to dehydroascorbate and even ascorbate, as evidenced in the malaria-parasitized mouse red cell [Stocker *et al.* (1986a)]. It is possible that there are coupling factors linking extra-cellular antioxidant potential with intracellular needs.

7

Bone minerals and fat-soluble vitamins

D. R. FRASER

Introduction

The function of bone as a tissue of land vertebrates is primarily mechanical. The bony elements of the skeleton provide an articulated, rigid framework which enables locomotion by the coordinated contraction and relaxation of the attached musculature. The conformation of different species and of individuals of those species, and the final stature at maturity are all determined by the skeletal structure. The bones of the head and the spine have an additional mechanical function of protecting the vulnerable soft tissue of the central nervous system against trauma. From an evolutionary point of view the skeleton became a substantial part of body mass with the transition of vertebrates from water to land. The skeletons of early giant extinct amphibians such as *Eryops*, up to 1.5 m in length, were massive in comparison to those of fish of a comparable size. This development of skeletal mass is clearly associated with the mechanical requirement of supporting the body without the help of buoyancy from water.

An apparently minor role of the skeleton is to serve as a store of calcium. Again, with the appearance of land vertebrates, the supply of calcium had to come entirely from the diet instead of from that infinite store dissolved in the ambient water of aquatic vertebrates. An internal calcium store could therefore be of use to land vertebrates to meet particular demands in reproduction and when the dietary supply of calcium is inadequate. However, the significance of bone as a general reserve of calcium for vertebrates is difficult to evaluate. In birds, bone mineral additional to that required for mechanical strength is laid down in the medullary cavity of long bones and this is resorbed to supply calcium for egg-shell formation (Kyes & Potter, 1934; Hurwitz & Bar, 1971). Studies in women indicate that bone mineral mass decreases by 2–3% over 100 days of lactation (Atkinson & West, 1970; Lamke *et al.*, 1977) and lactating dairy cows also lose mineral from bone (Ramberg *et al.*, 1970). Nevertheless, because of its primary role as a mechanical support, bone is unlikely to provide a substantial reserve of calcium, as extensive mineral mobilization would inevitably reduce its structural strength.

Specific nutritional effects on bone

To fulfil its mechanical role, each bone in the skeleton has to be an appropriate size, of correct configuration, and to be strong enough to resist fracturing. Failure to achieve adequate size, shape and strength can result from malnutrition. With a prolonged low plane of nutrition, bone, like other tissues, will not grow and stature at maturity will be below the genetic potential (Dickerson & McCance, 1961; Nakamoto & Miller, 1979). Deficiency of the mineral elements of bone could therefore be expected to interfere more specifically with the development in size, shape or strength of growing bone.

In rats, a dietary deficiency of calcium during growth causes undermineralization of the skeleton but growth rate is not affected until the bone mineral content is less than 50% of that laid down when the dietary calcium supply is adequate (Moore *et al.*, 1963). The significance of the supply of calcium in the development of bone in other species has not been extensively studied. In human populations receiving an intake of calcium well below the recommended value, bone growth appears to be unimpaired and the structure and strength appear to be normal (Walker, 1972). It is likely with a persistent low intake that the intestinal absorption capacity for calcium is greatly enhanced.

Dietary phosphorus deficiency, on the other hand, has a marked impact on growth. Because phosphorus is a major component in the synthesis of nucleic acids, proteins and phospholipids, as well as in the utilization of chemical energy, any inadequacy in the supply of phosphorus will inevitably have a profound effect on the growth of all tissues. Hence, experimental phosphorus deficiency has a more pronounced effect on skeletal growth than does deficiency of calcium (Field *et al.*, 1975).

The discovery that vitamin D could prevent and cure the bone disease of rickets (Mellanby, 1918; McCollum *et al.*, 1922) was the main basis for the concept that nutritional factors had specific roles in the formation of bone. Although this concept has been held by nutritionists for most of this century it is now clear that for vitamin D at least, it is erroneous. For vitamin D is not, under natural conditions, a nutrient. Apart from egg-yolk, some types of fatty fish, and to some extent milk fat, the diet for humans is a trivial source of vitamin D (for review see Fraser, 1983). The same applies to domestic animals and other land vertebrates. It is only those species housed away from sunlight, such as intensively-reared pigs and poultry, which require vitamin D to be supplied by man and this is done most conveniently by fortifying the diet. The seasonal variation of vitamin D status in humans and the ineffectiveness of the usual daily intake of 2.5 μg in influencing that status, indicates that vitamin D is obtained mainly by exposure to solar ultraviolet irradiation. A nutritional definition for vitamin D has not only misled us into ascribing a class of nutrients which specifically affect bone, it has also misled us when trying to discover the function of vitamin D in the growth of bone.

Vitamin D is a product of the photochemical cleavage of the 9,10 carbon-carbon bond of 7-dehydrocholesterol in skin. The vitamin D structure is then metabolically transformed to 1,25-dihydroxyvitamin D [1,25$(OH)_2$D] which is now known to be a steroid hormone (Kodicek, 1974), influencing the function of many different cell types. The actual regulatory role of 1,25$(OH)_2$D, although extensively investigated in recent years, is still not understood. Rather than being a specific bone-growth-promoting nutrient, vitamin D is now seen to be a precursor of a hormone which affects many physiological systems, perhaps by regulating calcium homoeostasis of cells. Indeed calcium, while a major component of bone mineral, also has a central role as an intracellular messenger in cellular control mechanisms (Rasmussen & Barrett, 1984). Thus deficiency of either vitamin D or calcium may have as much significance for extra-skeletal tissues as for the growth and development of bone.

Although the classification of vitamins A, D, E and K as a group, because of their lipophilic properties, has only chemical rather than biological justification, it is nevertheless curious that three of them appear to have specific actions in bone. In vitamin A deficiency, there is defective remodelling of bone during growth which leads to constriction of the brain cavity, the spinal canal and bony foramina through which peripheral nerves pass (for review see Barnicot & Datta, 1972). Hypervitaminosis A also affects the skeleton, inhibiting bone growth (Wolbach & Hegsted, 1965) and causing thinning and fracture of long bones (Dingle & Lucy, 1965). As with all the systemic functions of vitamin A, the actual molecular mechanism of its effect in bone remains unknown.

The role of vitamin K in the function of the plasma clotting proteins is to promote the post-translational carboxylation of glutamic acid residues to form γ-carboxyglutamate (Gla) (Nelsestuen & Suttie, 1973; Stenflo *et al.*, 1974). This modification enables these proteins to bind Ca^{2+} required for activation of the haemostatic process. Another vitamin-D-dependent Gla-containing protein, osteocalcin or bone Gla protein, has been isolated from bone (Hauschka *et al.*, 1975; Price *et al.*, 1976). The role of this calcium-binding bone protein has not been identified but its location in the extracellular matrix and its synthesis by osteoblasts suggests that it has some function in mineralization. Rats with long-term inhibition of vitamin K action by warfarin treatment have a bone defect which results in fusion of epiphyseal growth plates and consequent cessation of longitudinal bone growth (Price *et al.*, 1982). In normal rats the epiphyseal growth plates remain throughout life.

Although vitamin D has functions in most types of cell, the signs of vitamin D deficiency are seen most readily in bone. In growing animals and children, deficiency produces a disturbance of bone formation at the endochondral centres of ossification. In adults after epiphyseal fusion has occurred vitamin D deficiency results in impaired mineralization of the new bone produced during bone turnover. At all ages the characteristic histological feature of vitamin D deficiency is the accumulation of osteoid on bone surfaces with a markedly decreased proportion of calcification fronts.

This mineralization defect is typical of vitamin D deficiency but in very young children a similar pathological state is caused by a gross undersupply of dietary calcium (Maltz *et al.*, 1970; Kooh *et al.*, 1977; Pettifor *et al.*, 1978). Another special case is the osteopoenia or 'rickets' of premature, low-birth-weight children (Brooke & Lucas, 1985). Although vitamin D deficiency may be a contributory factor in the undermineralization of bone (Hillman *et al.*, 1985) the main cause of osteopoenia of prematurity is probably a deficiency of the mineral substrates. Breast milk will only supply a proportion of the calcium and phosphorus normally acquired by the fetus during the last trimester of pregnancy and supplementation with these minerals is necessary for bone mineralization in premature infants (Greer *et al.*, 1982a). Because of the utilization of phosphorus for soft tissue growth it is important that phosphorus intake is sufficiently high to enable calcium to be deposited as hydroxyapatite in bone (Senterre *et al.*, 1983). If the supply of phosphorus is inadequate, calcium absorbed from the diet is lost in urine. Thus for optimum bone mineralization, premature infants of less than 2000 g body weight require up to 200 mg Ca/kg body wt./day and a Ca:P dietary ratio of between 1.5 and 2 (Greer *et al.*, 1982b).

Disorders of bone formation during growth

In comparison to the human, the rate of increase in body weight of most domestic animals during growth is extremely rapid. For example, Great Dane dogs have a growth rate which is 20-fold higher than that of the human child (Hazewinkel *et al.*, 1985). If dietary calcium and phosphorus are not supplied in appropriate amounts or if the coordinated control of bone growth is disturbed during periods of rapid gain in body weight, then bone malformation will result. Hence rapidly growing species may demonstrate the effects of inappropriate nutrition on the growth of bone more readily than is apparent in the human.

Rapidly growing broiler chickens are susceptible to leg weakness related to tibial dyschondroplasia. In this condition the prehypertrophic cartilage of the proximal tibial growth plate persists so that a non-vascular cartilaginous 'plug' grows down the medullary cavity and endochondral bone formation becomes grossly distorted (Sauveur & Mongin, 1978). Although the condition is thought to have multiple causes, it is likely that nutritional factors are paramount in its aetiology. The incidence of the abnormality increases with an increase in dietary chloride level and this effect can be countered by raising the dietary levels of sodium, potassium or calcium (Simons *et al.*, 1987; Hulan *et al.*, 1987). These effects on bone growth appear to be related to changes in the acid-base balance of the birds, and the incidence of dyschondroplasia is increased by metabolic acidosis.

In rats and chickens, acidosis results in decreased circulating levels of 1,25$(OH)_2$D (Lee *et al.*, 1977; Sauveur *et al.*, 1977) and in humans chronic metabolic acidosis may lead to hyperparathyroidism (Coe *et al.*, 1975) and osteomalacia (Cunningham *et al.*, 1982). In chickens, an elevated secretion rate of growth hormone has also been related to the development of tibial dyschondroplasia (Vasilatos-Younken & Leach, 1986). It is therefore possible that tibial dyschondroplasia in growing chickens results from a combination of acid-base imbalance and hormonal imbalance that together disturb the orderly transition of epiphyseal cartilage into bone. Thus, during rapid growth, nutritional factors may modify the secretion of hormones which are regulating endochondral ossification and may in this way give rise to metabolic bone disease.

Rapid growth of pigs, dogs and horses may also be associated with abnormal bone development. In all these species disorderly endochondral ossification has been described and this gives rise to bone pain, deformity, abnormal gait and reduced mobility. Although these abnormalities are considered to be peculiar to each species it is remarkable how similar are the predisposing factors and the bone pathology between them all. In the pig (Woodard *et al.*, 1987a & b), dog (Hedhammar *et al.*, 1974; Hazewinkel *et al.*, 1985) and horse (Bridges *et al.*, 1984; Knight *et al.*, 1985), osteochondrosis is described with increased thickness and retention of epiphyseal cartilage, focal chondrocyte necrosis, disarranged metaphyseal bone trabeculae, protrusion of a chondroid core into the metaphysis and delayed remodelling of cortical bone. If the ossification defect persists, the epiphyses become swollen and the weakened metaphyses exhibit microfractures and attempts at repair with callus formation. Osteochondrosis dessicans can develop as the epiphyseal bone becomes unable to support the articular cartilage, which then becomes partially detached and fragments may break free into the joint space.

In all species the condition is more severe in large animals growing rapidly on a high plane of nutrition. Although there is no agreement on the mechanism by which nutrition may cause osteochondrosis, an elegant explanation has been proposed for the dog (Hedhammar *et al.*, 1974). Osteochondrosis appears to be more common in larger breeds fed an excess of dietary calcium at a time of rapid growth. The animals tend to be slightly hypercalcaemic with a consequent fall in the production of parathyroid hormone and an increase in that of calcitonin. Calcitonin stimulates the proliferation of chondroblasts and increases chondrogenesis while parathyroid hormone enhances bone remodelling and promotes cartilage maturation during osteogenesis. In osteochondrosis, the excessive production of immature epiphyseal cartilage along with diminished bone remodelling is compatible with the hormonal imbalance postulated to be induced by the high calcium diet. It is likely that $1,25(OH)_2D$ production would also be decreased and lower levels of this hormone may contribute to the osteochondrotic condition.

A reduction in growth rate by restricting food intake and a decrease in the supply of dietary calcium have both been found to prevent and correct osteochondrosis in dogs. Similarly for pigs and horses, decreasing the rate of growth is also effective in preventing this developmental abnormality of bone. Although the capacity for calcium absorption can be adaptively increased in calcium deficiency by a $1,25(OH)_2D$-dependent mechanism, there is, in effect, no upper limit for calcium absorption when a large amount is supplied (Heaney *et al.*, 1975). Most assessments of human calcium requirements have noted the relatively small proportion (30–40%) of dietary calcium absorbed in balance studies in well-nourished humans. Consequently, the recommended dietary intakes for children range from 500 to 1400 mg per day (I.U.N.S. Report, 1982). No apparent consideration has been given to any possible deleterious effects of high calcium intakes in rapidly growing children. However, at least one report notes that skeletal deformities are more common in children during rapid growth (Dluzniewska *et al.*, 1965). The observations about osteochondrosis in domestic animals could well have some relevance to the development of bone in children.

Calcium: phosphorus dietary ratio

Apart from the absolute dietary levels of calcium and phosphorus for optimum bone development, the ratio of the two elements to each other is also important for most domestic animals. Nutritional secondary hyperparathyroidism occurs in the horse (Krook & Lowe, 1964), dog (Saville *et al.*, 1969), cat (Krook *et al.*, 1963), pig (Brown *et al.*, 1966) and rat (Anderson & Draper, 1972) if there is excess phosphorus in relation to calcium in the diet. For most species the dietary Ca:P ratio should be between 1:1 and 2:1 to avoid hyperparathyroid bone disease.

However, in human populations where meat is a major part of the diet the Ca:P ratio can be as wide as 1:4 without apparently causing hyperparathyroidism or having any other deleterious effect on bone (Spencer *et al.*, 1978). A similar observation has been made on non-human primates (Anderson *et al.*, 1977) so it may be that in primates as a group, calcium availability and calcium retention are independent of the supply of dietary phosphorus. Further evidence for this is the failure of long-term phosphorus supplementation to affect mineral deposition or the remodelling of bone (Heaney & Recker, 1987). In contrast, long-term phosphorus supplementation of the diet of dogs has been found to stimulate bone formation (Harris *et al.*, 1976).

Dietary calcium and osteoporosis

A decrease in bone mass occurs with advancing age in both men and women but the rate of loss is more rapid in women after the menopause. The cause of this loss is an imbalance between the formation of bone by osteoblasts and its resorption by osteoclasts during bone turnover and remodelling. The accelerated rate of bone loss in post-menopausal women is related to oestrogen deficiency and can be prevented by oestrogen replacement therapy (Nordin *et al.*, 1980). The importance of osteoporotic bone loss, especially the accelerated loss after the menopause, lies in its association with an increased risk of symptomatic fractures of the vertebral bodies, wrist, or neck of the femur in response to minimal trauma.

Despite years of research, the specific biochemical mechanism causing osteoporosis of the elderly is unknown. However, because bone turnover is faster in osteoporosis and because there is a negative calcium balance, much attention has been devoted to the idea that osteoporosis is a nutritional calcium deficiency disease. One corollary of this concept is that if high bone mass could be achieved in early adult life, by a high calcium intake during growth, then the clinical effects of osteoporosis could be delayed. A second corollary is that a high calcium intake when osteoporosis is already apparent would prevent further loss of bone.

There is little evidence to support the view that the level of dietary calcium intake has any significant influence in either the prevention or treatment of osteoporosis. Calcium supplementation trials have shown either no effect (Nilas *et al.*, 1984; Riis *et al.*, 1987) or minimal inhibition of bone loss (Recker *et al.*, 1977; Horsman *et al.*, 1977). Where calcium supplements have had some effect on the rate of bone loss it is likely that this was mediated indirectly by suppression of parathyroid hormone secretion rather than by a direct action on the bone itself.

The lack of progress made in understanding the mechanism of osteoporosis might be attributed to two characteristics of research in this field: (1) the definition of osteoporosis as a problem of calcium balance and (2) the lack of a suitable animal model with which to investigate the mechanism.

It is notable that clinical osteoporosis, as a spontaneous disease, is a problem apparently peculiar to the human species. Experiments attempting to induce osteoporosis in dogs by ovariectomy have shown a fall in osteoblast activity (Malluche *et al.*, 1986). Nevertheless, it is overwhelmingly apparent that the many millions of ovariectomized pet dogs throughout the world do not suffer from osteoporotic fractures. In contrast to women, the female dog has a low circulating oestrogen level which rises once or twice a year at oestrus. Perhaps the monthly rise and fall of plasma oestrogen in women induces a particular dependence on oestrogen for bone cell function. This dependence could give rise to defective control of bone turnover with the onset of oestrogen deficiency at the menopause. The human species is unique in comparison to domestic animals in that individuals survive for many years beyond the period of reproduction. Chronic diseases of old age, such as osteoporosis, may also be unique to the human and an experimental animal model may be difficult to find.

Calcium deprivation and induced vitamin D deficiency

With the discovery of vitamin D and the subsequent widespread supplementation with this presumed 'nutrient' and, in particular, with the increased exposure of urban children to solar ultraviolet light, the incidence of vitamin D deficiency rickets declined and apparently disappeared as a problem of community health. However, many independent reports over the past 20 years indicate that rickets still occurs in Algeria, Libya, Morocco and Tunisia (Joint FAO/WHO Report, 1967), Egypt (Lawson *et al.*, 1987), Ethiopia (Hojer *et al.*, 1977), Greece (Lapatsanis *et al.*, 1968), Iran (Salimpour, 1975), Iraq (El-Radhi *et al.*, 1982), Saudi Arabia (Elidrissy & Sedrani, 1980) and in the Indian subcontinent (DHSS Report on Health and Social Subjects, 1980). In the Mediterranean and Middle Eastern countries it appears that the incidence of clinical vitamin D deficiency has been roughly 10–20% from 1965 onwards. It is remarkable that rickets is still common in countries where solar ultraviolet light is deemed to be plentiful.

Rickets also began to reappear in the U.K. in the 1960s in children of Asian immigrants (Dunnigan *et al.*, 1962). The reason for the particular susceptibility of the Asian children to rickets was unknown. There was no apparent difference in their exposure to sunlight nor in their intake of dietary vitamin D when compared to Caucasian children in the same environment (Dunnigan *et al.*, 1975; O'Hara-May & Widdowson, 1976; Hunt *et al.*, 1976). A recent analysis of the problem has concluded that although limited exposure to sunlight was an important aetiological feature, dietary factors also contributed to the appearance of vitamin D deficiency disease (Henderson *et al.*, 1987). These factors were a vegetarian diet (Dent & Gupta, 1975) and one with a high content of whole-meal flour (Wills *et al.*, 1972; Robertson *et al.*, 1981; Henderson *et al.*, 1987). Hence some mechanism other than just the supply of vitamin D was inducing clinical vitamin D deficiency.

From studies in rats, it is now postulated that that mechanism involves a low supply or low availability of dietary calcium. Calcium deprivation promotes mild hyperparathyroidism which stimulates the production of $1,25(OH)_2D$. The extra $1,25(OH)_2D$ is now known to enhance the metabolic inactivation of 25 hydroxyvitamin D [25(OH)D] in the liver (Clements *et al.*, 1987a). This enhanced destruction is not thought to be a mechanism for regulating hepatic vitamin D metabolism, but appears more likely to be secondary to some other primary effect of 1,25$(OH)_2$D on liver function. Evidence for this mechanism of inducing vitamin D deficiency has now also been obtained in humans (Clements *et al.*, 1987b). It is also evident that mild hyperparathyroidism, which would lead to enhanced inactivation of 25(OH)D, occurs frequently in Asian immigrants in the U.K. (Stephens *et al.*, 1982).

Vitamin D deficiency is also found in several clinical conditions characterized by hyperparathyroidism (Stanbury, 1981) or calcium malabsorption. These conditions include gastrointestinal disease (Dibble *et al.*, 1984) intestinal resection (Compston *et al.*, 1978), jejunoileal bypass (Teitelbaum *et al.*, 1977), gastrectomy (Nilas *et al.*, 1985), chronic liver disease (Dibble *et al.*, 1984), anticonvulsant therapy (Silver *et al.*, 1974), and gross obesity (Bell *et al.*, 1985). In all of these abnormal states, parathyroid hormone secretion is raised with a consequent increase in 1,25$(OH)_2$D production. It is therefore likely that vitamin D deficiency which occurs in these clinical states is a result of enhanced hepatic inactivation of 25(OH)D under the influence of 1,25$(OH)_2$D.

This process of enhanced inactivation provides a unified explanation for vitamin D deficiency related to calcium deprivation, either from dietary insufficiency or from disease. Therefore, an adequate supply of calcium may be as important for ensuring normal vitamin D endocrine function as it is for mineralization in the growth and maintenance of the skeletal system.

References

Anderson, G. H. & Draper, H. H. (1972): Effect of dietary phosphorus on calcium metabolism in intact and parathyroidectomized adult rats. *J. Nutr.* **102**, 1123–1132.

Anderson, M. P., Hunt, R. D., Griffiths, H. J., McIntyre, K. W. & Zimmerman, R. E. (1977): Long-term effect of low dietary calcium:phosphate ratio on the skeleton of *Cebus albifrons* monkeys. *J. Nutr.* **107**, 834–839.

Atkinson, P. J. & West, R. R. (1970): Loss of skeletal calcium in lactating women. *J. Obstet. Gynaecol. Br. Cwlth.* **77**, 555–560.

Barnicot, N. A. & Datta, S. P. (1972): In *Biochemistry and Physiology of Bone*, Vol. 2 ed G. H. Bourne, pp. 197–215. New York: Academic Press.

Bell, N. H., Epstein, S., Greene, A., Shary, J., Oexmann, M. J. & Shaw, S. (1985): Evidence for alteration of the vitamin-D-endocrine system in obese subjects. *J. Clin. Invest.* **76**, 370–373.

Bridges, C. H., Womack, J. E., Harris, E. D. & Scrutchfield, W. L. (1984): Consideration of copper metabolism in osteochondrosis of suckling foals. *J. Am. Vet. Med. Assoc.* **185**, 173–178.

Brooke, O. G. & Lucas, A. (1985): Metabolic bone disease in preterm infants. *Archs Dis. Childhood* **60**, 682–685.

Brown, W. R., Krook, L. & Pond, W. G. (1966): Atrophic rhinitis in swine: etiology, pathogenesis and prophylaxis. *Cornell Vet.*, Suppl. 1, **56**, 1–128.

Clements, M. R., Johnson, L. & Fraser, D. R. (1987a): A new mechanism for induced vitamin D deficiency in calcium deprivation. *Nature* **324**, 62–65.

Clements, M. R., Davies, M., Fraser, D. R., Lumb, G. A., Mawer, E. B. & Adams, P. H. (1987b): Metabolic inactivation of vitamin D is enhanced in primary hyperparathyroidism. *Clin. Sci.* **73**, 659–664.

Coe, F. L., Firpo, J. J., Hollandsworth, D. L., Segil, L., Canterbury, J. M. & Reiss, E. (1975): Effect of acute and chronic metabolic acidosis on serum immunoreactive parathyroid hormone in man. *Kidney Internat.* **8**, 262–273.

Compston, J. E., Ayers, A. B., Horton, L. W. L., Tighe, J. R. & Creamer, B. (1978): Osteomalacia after small intestinal resection. *Lancet* **i**, 9–12.

Cunningham, J., Fraher, L. J., Clemens, T. L., Revell, P. A. & Papapoulos, S. E. (1982): Chronic acidosis with metabolic bone disease. Effect of alkali on bone morphology and vitamin D metabolism. *Am. J. Med* **73**, 199–204.

Dent, C. E. & Gupta, M. M. (1975): Plasma 25-hydroxyvitamin-D levels during pregnancy in Caucasians and in vegetarian and non-vegetarian Asians. *Lancet* **ii**, 1057–1060.

DHSS Report on Health and Social Subjects No. 19 (1980): *Rickets and osteomalacia. Report on the working party on fortification of food with vitamin D.* London: Her Majesty's Stationery Office.

Dibble, J. B., Sheridan, P. & Losowsky, M. S. (1984): A survey of vitamin-D deficiency in gastrointestinal and liver disorders. *Q. J. Med.* **53**, 119–134.

Dickerson, J. W. T. & McCance, R. A. (1961): Severe undernutrition in growing and adult animals. 8. The dimensions and chemistry of the long bones. *Br. J. Nutr.* **15**, 567–576.

Dingle, J. T. & Lucy, J. A. (1965): Vitamin A, carotenoids and cell function. *Biol. Rev.* **40**, 422–461.

Dluzniewska, K., Obtulowicz, A. & Koltek, K. (1965): On the relationship between diet, rate of growth and skeletal deformities in school children. *Folia Medica Craciviensia* **7**, 115–126.

Dunnigan, M. G., Paton, J. P. J., Haase, S., McNicol, G. W., Gardner, M. D. & Smith, C. M. (1962): Late rickets and osteomalacia in the Pakistani community in Glasgow. *Scot. Med. J.* **7**, 159–167.

Dunnigan, M. G., Childs, W. C., Smith, C. M., McIntosh, W. B. & Ford, J. A. (1975): The relative roles of ultraviolet deprivation and diet in the aetiology of Asian rickets. *Scot. Med. J.* **20**, 217–218.

Elidrissy, A. T. H. & Sedrani, S. H. (1980): Infantile vitamin D deficiency rickets in Riyadh. *Calc. Tiss. Int.* **33**, 47–52.

El-Radhi, A. S., Majeed, M., Mansour, N. & Ibrahim, M. (1982): High incidence of rickets in children with wheezy bronchitis in a developing country. *J. Roy. Soc. Med.* **75**, 884–887.

Field, A. C., Suttle, N. F. & Nisbet, D. I. (1975): Effect of diets low in calcium and phosphorus on the development of growing lambs. *J. Agr. Sci.* **85**, 435–442.

Fraser, D. R. (1983): The physiological economy of vitamin D. *Lancet* **i**, 969–972.

Greer, F. R., Steichen, J. J. & Tsang, R. C. (1982a): Calcium and phosphate supplements in breast milk-related rickets. *Am. J. Dis. Children* **136**, 581–583.

Greer, F. R., Steichen, J. J. & Tsang, R. C. (1982b): Effects of increased calcium, phosphorus, and vitamin D intake on bone mineralization in very low-birth-weight infants fed formulas with Polycose and medium-chain triglycerides. *J. Pediatr.* **100**, 951–955.

Harris, W. H., Heaney, R. P., Davis, L. A., Weinberg, E. H., Coutts, R. D. & Schiller, A. L. (1976): Stimulation of bone formation *in vivo* by phosphate supplementation. *Calcif. Tissue Res.* **22**, 85–98.

Hauschka, P. V., Lian, J. B. & Gallop, P. M. (1975): Direct identification of the calcium-binding amino acid γ-carboxyglutamate, in mineralized tissue. *Proc. Natl. Acad. Sci. U.S.A.* **72**, 3925–3929.

Hazewinkel, H. A. W., Goedegebuure, S. A., Poulos, P. W. & Wolvekamp, W. T. C. (1985): Influence of chronic calcium excess on skeletal development of growing Great Danes. *J. Amer. An. Hosp. Assoc.* **21**, 377–391.

Heaney, R. P., Saville, P. D. & Recker, R. R. (1975): Calcium absorption as a function of calcium intake. *J. Lab. Clin. Med.* **85**, 881–890.

Heaney, R. P. & Recker, R. R. (1987): Calcium supplements: anion effects. *Bone and Mineral* **2**, 433–439.

Hedhammar, A., Wu, F. M., Krook, L., Schryver, H. F., de Lahunta, A., Whalen, J. P., Kallfelz, F. A., Nunez, E. A., Hintz, H. F., Sheffy, B. E. & Ryan, G. D. (1974): Overnutrition and skeletal disease. An experimental study in growing Great Dane dogs. *Cornell Vet.* **64**, Suppl. 5, 1–160.

Henderson, J. B., Dunnigan, M. G., McIntosh, W. B., Abdul-Motaal, A. A., Gettinby, G. & Glekin, B. M. (1987): The importance of limited exposure to ultraviolet radiation and dietary factors in the aetiology of Asian rickets: a risk-factor model. *Q. J. Med.* **63**, 413–425.

Hillman, L. S., Hoff, N., Salmons, S., Martin, L., McAlister, W. & Haddad, J. (1985): Mineral homeostasis in very premature infants: serial evaluation of serum 25-hydroxyvitamin D, serum minerals, and bone mineralization. *J. Pediatr.* **106**, 970–980.

Hojer, B., Gebre-Medhin, M., Sterky, G., Zetterstrom, R. & Daniel, K. (1977): Combined vitamin D deficiency rickets and protein energy malnutrition in Ethiopian infants. *J. Trop. Paediat.* **23**, 73–79.

Horsman, A., Gallagher, J. C., Simpson, M. & Nordin, B. E. C. (1977): Prospective trial of oestrogen and calcium in postmenopausal women. *Br. Med. J.* **2**, 789–792.

Hulan, H. W., Simons, P. C. M., van Schagen, P. J. W., McRae, K. B. & Proudfoot, F. G. (1987): Effect of dietary cation-anion balance and calcium content on general performance and incidence of leg abnormalities of broiler chickens. *Can. J. Anim. Sci.* **67**, 165–177.

Hunt, S. P., O'Riordan, J. L. H., Windo, J. & Truswell, A. S. (1976): Vitamin D status in different subgroups of British Asians. *Br. Med. J.* **2**, 1351–1354.

Hurwitz, S. & Bar, A. (1971): The effect of pre-laying mineral nutrition on the development, performance, and mineral metabolism of pullets. *Poult. Sci.* **50**, 1044–1055.

I.U.N.S. Report by Committee 1/5 (1982): Recommended dietary intakes around the world. *Nutr. Abstr. Rev.* **53**, 939–1015.

Joint FAO/WHO Expert Committee on Nutrition (1967): Seventh report, *Rickets*, pp. 31–34.

Knight, D. A., Gabel, A. A., Reed, S. M., Emberton, R. M., Tyznik, W. J. & Bramlage, L. R. (1985): Correlation of dietary mineral to incidence and severity of metabolic bone disease in Ohio and Kentucky. *Proc. 31st Mt. Am. Ass. Equine Pract.* pp. 445–461.

Kodicek, E. (1974): The story of vitamin D from vitamin to hormone. *Lancet* **i**, 325–329.

Kooh, S. W., Fraser, D., Reilly, B. J., Hamilton, J. R., Gall, D. G. & Bell, L. (1977): Rickets due to calcium deficiency. *New Engl. J. Med.* **297**, 1264–1266.

Krook, L., Barrett, R. B., Usui, K. & Wolke, R. E. (1963): Nutritional secondary hyperparathyroidism in the cat. *Cornell Vet.* **53**, 224–240.

Krook, L. & Lowe, J. E. (1964): Nutritional secondary hyperparathyroidism in the horse. *Path. Vet.*, Suppl. **1**, 1–98.

Kyes, P. & Potter, T. S. (1934): Physiological marrow ossification in female pigeons. *Anat. Rec.* **60**, 377–379.

Lamke, B., Brundin, J. & Moberg, P. (1977): Changes of bone mineral content during pregnancy and lactation. *Acta Obstet. Gynecol. Scand.* **56**, 217–219.

Lapatsanis, P., Deliyanni, V. & Doxiadis, S. (1968): Vitamin D deficiency rickets in Greece. *J. Pediat.* **73**, 195–202.

Lawson, D. E. M., Cole, T. J., Salem, S. I., Galal, O. M., El-Meligy, R., Abdel-Azim, S., Paul, A. A. & El-Husseini, S. (1987): Aetiology of rickets in Egyptian children. *Hum. Nutr: Clin. Nutr.* **41C**, 199–208.

Lee, S. W., Russell, J. & Avioli, L. V. (1977): 25-Hydroxycholecalciferol to 1,25-dihydroxycholecalciferol: conversion impaired by systemic metabolic acidosis. *Science* **195**, 994–996.

Malluche, H. H., Faugere, M.-C., Rush, M. & Friedler, R. (1986): Osteoblastic insufficiency is responsible for maintenance of osteopenia after loss of ovarian function in experimental beagle dogs. *Endocrinology* **119**, 2649–2654.

Maltz, H. E., Fish, M. B. & Holliday, M. A. (1970): Calcium deficiency rickets and the renal response to calcium infusion. *Pediatrics* **46**, 865–870.

McCollum, E. V., Simmonds, N., Becker, J. E. & Shipley, P. G. (1922): Studies on experimental rickets. XXI. An experimental demonstration of the existence of a vitamin which promotes calcium deposition. *J. Biol. Chem.* **53**, 293–312.

Mellanby, E. (1918): The part played by an 'accessory factor' in the production of experimental rickets. *J. Physiol.* **52**, xi–xii.

Moore, T., Impey, S. G., Martin, P. E. N. & Symonds, K. R. (1963): Meat diets. II. Effect of the age of rats on their ability to withstand the low calcium intake induced by a diet of minced beef. *J. Nutr.* **80**, 162–170.

Nakamoto, T. & Miller, S. A. (1979): The effect of protein-energy malnutrition on the development of bones in newborn rats. *J. Nutr.* **109**, 1469–1476.

Nelsestuen, G. L. & Suttie, J. W. (1973): The mode of action of vitamin K. Isolation of a peptide containing the vitamin K-dependent portion of prothrombin. *Proc. Natl. Acad. Sci. U.S.A.* **70**, 3366–3370.

Nilas, L., Christiansen, C. & Rødbro, P. (1984): Calcium supplementation and postmenopausal bone loss. *Br. Med. J.* **289**, 1103–1106.

Nilas, L., Christiansen, C. & Christiansen, J. (1985): Regulation of vitamin D and calcium metabolism after gastrectomy. *Gut* **26**, 252–257.

Nordin, B. E. C., Heyburn, P. J., Peacock, M., Horsman, A., Aaron, J., Marshall, D. & Crilly, R. G. (1980): Osteoporosis and osteomalacia. *Clin. Endocrinol. Metab.* **9**, 177–205.

O'Hara-May, J. & Widdowson, E. M. (1976): Diets and living conditions of Asian boys in Coventry with and without signs of rickets. *Brit. J. Nutr.* **36**, 23–36.

Pettifor, J. M., Ross, P., Wang, J., Moodley, G. & Cowper-Smith, J. (1978): Rickets in children of rural origin in South Africa: is low dietary calcium a factor? *J. Pediat.* **92**, 320–324.

Price, P. A., Otsuka, A. S., Poser, J. W., Kristaponis, J. & Raman, N. (1976): Characterization of a γ-carboxyglutamic acid-containing protein from bone. *Proc. Natl. Acad. Sci. U.S.A.* **73**, 1447–1451.

Price, P. A., Williamson, M. K., Haba, T., Dell, R. B. & Lee, W. S. S. (1982): Excessive mineralization with growth plate closure in rats on chronic warfarin treatment. *Proc. Natl. Acad. Sci. U.S.A.* **79**, 7734–7738.

Ramberg, C. F., Mayer, G. P., Kronfeld, D. S., Phang, J. M. & Berman, M. (1970): Calcium kinetics in cows during late pregnancy, parturition, and early lactation. *Am. J. Physiol.* **219**, 1166–1177.
Rasmussen, H. & Barrett, P. Q. (1984): Calcium messenger system: an integrated view. *Physiol. Rev.* **64**, 938–984.
Recker, R. R., Saville, P. D. & Heaney, R. P. (1977): Effect of estrogens and calcium carbonate on bone loss in postmenopausal women. *Ann. Intern. Med.* **87**, 649–656.
Riis, B., Thomsen, K. & Christiansen, C. (1987): Does calcium supplementation prevent postmenopausal bone loss? A double-blind, controlled clinical study. *New Engl. J. Med.* **316**, 173–177.
Robertson, I., Ford, J. A., McIntosh, W. B. & Dunnigan, M. G. (1981): The role of cereals in the aetiology of nutritional rickets: the lesson of the Irish National Nutrition Survey 1943–8. *Brit. J. Nutr.* **45**, 17–22.
Salimpour, R. (1975): Rickets in Tehran. Study of 200 cases. *Archs Dis. Childhood* **50**, 63–66.
Sauveur, B., Garabedian, M., Fellot, C., Mongin, P. & Balsan, S. (1977): The effect of induced metabolic acidosis on vitamin D_3 metabolism in rachitic chicks. *Calcif. Tissue Res.* **23**, 121–124.
Sauveur, B. & Mongin, P. (1978): Tibial dyschondroplasia, a cartilage abnormality in poultry. *Ann. Biol. Anim. Bioch. Biophys.* **18**, 87–98.
Saville, P. D., Krook, L., Gustafsson, P. D., Marshall, J. M. & Figarola, F. (1969): Nutritional secondary hyperparathyroidism in the dog: morphologic and radioisotope studies with treatment. *Cornell Vet.* **59**, 155–167.
Senterre, J., Putet, G., Salle, B. & Rigo, J. (1983): Effects of vitamin D and phosphorus supplementation on calcium retention in preterm infants fed banked human milk. *J. Pediatr.* **103**, 305–307.
Silver, J., Davies, T. J., Kupersmitt, E., Orme, M., Petrie, A. & Vajda, F. (1974): Prevalence and treatment of vitamin D deficiency in children on anticonvulsant drugs. *Archs Dis. Childhood* **49**, 344–350.
Simons, P. C. M., Hulan, H. W., Teunis, G. P. & van Schagen, P. J. W., (1987): Effect of dietary cation-anion balance on acid-base status and incidence of tibial dyschondroplasia of broiler chickens. *Nutr. Rep. Int.* **35**, 591–600.
Spencer, H., Kramer, L., Osis, D. & Norris, C. (1978): Effect of phosphorus on the absorption of calcium and on the calcium balance in man. *J. Nutr.* **108**, 447–457.
Stanbury, S. W. (1981): Vitamin D and hyperparathyroidism. *J. Roy. Coll. Phys. London* **15**, 205–217.
Stenflo, J., Fernlund, P., Egan, W. & Roepstorff, P. (1974): Vitamin K dependent modifications of glutamic acid residues in prothrombin. *Proc. Natl. Acad. Sci. U.S.A.* **71**, 2730–2733.
Stephens, W. P., Klimiuk, P. S., Warrington, S., Taylor, J. L., Berry, J. L. & Mawer, E. B. (1982): Observations on the natural history of vitamin D deficiency amongst Asian immigrants. *Q. J. Med.* **51**, 169–188.
Teitelbaum, S. L., Halverson, J. D., Bates, M., Wise, L. & Haddad, J. G. (1977): Abnormalities of circulating 25-OH vitamin D after jejunoileal bypass for obesity and evidence of an adaptive response. *Ann. Internal. Med.* **86**, 289–293.
Vasilatos-Younken, R. & Leach, R. M. (1986): Episodic patterns of growth hormone secretion and growth hormone status of normal and tibial dyschondroplastic chickens. *Growth* **50**, 84–94.
Walker, A. R. P. (1972): The human requirements of calcium: should low intakes be supplemented? *Am. J. Clin. Nutr.* **25**, 513–530.
Wills, M. R., Day, R. C., Phillips, J. B. & Bateman, E. C. (1972): Phytic acid and nutritional rickets in immigrants. *Lancet* **i**, 771–773.
Wolbach, S. B. & Hegsted, D. M. (1965): Hypervitaminosis A and the skeleton of growing chicks. *Archs Path.* **54**, 30–38.
Woodard, J. C., Becker, H. N. & Poulos, P. W. (1987a): Effect of diet on longitudinal bone growth and osteochondrosis in swine. *Vet. Pathol.* **24**, 109–117.
Woodard, J. C., Becker, H. N. & Poulos, P. W. (1987b): Articular cartilage blood vessels in swine osteochondrosis. *Vet. Pathol.* **24**, 118–123.

* * * * *

Discussion

Dr Elia pointed out that osteochondrosis which Fraser had mentioned as occurring in the pig, horse and dog also occurred in children, and this did not seem to be associated with any systemic disturbance of calcium. *Professor Fraser* thought that the condition in animals and man might be related and suggested that as far as calcium feeding in man was concerned no-one had looked at the small endocrine changes associated with such feeding.

Professor Beynen asked if the calcium:phosphorus ratio has any influence on soft tissue calcification or renal function in primates, and *Fraser* replied that calcium and phosphorus can be excreted quite easily in primates and therefore there are no problems except for those individuals who have renal disorders.

Dr Ingram suggested that there might be an animal model of osteoporosis in certain strains of mice that showed a menopause. *Fraser* noted this with interest and also commented that experiments on rats after ovariectomy have tended to be for a short term only.

Professor Van Soest wondered whether high-fibre diets and wholemeal raised any problems with the absorption of calcium. *Fraser* said that cereal fibre given in large amounts did indeed lead to negative calcium balance and the report in the British Journal of Nutrition several years ago showed that this also enhanced the removal of vitamin D from the plasma. This could possibly give rise to vitamin D deficiency by the mechanism which he had outlined in his talk.

Dr Whitehead wondered whether there was enough information available to express a range of RDA for calcium, both minimum and maximum, to which *Fraser* replied that there was not and that there was not even any indication of minimum requirements because of the ability of man to adapt to low calcium intakes.

Professor James raised the question of osteoporosis, reminding us that it was a matrix problem and not necessarily a calcium problem. As a recent report had shown, lacto-ovo-vegetarians can sustain their bone mass throughout life and there was a reduced calcium output on this high vegetable diet. It has also been reported that the testosterone and oestrogen levels in the blood tended to rise in these individuals; adding 3 mg boron instead of fruit and vegetables with a similar boron content led to a fall in urinary calcium and a rise in circulating sex hormone levels. At the Rowett Institute studies had shown that molybdenum and boron can bind sex hormones and alter their metabolism and the reproductive function of cattle and rodents. Altering the sex hormone status of rats by ovariectomy led to a rise in bone matrix turnover as measured by the urinary excretion of cross links of bone-specific collagen. Thus the boron which is present in relatively high quantities in vegetables could first of all have an effect on the sex hormone levels, which in turn will affect matrix turnover. The calcium deficiency which eventually develops in the elderly may then be secondary to inadequate boron intakes from fruit and vegetables.

Professor Care noted that rickets still occurred in sunny countries such as those in Asia and round the Mediterranean basin and he wondered whether similar findings were found in the Gambia where there was adequate sunshine and low calcium intake. *Dr Ann Prentice* answered this question by saying that there were some reports suggesting this was so and that they were currently studying the problem.

Professor Goldspink remarked on the fact that calcitonin was being marketed for treatment of cases of acute osteoporosis. Is there any evidence that this is of any value? *Dr Fraser* said that this was one of many attempts to treat osteoporosis and several of the findings seemed to be paradoxical.

8

Comparative salt and water metabolism

R. YAGIL

Introduction

The 'milieu interieur', as referred to by Claude Bernard, applies to the environment within an animal's body; an environment that must be retained more or less unchanged in all animals, from the one-celled paramecium to the multi-celled, multi-organed animal *Homo sapiens*, where the internal environment has also been referred to as 'the sea within us' (Bricker, 1975). Maintaining a more or less similar internal environment in all animals is a gigantic task considering that animals inhabit water, both fresh and saline; live on land, from areas that vary from the luxuriant to those of extreme aridity and they even live temporarily in the air. Animals live in cold and hot climates and must cope with continuous environmental change, both daily and seasonal.

In the maintenance of the milieu interieur there must be a regulation of both intakes and losses of all substances to and from the body. Water is an essential constituent of all living things. It is the universal biological solvent, the diffuse phase in which most of the cellular reactions of metabolism occur, and the most necessary to life of all environmental constituents. There have been numerous migrations of animals from water to land in the course of evolution, but only a few animal species have been successful in maintaining themselves entirely free of water. Insects have made a successful migration from water although some of them still return to water for part of their life cycle. Birds and mammals return to a watery medium for the embryonic life cycle. Over 60% of the earth's surface is covered by ocean water and only approximately 1% by fresh water. Although the desert camel and the marine-living whale seem 'oceans apart' in the salt and water stresses that affect them, they must both overcome an excess of salt and a dearth of drinking water.

Sodium, potassium and chloride are the dominant inorganic constituents of the body fluids of animals (Mackay, 1979). These three elements are the determining factors in the normal functioning of the milieu interieur due to their primary biological, physical and chemical properties when in solution and to the properties which they confer on the solution in which they are dissolved. In animals with body fluid compartments, sodium and chloride are mainly found in the extracellular fluid compartments, while potassium is mainly found in the intracellular fluid. The electrolytes are maintained in their specific compartments by active transport systems which are located in the cell membrane.

Sodium and chloride concentrations in seawater are equal to, or even exceed, the concentrations of these constituents in the tissues of most animals living in the marine environment. While marine invertebrates have internal sodium and chloride concentrations similar to those in the water, marine vertebrates generally have lower internal sodium and chloride concentrations than sea water. The internal potassium concentrations in both marine invertebrates and vertebrates are lower than the levels in the sea, and so special potassium excretory mechanisms are required.

The two main processes which affect the interior equilibrium are intake of substances on the one hand, and losses of substances on the other. Neural and hormonal control of these processes guarantee homoeostasis.

Most of the mammals that are not terrestrial are marine, and to a certain degree these are exposed to the same fresh water scarcity as desert mammals. The platypus and the South American opossum are the only mammals that inhabit fresh water (Bentley, 1971).

Uptake of salt and water

Water is normally taken up orally, or through the outer layers of the body, or via the food. Some of the lower animals even utilize water vapour as a source of water. In addition to the intake of fluid the oxidation of food results in the formation of water; one gram of protein yields about 0.4 ml of water, a gram of carbohydrate yields approximately 0.56 ml of water, and one gram of fat yields about 1.07 ml of water. Metabolic water obtained from the oxidation of fat makes flying insects independent of external water sources (Cockbain, 1961). The relatively large production of metabolic water obtained from the burning of fat led to the erroneous assumption that the hump-fat of the dromedary was a source of water in times of water deprivation (Leonard, 1894). This was shown not to be the case as the hump remains unaffected during long periods without drinking water (Yagil *et al.*, 1974). In addition, when comparing the water per calorie, in terms of oxidative energy, metabolism of lipids offers no advantages over metabolism of carbohydrates (Quinton, 1979). Therefore utilizing hump fat would cost the camel more water lost through the lungs to provide the oxygen needed for metabolism, than would be gained from its metabolism (Schmidt-Nielsen, 1964).

Although whales and seals can excrete urine that is more concentrated than sea water (Schmidt-Nielsen, 1983), there is no evidence that they drink water in addition to that taken up involuntarily while feeding (Haines *et al.*, 1974). They obtain about 30% free water from ingested sea water (Schmidt-Nielsen, 1983).

Oral ingestion of fluid via food or via drinking on the one hand, and excretion of fluid and salts by the kidneys on the other, regulate the water metabolism. There are no specialized accessory organs in mammals, such as nasal or rectal glands, or specialized salt cells, to help in the regulation of salt or water.

Thirst

Drinking is determined by the environmental temperature and humidity; the hotter and drier the air, the greater the thirst drive. The thirst sensation is, of course, affected by the great amounts of water lost for evaporative cooling and by drinking. In such conditions the jerboa, the antelope jackrabbit and the pocket mouse, which have adapted to insufficient drinking water, refuse to drink even when severely dehydrated (Ghobrial & Nour, 1975). Many mammals drink more than is physiologically required, necessitating the action of the kidneys to maintain a strict water equilibrium.

Man is one of the few mammals known to deny himself drinking water voluntarily in a hot environment, leading to losses of up to 4% of the body water pool (Berlyne *et al.*, 1976). Thirst is controlled by centres in the hypothalamus, angiotensin II being considered the vital link in the control of water intake.

The type of drinking water also determines the amount drunk: dromedaries increase their daily consumption from 3 litres a day to 5–12 litres per day when drinking water is changed from tap water to water containing 5.5% NaCl (Maloiy, 1972), while the marsh mouse decreased its water intake by 55% when presented with saltwater (Fisher, 1962). The Somali donkey increased its drinking slightly when salinity was increased to 1%, after which there was a decline in drinking (Maloiy, 1972). When sea water instead of fresh water was given to rats in gradually increasing concentrations, drinking increased until the concentration reached 50% (Etzion & Yagil, 1987). At higher concentrations there was a steady decline in drinking. The animals drunk virtually nothing when acutely exposed to undiluted sea water.

The ability to replenish lost water by dehydrated mammals has been classified as being either 'rapid' or 'slow' (Adolph, 1982). The dog, sheep, goat, burro and camel appear among the fast drinkers while man, rat and guinea pig are slow drinkers. Dogs dehydrated for 24 hrs replaced water deficit in 5 min (Ramsay *et al.*, 1977) while rats deprived of water overnight required more than 3 hours to reestablish homoeostasis; in man water replenishment is also gradual (Adolph, 1982). Sheep are not fast drinkers, as was originally thought (Laden *et al.*, 1987), and although goats and dogs are fast drinkers they do not absorb the water rapidly into their blood (Ramsay *et al.*, 1977; Shkolnik *et al.*, 1980). A rapid absorption of water into the blood in these animals would lead to massive haemolysis and death. The camel, however, has extremely resistant red blood cells (Yagil *et al.*, 1974) and therefore the desert camel is able to drink amounts of water ranging up to 200 litres within 3 minutes (Yagil *et al.*, 1974), and to absorb this water into the blood stream within a few hours (Etzion *et al.*, 1984). Although Hoppe *et al.* (1975) claimed that the camel does not absorb water rapidly, the serial changes in haematocrit following drinking indicate that absorption is indeed rapid.

In isotope studies, tritiated water was given orally in identical minute-volumes to camels allowed water *ad libitum*, to camels dehydrated for 10 days, and to rehydrated animals.

The dehydrated camel circulates water with urea from its kidneys to the rumen and back to the blood and kidneys in a continuous circle, guaranteeing a normal appetite and a source of water for metabolism (Yagil, 1985). This phenomenon is the secret of the camel's survival and is based on the following: (1) the camels prefer to eat salty green fodder, which is the source of water and protein as well as salt. (2) In the rumen the flora degrade the food to form microbial protein. (3) In the intestines the salt, and accompanying water, are absorbed under hormonal control of aldosterone. (4) The protein is absorbed as amino acids and degraded in the normal metabolism, forming urea as the end waste product. (5) In the kidneys urea and water are selectively reabsorbed while the salt is excreted in a concentrated urine. (6) The urea and water pass into the rumen where the water maintains the optimal environment for fermentation and the urea is reutilized for the formation of further microbial protein. (7) Water and protein reach the intestines.

In this manner there is a continual recycling of water and urea (protein), salt being the limiting factor in the cycle as it is continuously being excreted. It is now clear why the camel has such a dependence on salt in its diet (Yagil, 1985) and why it has the lowest water turnover of all ruminants (Macfarlane & Siebert, 1967). Other ruminants are also capable of urea recycling but losses of water for cooling diminish the alimentary water, interrupting the cycle and ending in depressed appetite.

Food is an important component of the water metabolism as well as providing essential nutrients, especially in arid and semi-arid regions. Fresh vegetation contains about 90% water, as do cacti and roots of desert plants (Ghobrial & Nour, 1975). Some animals do not drink as long as their food is lush. This is true for camels in winter (Yagil, 1985), and for arid and semi-arid rodents (Yousef *et al.*, 1972) and even sheep (Macfarlane & Howard, 1970). Some carnivorous animals rely on their prey for their liquid requirements. Gazelles can maintain their water balance even on dry fodder which contains less than 1% water, if they graze at night when there is an increase of 30–40% water content in the food due to the increase in air humidity to 85% (Taylor, 1972).

All animals require a source, dietary or otherwise, of the electrolytes, sodium, potassium and chloride. These electrolytes are available to animals in a variety of foods, water and soils. In general potassium is readily available, since it is the main electrolyte of the intracellular fluid of plants. Sodium and chloride are normally present in only small quantities in most terrestrial and freshwater plants; saltbushes being one of the exceptions (LeHouerou, 1978), containing unusually large amounts of salts, as the name signifies. The salt content of food, particularly that eaten by herbivorous terrestrial and freshwater animals, appears to be insufficient to meet the animals' daily requirements, so supplementary sources are required.

Practically all freshwater animals have evolved mechanisms for actively taking up salt from their environment (Mackay, 1979) either via their gills or even through their body surface. Marine mammals, in contrast, are confronted by an excess of salts and in order to limit their intake the salt water is not readily drunk. Large terrestrial mammals actively seek salt. For example the one-humped desert camel's basic physiological adaptive mechanisms are dependent on a large salt intake (Yagil, 1985). This is achieved by eating the normally salty browse or by eating salty soils or drinking brackish water. Man is so dependent on salt in his diet that payment for labour is still referred to as 'salary', a word derived from the Greek word 'saluris'—salt.

Seals and whales are carnivorous. Fish-eating mammals obtain food with a relatively low salt content and high protein content, while crab- and clam-eating animals take up food which is isosmotic with sea water. The baleen whale eats crustacean plankton which have a high salt content. Similarly, the herbivorous dugongs and manatees have a high salt intake which is typical of the feed which is available to them.

Mammals, like birds and terrestrial insects, must satisfy all their electrolyte requirements from their diet alone. When the salt content of the food increases above certain levels, drinking is initiated. Highly salty water, on the other hand, depresses the appetite.

Besides sodium, potassium and chloride, other important electrolytes include bicarbonate, phosphate, magnesium and calcium. Bicarbonate plays a decisive role in the acid-base metabolism, where reabsorption or formation of new bicarbonate neutralizes metabolic acids (Ganong, 1985). Calcium, phosphorus and magnesium are vital for bone formation and deficiency of the latter in the diet of cattle leads to hypomagnesaemic tetany (Houpt, 1984).

Metabolic water

In hot xerophylic habitats small size is the norm, where oxidative water production offers maximal advantage. The opposite is true for cold and wet environments; a large size affords relatively less heat loss due to a low surface to volume ratio. The exception to this rule is the camel (*C. dromedarius*), one of the largest animals living in a desert environment, and whose size affords many advantages over smaller animals (Yagil, 1985). Camels heat up more slowly than small animals and their long legs enable the animal to traverse great distances to find scarce food and water.

Oxidative water does not play a major role in the water balance of mammals, accounting for a maximum of 13–20% in man (Kleeman, 1972). The kangaroo rats and pocket mice which inhabit the deserts in North America live on dry food without any drinking water (Schmidt-Nielsen, 1983).

Losses from the body

Avenues of loss of water and salts from the body include the alimentary canal, kidney, sweat glands and in some animals, or some circumstances, passive diffusion across the respiratory and body surfaces. Some mammals lose large quantities of fluid in their faeces.

Evaporative water losses

Evaporation is of the greatest importance for maintaining thermostability in most mammals. Since all terrestrial animals lose water through cutaneous and respiratory evaporation without a proportional loss of salts, they must either make up the losses of water or must excrete excess salt (ie hypertonic excretions) in order to prevent haemoconcentration.

In evaporation each escaping water molecule must attain sufficient energy to disrupt the two hydrogen bonds. At a temperature of 37°C, 575 calories (2.4kJ) are absorbed in order to evaporate every ml of water. The specific properties of water make it the best medium for preventing drastic temperature changes of the milieu interieur (Quinton, 1979). In addition most homoeothermic animals have body temperatures between 37 and 40°C, the temperature range in which aqueous solutions of NaCl approach a maximum activity coefficient (Harned & Owens, 1958). Terrestrial animals lose a relatively small volume of water while transferring a significant amount of heat from the body to the environment. However, in absolute terms, much water can be lost by evaporative cooling, up to 4 litres an hour for man (Ingram & Mount, 1975).

The losses of body water occurring with evaporation have been divided into insensible and sensible (sweat) losses.

Insensible water losses. In cows and man respiratory water losses account for more than 79% of the insensible losses (Chew, 1965). Respiratory losses are determined by outer temperatures and humidity. More water is lost via the respiratory tract in active animals than those at rest (Raab & Schmidt-Nielsen, 1972). It must be noted that short shallow respiration is less efficient in extracting oxygen from the air and therefore increases the water loss per unit O_2 consumed.

In heat-loaded dogs, birds, gazelles and other panting animals there is a sudden increase in respiratory rate to a resonant frequency (Taylor, 1972; Stitt, 1976) and this increase is accompanied by an increase in respiratory water loss. Panting animals not only accrue water deficits but the alkalosis which can accompany hyperventilation can cause hypocalcaemic tetany by driving calcium into the bones. Respiratory water losses are greatly reduced in the dehydrated camel by depressing metabolism (Yagil *et al.*, 1979) which depresses respiratory rate (Schmidt-Nielsen *et al.*, 1963).

Elevation of body temperatures is a common mechanism of conserving water that would have been lost in maintaining a steady body temperature. Among the many animals which demonstrate physiological hyperthermia are the desert gazelle (Taylor, 1972), camel (Schmidt-Nielsen, 1964), and rat (Sod-Moriah & Yagil, 1973).

Sweat. Not all animals have the benefit of copious sweating as a cooling mechanism. In man the densest area of sweat glands is on the forehead, twice as many as other areas (Szabo, 1962). Recorded sweat rates in man range from 2 l/h (Dill *et al.*, 1976) to 4 l/h (Ingram & Mount, 1975). These high sweat rates allow man to have the highest tolerance of sustainable ambient temperatures (59°C). Zebu cattle only sweat at rates of about 140 ml/m^2 per hour (Macfarlane, 1964). Nevertheless the Zebu has more sweat glands than European cattle and is, therefore, better adapted to heat stress (Johnson, 1968).

It is important to note that effective sweat is hypotonic to plasma (Ganong, 1985). Sweating is an acquired mechanism, requiring time to become effective (Folk, 1966). As acclimatization occurs and sweating becomes profuse there is an accompanying fall in concentration of salt in the sweat, which becomes more hypotonic with respect to plasma (Quinton, 1979). Burros have many sweat glands and sweat profusely but also lose little salt in their sweat. Retaining blood salt is important in preventing vascular collapse which would occur if large volumes of isotonic fluid were lost from the ECF. Relatively large amounts of salt can still be lost in copious sweating and must be replaced.

When water is lost and salt is conserved in the extracellular fluid compartment (ECF), partial dehydration occurs in the larger intracellular fluid compartment (ICF) in order to preserve the equilibrium between the ICF and ECF. Severe cellular dehydration is prevented by excretion of salts in the urine. This fluid shift more than doubles the amount of water available for cooling. In cattle ECF conservation is accomplished by secreting isotonic sweat, which contains mainly potassium salts (MacFarlane, 1964).

Copious sweating is controlled by vasopressin and urea is secreted in the sweat. The ADH-controlled passage of water is similar to that occurring in the mammalian kidney (Yagil, 1985). Aldosterone accounts for the reabsorption of sodium and the excretion of potassium, as occurs in the intestines and kidneys.

In sheep, goats (Waites & Voglmayr, 1963), and equines (Robertshaw & Taylor, 1968) sweating is under direct nervous control. Sweating in most lower mammals is probably sympathetically innervated since it can be stimulated by injections of epinephrine and norepinephrine. In primates hypothalamic and peripheral sensors interact additively (Smiles *et al.*, 1976) to stimulate sweating via the sympathetic pathways. Eccrine glands are apparently under parasympathetic control (Sato, 1977).

Salivary water losses

Although losses of saliva could be considered as losses of salt and water from the alimentary canal the use of saliva for cooling is a special phenomenon.

Many rodents, rabbits, cats and even elephants cool themselves by evaporation of saliva from their fur or skin (Rodland & Hainsworth, 1974; Ghobrial & Nour, 1975). The salivary gland of rats exposed to chronic heat loads hypertrophies (Horowitz, 1976). In contrast man and most of the ruminants have a rapid decline in saliva in heat and when thirsty.

Faecal water losses

In the large ruminants faecal water losses can be substantial, 30–70 ml/kg per day (Macfarlane, 1964), compared with 2.1 ml/kg per day for man (Wolf, 1958). When drinking water is restricted, Somali donkeys reduce fecal water losses to 13 ml/kg per day (Maloiy, 1972); camels 4 ml/kg per day and sheep 8 ml/kg per day (Laden *et al.*, 1987). Australian marsupials reduce their faecal water losses by half. It must be noted that the reduction in water losses is not only due to less faecal mass as the appetite declines (Laden *et al.*, 1987), but especially to the increased salt and water absorption from the gut (Degen, 1977; Laden *et al.*, 1987; Maloiy, 1972) which is under the influence of aldosterone (Efstratopoulus *et al.*, 1974; Yagil & Etzion, 1979) and probably vasopressin (Robertson, 1983). Water is passively removed from the intestines with the hormonally-governed uptake of salts (Frizell *et al.*, 1976). When water is required, 95% of Na and 80% of the water entering the colon is absorbed (Kramer *et al.*, 1962).

Renal water losses

The mammalian kidneys perform various tasks which help maintain the physiological integrity of the milieu interieur (Gans & Mercer, 1984). These tasks are: balance of water and electrolytes; conservation of glucose and amino acids; and the elimination of the nitrogenous end-products of protein metabolism, excess hydrogen ions and complex organic compounds (both endogenous and exogenous). Erythropoietin and renin are hormones secreted by the kidneys.

In mammals the GFR tends to remain more or less static while the tubular reabsorption changes and this determines final urine production (Quinton, 1979). Because of the high metabolic rate of mammals there are high rates of filtration and therefore under normal conditions alterations in GFR are not the primary means of reducing water output. The absolute value of the GFR increases as a logarithmic function of body weight. In dehydrated camels (Yagil & Berlyne, 1977), reindeer (Valtonen & Eriksson, 1977) and desert kangaroos (Denny & Dawson, 1977) the GFR declines significantly to compensate for the lack of water, while in dehydrated man the GFR declines by only 8% (Renkin & Gilmore, 1973).

After filtration approximately 65–80% of the filtered water is reabsorbed as isotonic fluid in the proximal tubule.

In the loops of Henle concentration of the urine occurs, each species having its own specific concentrating capabilities. In some species the thin, descending portion of the loop may go as far as the papilla before turning upward and then becoming the thick ascending limb of the loop.

The mammalian kidney relies significantly upon urea trapping in the medulla when establishing cortical-medullary concentration gradients (Kokko & Tisher, 1976). Unlike mammals with their ability to concentrate their blood urea, birds are virtually incapable of doing so, which accounts for their inability to concentrate their urine.

Anion reabsorption takes place in the proximal portion of the distal tubules while cation reabsorption occurs in the distal segment (Quinton, 1979).

The final volume of water lost as urine is determined mainly by the water permeability of the cells in the distal tubule and collecting ducts.

The connection between body water status and tubular function is vividly demonstrated in marine mammals; the dolphin has decreased tubular reabsorption following eating, corresponding to the uptake of water and nitrogen. In contrast the tubular reabsorption increases greatly when food is restricted for a day and water is therefore scarce (Malvin & Rayner, 1968).

Mammals that are close to fresh water, eg the beaver, do not have long loops of Henle and so lack the capability of concentrating their urine by increasing tubular reabsorption (Schmidt-Nielsen & O'Dell, 1961). The reindeer also lacks tubular reabsorptive capabilities, which makes the animal susceptible to dehydration (Valtonen & Eriksson, 1977).

In dormant bears tubular reabsorption of water decreases but since the GFR decreases as well, urine excretion is virtually unchanged (Brown *et al.*, 1971). However there is almost complete reabsorption of water and urea in the bladder (Nelson *et al.*, 1975).

Hormonal control of water and salt metabolism

In mammals there is hormonal control of salt and water uptake and losses. Thirst is controlled through centres situated in the ventromedial and anterior regions of the hypothalamus which act via aldosterone-ADH. Angiotensin appears to be the link between ECF volume sensors, thirst drive and aldosterone (Ganong, 1985).

Aldosterone, secreted from the adrenal cortex, causes the absorption of salt from the intestines and the reabsorption of salt from the kidneys and sweat glands (Efstratopoulus *et al.*, 1974; Yagil & Etzion, 1979). The stimuli for secretion of aldosterone come either from the renin-angiotensin axis or via the adenohypophysis-ACTH axis (Houpt, 1984). Prolactin, although associated mainly with milk secretion, has an aldosterone-like effect on the intestines (Mainoya, 1981) and kidneys in male as well as female animals.

Vasopressin is a neural secretion which is formed in the hypothalamus and descends along axons to the neurohypophysis (Gans & Mercer, 1984). In high concentration vasopressin acts like oxytocin and *vice versa*. Vasopressin release is sparked off by increased blood osmolality or decline in volume of ECF. These stimuli also act on the thirst centre, along with intracellular Na (Andersson, 1977). ECF volume is monitored in the left atrium by stretch receptors and by pressure receptors in the carotid sinus (Koushanpour, 1976). Vasopressin acts on the distal convoluted tubule to reabsorb water and on the collecting duct to reabsorb water and urea (Quinton, 1979). There are vasopressin receptors in intestinal mucosa which strongly suggests that vasopressin acts on the intestines (Robertson, 1984).

Plasma volumes are elevated in man exposed to extreme heat (Folk, 1966), in dehydrated camels (Yagil *et al.*, 1974), and in dehydrated dogs (R. Yagil, unpublished data). This phenomenon can only be explained by the intestinal movement of water into the blood. More severe dehydration leads to an increased haematocrit (Yagil, 1985). Mine workers in South Africa injected with vasopressin had decreased haematocrit (Senay *et al.*, 1980), confirming the dilution of blood under the influence of vasopressin as suggested in the camel (Yagil & Etzion, 1979).

Angiotensin-renin have great effect on renal water metabolism. Angiotensin II stimulates vasopressin release (Ulrich *et al.*, 1975), and decreases renal blood flow by constricting glomerular arterioles (Leyssac, 1976). The renal sympathetic innervation causes decrease in GFR (Stein *et al.*, 1973) which in turn causes the secretion of renin (Coote *et al.*, 1972).

Parathyroid hormone (PTH) determines the rate of calcium and phosphate absorption from the gut and their excretion from the kidneys. The passage of phosphate appears to carry water with it (Yagil, 1985). Thyroid hormones and growth hormone (GH) have trophic effects on the kidneys and in general directly affect the production of metabolic water. The permissive action of the steroids, secreted from the adrenal cortex, are essential for maximal rates of water excretion.

Lactation

Although lactation is not normally considered in the context of salt and water metabolism, losses of water and electrolytes can be substantial. Women may secrete approximately 1 litre of milk a day (Lawrence, 1980), cows can produce 70 litres a day and camels 40 litres a day (Yagil, 1987).

Although the very high fat content of seal and whale milk was considered a physiological mechanism for reducing water losses (Folk, 1966; Schmidt-Nielsen,

1983), diluted milk is the physiological mechanism for the survival of desert mammals (Yagil & Etzion, 1987). In severely dehydrated camels, partially dehydrated cows, and Bedouin women, diluted milk is secreted in response to water deficiency. Even the harp seal, which normally secretes milk with a high fat content, secretes diluted milk when its young requires fluid in a certain stage of its development (Lavigne *et al.*, 1982). The high fat content in marine mammalian milk is a source of energy and a basis for depositing blubber for insulation and not a water-conserving mechanism. Milk of dehydrated camels not only contains more water but also more salt and urea. As previously described, the salt is necessary to guarantee salt and water absorption from the intestines and the urea is an additional source of nitrogen for the suckling animal. Young camels are, therefore, virtually immune to the scarcity of external water sources. High fat in the milk of dehydrated animals will occur when ECF fluid volume has declined to such a degree that insufficient remains for the milk. The connection between water and salt metabolism on the one hand and lactation on the other was vividly demonstrated when heat-acclimatized laboratory rats secreted diluted milk after being injected with either vasopressin or aldosterone (Yagil & Etzion, 1987).

A large production of milk in cows can lead to such great losses of calcium that the animal falls in a convulsive state known as 'milk fever' (Houpt, 1984).

Urea metabolism

I shall make special mention of urea metabolism since it is probable that uraemia could be of great physiological benefit under certain circumstances, though normally considered pathological in man.

Marine sharks and rays accumulate urea in their bodies as a means of trapping body water (Goldstein *et al.*, 1968). The same phenomenon is found in the cocoon stage of the African lungfish, *Protopterus*, which can remain in estivation for 3 years until rain again vitalizes the animal (Smith, 1959).

Hibernating bears also have physiological uraemia with increased bladder urea and water reabsorption (Nelson *et al.*, 1975). As previously discussed the secret of the camel's ability to survive long periods without drinking water is mainly determined by the circulation of urea and water from the kidneys to the stomachs and back to the kidneys (Yagil, 1985), as well as by urea increasing in the milk when drinking water is unavailable (Yagil & Etzion, 1980).

In mammalian metabolism, urea accompanies the water reabsorbed from the collecting ducts of the nephron and is excreted in sweat (Ingram & Mount, 1975). The passage of urea and water is controlled by vasopressin. This is a noteworthy fact as a lack of dietary protein makes urine concentration impossible. Urea concentration in the medullary interstitium is vital for urine concentration. Therefore it is reasonable to assume that in a healthy man uraemia is a sign of the need to retain blood water rather than a sign of kidney problems.

Exceptional intakes of salts and water and the effects on homoeostasis

In an attempt to utilize marginal areas for fodder crop production, salt bushes were grown on sea water (Pasternak & Benjamin, 1983). However, feeding sheep with this highly salty fodder proved unsuccessful, as it did for goats (O'Leary, 1985). It was postulated that the salt load was too great for the animals to handle. Experiments proved that sheep would eat the highly salty vegetation under certain conditions (personal observations) which were: (1) when the animals had just been weaned and had no taste preferences for other food; (2) when drinking water was available *ad libitum*; and (3) when shade was available during the heat of the day so the animals could lie down and cool off.

Under these conditions the animals were able to eat the sea-irrigated fodder, consuming up to 5 kg per animal daily. This necessitated the excretion of large volumes of diluted urine. Urinary excretion of salt was such that blood osmolality and haematocrit remained normal. The faeces changed from the consistency of cattle faeces to pellets, though these still formed a mass of faecal material rather than individual pellets. It was adequately demonstrated that a large salt load in food was no stress to the sheep as long as water was not required for cooling and was adequate for renal excretion of salts.

In another experiment (Yagil *et al.*, 1988) it was found that in the heat of summer sheep showed signs of dehydration after 3 hours of grazing although they had left the pens at 6 a.m. when it was relatively cool. The sheep had increased body temperatures and had lost weight. The haematocrit was lower than normal (as shown to occur when water is absorbed from the intestines). The animals actively sought shade and following drinking their weight increased to equal the amount of food eaten.

The large uptake of salts was gradual in sheep and was therefore not as stressful as swallowing sea water in man (Yagil *et al.*, 1983). Accidental swallowing of sea water causes a flow of fluid into the intestines, causing increased haematocrit and a temporary shutdown of the kidneys (Grausz *et al.*, 1971; Oren *et al.*, 1982). It is possible that the intestines rather than the kidneys limit man's capability to utilize sea water for drinking. This is true only up to a point. In rats given saline water in increasing concentrations until pure sea water was presented, water intake was greatly depressed after 50% sea water was given (Etzion *et al.*, 1987). It was surmised that the renal response to the salinity was the limiting factor in drinking the highly saline water. The biggest possible salt stress to the human organism occurs with swallowing of Dead Sea Water (Yagil *et al.*, 1983). It has been found that following the swallowing of as little as a half a glass (100 ml) of Dead Sea water there is total disruption of normal metabolism. The mucosa of the intestines are destroyed, either by the enormous osmotic load in the water or by the bromide, which is present in large concentrations. The bromides and the magnesium (which is also present in high concentrations) act synergistically as potent tranquillizers resulting in coma and depressed respiration of such a degree that artificial respiration is required. Only if the kidneys are sufficiently normal can the salt load be excreted. If there is an impaired renal function, death occurs after a few days.

Conclusions

Maintenance of salt and water equilibrium in man and animals is a complex activity. Environmental stresses, such as heat, cold, dehydration, lactation and malnutrition, affect the intake and losses of water and salt from the body. Endocrine control is based on maintaining blood pressure and cell viability of the most important organs of the body.

References

Adolph, E. F. (1982): Termination of drinking. Satiation. *Fed. Proc.* **41**, 2533–2535.

Andersson, B. (1977): Regulation of body fluids. *Annu. Rev. Physiol.* **39**, 185–200.

Bentley, P. J. (1971): *Endocrines and osmoregulation: a comparative account of the regulation of water and salt in vertebrates.* pp. 106–107. New York: Springer.

Berlyne, G. M., Yagil, R., Goodwin, S. & Morag, M. (1976): Drinking habits and urine concentration of man in Southern Israel. *Isr. J. Med. Sci.* **12**, 765–769.

Bricker, N. S. (1975): *The sea within us. A clinical guide to fluid and electrolyte balances.* New York: Science & Medicine Publ. Co.

Brown, D. C., Mulhausen, R. O., Andrew, D. J. & Seal, U. S. (1971): Renal function in anesthetized dormant and active bears. *Am. J. Physiol.* **220**, 293–298.

Chew, R. M. (1965): Water metabolism in mammals. In *Physiological mammalogy. II. Mammalian reactions to stressful environments.* ed A. Mayer. New York: Academic Press.

Cockbain, A. J. (1961): Fuel utilization and duration of tethered flight in aphis fabae Scop. *J. Exp. Biol.* **38**, 163–174.

Coote, J. H., Johns, E. J., Macleod, V. H. & Singer, B. (1972): Effect of renal nerve stimulation renal blood flow and adrenergic blockade on plasma renin activity in the cat. *J. Physiol., Lond.* **226**, 15–36.

Degen, A. A. (1977): Fat-tailed Awassi and German Mutton Merino sheep under semi-arid conditions. 1. Total body water, its distribution and water turnover. *J. Agric. Sci. Cambr.* **88**, 693–698.

Denny, J. & Dawson, T. J. (1977): Kidney structure and function of desert kangaroos. *J. Appl. Physiol.* **42**, 636–642.

Depocas, F., Hart, J. S. & Fisher, H. D. (1971): Sea water drinking and water flux in starved and fed Harbor seals, *Phoca Vitulina. Can. J. Physiol. Pharmacol.* **49**, 53–56.

Dickson, W. M. (1984): Endocrinology, Reproduction and Lactation. In *Dukes' Physiology of domestic animals*, tenth edition, 761–797. Ithaca: Comstock Publ. Assoc.

Dill, D. B., Sohol, L. F. & Oddershede, I. B. (1976): Physiological adjustments of young men to five-hour desert walks, *J. Appl. Physiol.* **40**, 236–242.

Efstratopoulus, A. D., Peart, W. S. & Wilson, G. A. (1974): The effect of aldosterone on colonic potential difference and renal excretion in normal man. *Clin. Sci. Mol. Med.* **46**, 489–493.

Etzion, Z., Meyerstein, N. & Yagil, R. (1984): Tritiated water metabolism during dehydration and rehydration in the camel. *J. Appl. Physiol. Resp. Environm. Exercise Physiol.* **56**, 217–220.

Etzion, Z. & Yagil, R. (1987): Metabolic effects in rats drinking increasing concentrations of sea water. *Comp. Biochem. Physiol.* **86A**, 49–55.

Fisher, G. F. (1962): Ingestion of sea water by *Peromyscus maniculatus. J. Mammal.* **43**, 416–417.

Folk, G. E. Jr. (1966): *Introduction to environmental physiology.* 308 pp. Philadelphia: Lea & Febiger.

Frizell, R. A., Koch, M. J. & Schultz, S. G. (1976): Ion transport by rabbit colon. I. Active and passive components. *J. Memb. Biol.* **27**, 297.

Ganong, W. F. (1985): *Review of medical physiology*, 12th edn. Los Altos, Ca: Lange Medical Publ.

Gans, J. H. & Mercer, P. F. (1984): The kidneys. In *Dukes' Physiology of domestic animals*, tenth edition. 507–536. Ithaca: Comstock Publ. Assoc.

Ghobrial, L. I. & Nour, T. A. (1975): The physiological adaptions of desert rodents. In *Rodents in desert environments*, ed Parkash and Ghost, pp. 413–444. The Hague: Junk.

Goldstein, L., Oppelt, W. W. & Maren, T. H. (1968): Osmotic regulation and urea metabolism in the lemon shark *Negaprion brevirostris. Am. J. Physiol.* **215**, 1493–1497.

Grausz, T., William, J. C. & Early, E. (1971): Acute renal failure complicating submersion in sea water. *J. Am. Med. Ass.* **217**, 207–209.

Haines, H., Macfarlane, W. V., Setchell, C. & Howard, B. (1974): Water turnover and pulmocutaneous evaporation of Australian desert dasyuride and murids. *Am. J. Physiol.* **227**, 958–963.

Hall, W. G. & Blass, E. M. (1974): Orogastric, hydrational and behavioral controls of drinking following water deprivation in rats. *J. Comp. Physiol. Psychol.* **89**, 939–954.

Harned, H. S. & Owens, B. B. (1958): *Physical chemistry of electrolytic solutions*. New York: Reinhold.
Hoppe, P., Kay, N. B. & Maloiy, G. M. O. (1975): The rumen as a reservoir during dehydration and rehydration in the camel. *Proc. Physiol. Soc.* **254**, 76P–77P.
Horowitz, M. (1976): Acclimatization of rats to moderate heat: body water distribution and adaptability of the submaxillary salivary gland. *Pflugers Arch. Ges. Physiol.* **366**, 173–176.
Houpt, T. R. (1984): Water balance and excretion. In: *Dukes' Physiology of domestic animals*, tenth edition, pp. 486–506. Ithaca: Comstock Publ. Assoc.
Ingram, D. L. & Mount, L. E. (1975): *Man and animals in hot environments*, 185 pp. New York: Springer.
Johnson, K. G. (1968): Renal function in *Bos taurus* and *Bos indicus*—cross-bred cows under conditions of normal hydration and mild dehydration. *Res. Vet. Sci.* **12**, 438–447.
Kleeman, C. R. (1972): Water metabolism. In *Clinical disorders of fluid and electrolyte metabolism*, ed M. J. Maxwell and C. R. Kleeman. New York: McGraw-Hill.
Kokko, J. P. & Tisher, C. C. (1976): Water movement across nephron segments involved with the countercurrent multiplication system. *Kidney Int.* **10**, 64–81.
Koushanpour, E. (1976): *Renal physiology: principles and functions. An integrated analysis to renal-body fluid regulating systems*, pp. 401–406. Philadelphia: Saunders.
Kramer, P., Kearney, M. M. & Ingelfinger, R. J. (1962): The effect of specific foods and water loading on the ileal excreta of ileostomized human subjects. *Gastroenterology* **42**, 535.
Laden, S., Nehmadi, L. & Yagil, R. (1987): Dehydration tolerance in Awassi fat-tailed sheep. *Can. J. Zool.* **65**, 363–367.
Lavigne, D. M., Stewart, R. E. A. and Fletcher, F. (1982): Changes in composition and energy content of Harp Seal milk during lactation. *Physiol. Zool.* **55**, 1–9.
Lawrence, R. A. (1980): Breast feeding. A guide for the medical profession, pp. 1–72. London: Mosby.
L•Houerou, H. N. (1978): Resources and potential of native flora for fodder and sown pasture production in the arid semi-arid zones of North Africa. In *Arid land plant resources*, eds J. F. Goodin and O. K. Northington. Texas Univ. Lubbock: Proc. Int. Arid Land Conf. ICASLAS.
Leonard, A. G. (1894): *The Camel: Its uses and management*, 335 pp. London: Longmans Green.
Leyssac, P. P. (1976): The renin angiotensin system and kidney function. A review of contributions to a new theory. *Acta Physiol. Scand.* **442**, Suppl. pp. 1–52.
Macfarlane, W. V. (1964): Terrestrial animals in dry heat: Ungulates. In *Handbook of physiology, Section 4. Adaptation to environment*. ed D. B. Dill, pp. 509–539. Washington: American Physiological Society.
Macfarlane, W. V. & Howard, B. (1970): Water in the physiological ecology of ruminants. In: *The Physiology of digestion and metabolism in the ruminant*. ed A. T. Philipson, pp. 362–374. Aberdeen: Oriel Press.
MacFarlane, W. V. & Siebert, B. D. (1967): Hydration and dehydration of desert camels. *Aust. J. Exp. Biol. Med. Sci.* **45**, 29.
Mackay, W. C. (1979): Electrolytes. In *Nitrogen, electrolytes, water and energy metabolism. Comparative animal nutrition 3*. ed M. Rechcigl, Jr, pp. 80–99. Basel: S. Karger.
Mainoya, J. R. (1981): Colon absorption of water and NaCl in the rat during lactation and the possible involvement of prolactin. *Experimentia* **37**, 1083–1084.
Maloiy, G. M. O. (1972): Renal salt and water excretion in the camel. In *Comparative physiology of desert animals*, ed G. M. O. Maloiy, pp. 243–260. New York: American Press.
Malvin, R. L. & Rayner, M. (1968): Renal function and blood chemistry in Cetacea. *Am. J. Physiol.* **214**, 187–191.
Nelson, R. A., Jones, J. D., Wahner, H. W., McGill, D. B. & Code, C. F. (1975): Nitrogen metabolism in bears: urea and metabolism in summer starvation and in winter sleep and role of urinary bladder in water and nitrogen conservation. *Mayo Clin. Proc.* **50**, 141–146.
O'Leary, J. M. (1985): *Saline environments and halophylic crops*. Tucson, Arizona: Proc. Int. Conf. Arid Lands Today and Tomorrow.
Oren, A., Etzion, Z., Broitman, D. & Yagil, R. (1982): Renal involvement following near drowning in the sea. *Comp. Biochem. Physiol. 73A*, 175–179.
Pasternak, D., Danon, A., Aronson, J. A. & Benjamin, R. W. (1983): *Fodder production with saline water*. Beersheva: Annual Report Ben-Gurion University of the Negev.
Quinton, P. M. (1979): Comparative Water Metabolism in Animals: Protozoa to Man. In *Nitrogen, electrolytes, water and energy metabolism. Comp. Anim. Nutr. Vol. 3*, ed M. Rechcigl, Jr, pp. 100–123. Basel: S. Karger.
Raab, J. L. & Schmidt-Nielsen, K. (1972): Effect of running on water balance of the kangaroo rat. *Am. J. Physiol.* **222**, 1230–1235.

Ramsay, D. J., Rolls, B. J. & Wood, R. J. (1977): Thirst following water deprivation in dogs. *Am. J. Physiol.* **232**, 93–100.

Renkin, E. M. & Gilmore, J. P. (1968): Glomerular filtration. In *Handbook of physiology, section 8, Renal physiology*, ed J. Orloff, R. W. Berliner and S. R. Geiger, pp. 185–248. Washington: American Physiological Society.

Robertshaw, K. W. & Taylor, C. R. (1968): *The control of sweating gland function in equines*, pp. 370. Washington: Proc. Int. Union Physiol. Sci. XXIV Int. Congr. vol. 7.

Robertson, G. L. (1984): Abnormalities of thirst regulation. *Kidney Intl.* **25**, 460–469.

Rodland, K. D. & Hainsworth, F. R. (1974): Evaporative water loss and tissue dehydration of hamsters in the heat. *Comp. Biochem. Physiol.* **49**, 331–334.

Sato, K. (1977): The physiology, pharmacology and biochemistry of the eccrine sweat gland. *Rev. Physiol. Biochem. Pharmacol.* **79**, 51–131.

Schmidt-Nielsen, K. (1964): *Desert animals. Physiological problems of heat and water*, 277 pp. Oxford: Clarendon Press.

Schmidt-Nielsen, K. (1983): *Animal physiology: Adaptation and environment*, 3rd edition. Cambridge: Cambridge University Press.

Schmidt-Nielsen, K., Crawford, E. C., Newsome, A. E. & Rawson, K. S. (1963): The metabolic rate of camels. *Fed. Proc.* **22**, 176–179.

Schmidt-Nielsen, K. & O'Dell, R. (1961): Structure and concentrating mechanism in the mammalian kidney. *Am. J. Physiol* **200**, 1119–1124.

Senay, L. C. Jr., Wolfswinkel, J., Jooste, P. & Striydom, N. B. (1980): *An apparent relationship between ADH and haemodilution during exercise and heat exposure*, Vol. 14, p. 694. Budapest, Hungary: Proc. Intl. Congr. Physiol. Sci.

Shkolnik, A., Maltz, E. & Chosniak, I. (1980): The role of the ruminants' digestive tract as a water reservoir. In *Digestive physiology and metabolism in ruminants*, ed Y. Ruckebusch and P. Thivend, pp. 731–742. Lancaster: Medical Techn. Press.

Smiles, K. A., Elizondo, R. S. & Barney, C. C. (1976): Sweating responses during changes of hypothalamic temperature in the rhesus monkey. *J. Appl. Physiol.* **40**, 653–657.

Smith, H. W. (1959): The kidney structure and function in health and disease, 1049 pp. New York: Oxford Univ. Press.

Sod-Moriah, U. A. & Yagil, R. (1973): Hyperthermia in heat-adapted female rats. *Comp. Biochem. Physiol.* **46A**, 487–490.

Stein, J. H., Boonjarern, S., Mauk, R. C. & Ferris, T. F. (1973): Mechanism of the redistribution of renal cortical blood flow during haemorrhagic hypotension in the dog. *J. Clin. Invest.* **52**, 39.

Stitt, J. T. (1976): The regulation of respiratory evaporative heat loss in the rabbit. *J. Physiol., Lond.* **258**, 157–171.

Szabo, G. (1962): The number of eccrine sweat glands in human skin. In *Advances in biology of skin*, Vol. 3, ed W. Montagna, R. A. Ellis and A. F. Silver. Oxford: Pergamon Press.

Taylor, C. R. (1972): The desert gazelle: a paradox resolved. In *Comparative physiology of desert animals*, ed G. M. O. Maloiy, pp. 215–228. New York: Academic Press.

Uhlich, E., Weber, P., Eigler, J. & Groschel-Stewart, U. (1975): Angiotensin stimulated AVP-release in humans. *Klin. Wschr.* **53**, 177–180.

Valtonen, M. & Eriksson, L. (1977): Response of reindeer to water loading, water restriction and ADH. *Acta Physiol. Scand.* **100**, 340–346.

Waites, G. M. H. & Voglmayr, J. K. (1963). The functional activity and control of the apocrine sweat glands of the scrotum of the ram. *Aust. J. Agric. Res.* **14**, 753–765.

Wolf, A. V. (1958): *Thirst.* Springfield, Illinois: Thomas.

Yagil, R. (1985): The desert camel: comparative physiological adaptation. In *Comparative animal nutrition* Vol. 5, 163 pp. Basel: S. Karger.

Yagil, R. (1986): The camel: self-sufficiency in animal protein in drought-stricken areas. *Wld Animal Rev.* **57**, 2–11.

Yagil, R. (1987): Camel milk—a review. *Int. J. Anim. Sci.* **2**, 81–99.

Yagil, R., Amir, H., Abu-Rabiya, Y. & Etzion, Z. (1987): Dilution of milk: a physiological adaptation of mammals to water stress? *J. Arid Env.* **11**, 243–247.

Yagil, R. & Berlyne, G. M. (1977): Glucose loading and dehydration in the camel. *J. Appl. Physiol. Resp. Environm. Exercise Physiol.* **421**, 680–683.

Yagil, R. & Etzion, Z. (1979): Antidiuretic hormone and aldosterone in the dehydrated and rehydrated camel. *Comp. Biochem. Physiol.* **63A**, 275–278.
Yagil, R. & Etzion, Z. (1980): The effect of drought conditions on the quality of camels' milk. *J. Dairy Res.* **47**, 159–166.
Yagil, R., Etzion, Z. & Ganani, J. (1979): Camel thyroid metabolism: effect of season and dehydration. *J. Appl. Physiol.* **45**, 540–544.
Yagil, R., Etzion, Z. & Oren, A. (1983): Physiology of drowning. A mini-review. *Comp. Biochem. Physiol.* **74A**, 189–193.
Yagil, R., Etzion, Z., Oren, A. & Keynan, A. (1981): The role of magnesium in drownings in the Dead Sea. *Comp. Biochem. Physiol.* **71A**, 99–106.
Yagil, R., Sod-Moriah, U. A. & Meyerstein, N. (1974): Dehydration and camel blood, I, II, III. *Am. J. Physiol.* **226**, 298–308.
Yagil, R., van Creveld, C., Oren, T. & Rogel, A. (1988): Responses of Awassi sheep and goats to grazing in the summer. *Int. J. Anim. Sci.* (in press.)
Yorio, T. & Bentley, P. J. (1976): Asymmetrical permeability of the integument of tree frogs (Hylidae). *J. Exp. Biol.* **67**, 197–204.
Yousef, M. K., Horvath, S. M. & Bullard, R. W. (1972): *Physiological adaptations: desert and mountain.* New York: Academic Press.

* * * * *

Discussion

Dr Tomkins said that in Third World countries children in the heat were given not only breast milk but additional water, and that this water was as often as not contaminated with pathogens which give rise to disease in the infants. He enquired whether it was necessary to give this additional water to children in hot climates. *Professor Yagil* quoted a WHO study examining the composition of milk in three groups of African women, an urban group, a group of well-off rural women and a group of poor rural women who had to work during the day. He noted with interest that this study had not examined the water content of milk, but as the fat content was low he felt that the milk was probably diluted under these circumstances and he agreed that there was no need to give water to infants in addition to breast milk. *Dr Tomkins* in a second question wondered why malnourished children have difficulty in excreting sodium through the kidney but have no problems in sodium excretion through the gut. *Professor Yagil* postulated that the thyroid depression under these circumstances may have some effect on aldosterone but that he would need notice of this question.

Dr Prentice noticed that in the Gambia women work during Ramadan and for 15 hours have no intake of water of any kind and yet the lactation seemed to continue successfully. He noted a similar decrease in lactose and increase in sodium and chloride concentration to that seen in the camels. Initially he had assumed that this was a defect but he now wondered whether this was an example of physiological adaptation of the breast milk composition. He also noted that in these women they tended to be overhydrated in the morning and wondered therefore whether the milk was more dilute. *Professor Yagil* noted that the raised concentration of sodium and chloride in the milk which may occur under these circumstances was useful in that the infant also lost sodium during the heat and so would require this extra sodium from the milk. He also made the observation that the vitamin C content of camels' milk was very high and for this reason it was difficult to make any milk products such as cheese.

Dr Speakman asked whether the volumes of milk produced by camels in dehydration and in hydrated conditions were known. The difference in the percentage of water in milk between the hydrated and dehydrated states would amount to a difference in water intake of only one litre every 24 hours. He wondered therefore if the primary response to water requirements of the young was to alter the volume of water delivered in the milk and the change in percentage water content was thus a secondary consequence to the delivery of a fixed amount of energy in a varying volume of water. *Professor Yagil* mentioned that there was no change in the blood chemistry of the baby camel that was entirely living on breast milk in a severe dehydration environment and therefore he presumed that there was sufficient water in camels' milk for the infant.

9

The variability of energy metabolism in man

J. C. WATERLOW

Introduction

Three years ago the Rank Prize Funds organized a symposium on Nutritional Adaptation in Man (Blaxter & Waterlow, 1985). At the present time there is a particularly strong interest in the capacity of man to adapt to low energy intakes. The concept of adaptation implies a range of different sustainable states, each perhaps with its cost. A starting-point from which to attack the problem would be a better knowledge of human variability, because without the capacity to vary there is no scope for adaptation. The single most important component of energy expenditure is the basal metabolic rate (BMR) (World Health Organization, 1985). Therefore in this joint paper Professor Shetty is discussing the variability of BMR within and between individuals and Dr Henry the variations between different ethnic groups and habitats. As an introduction to these presentations about man, I am trying to look at variability in BMR against a wider background.

Variability of the BMR

I have been accustomed to think of the BMR as the sum of the inevitable energy costs of chemical processes essential for life, of which two that are probably the most important quantitatively are ion transport and protein turnover. Perhaps naively, I think of cell membranes as having a rather fixed structure, so that the rate of active ion transport needed to maintain the intracellular environment would normally be fixed. However, this simplistic view is being undermined by new information on possible variations in the number of sodium pumps on a cell membrane (eg Kjeldsen

Table 1. *Intra-individual variability of measurements of whole body protein synthesis with ^{15}N-glycine.*

Oral dose of tracer; mean of estimates from urea and ammonia

A. Two subjects studied 5 times in 6 months	Fern *et al.*, 1984
Coefficient of variation: Subject 1: 6.6%	
2: 7.7%	
B. Seven subjects studied twice.	Fern *et al.*, 1984
Mean difference between replicates: 9.8%	
C. Nine subjects studied twice.	Gann, 1988
Mean difference between replicates: 7.3%	

Table 2. *Inter-individual variability of measurements of whole body protein synthesis with ^{15}N-glycine.*

A. 12 subjects studied twice.
Between-subject range (g N/kg per day):
Study I (febrile): 0.26–1.26
Study II (normal): 0.21–0.76
Pearson's rank correlation = 0.89 $P<0.001$
(From Garlick *et al.*, 1980)

B. Nine subjects studied twice.
Between-subject range (gN/9 h):
Study I (on indomethacin): 7.35–19.4
Study II (1 week after stopping indomethacin: 8.7–19.5
Pearson's rank correlation = 0.97 $P<0.001$
(From Gann, 1988).
Relating the rates to lean body mass did not reduce the variability (Gann, personal communication).

et al., 1984). As regards protein turnover, many advantages have been proposed for this energetically wasteful process: increased plasticity, particularly during growth; flexibility of enzyme response; removal of damaged or miscoded proteins, etc, and we are gradually assembling information about its variability (see below).

The point of view of the classical physiologist is different. The BMR, at least in homoeothermic animals, varies as the surface area of the body. From this it is deduced that its main function is to compensate for heat loss and to maintain body temperature. How can we reconcile these two different views about the nature and function of the BMR? If protein turnover, for example, is so important, how can man get away with a turnover rate which, per kg, is 1/10 that of the rat? In what follows, since there is very little reliable information about total rates of ion transport in the whole body, I shall confine myself to protein turnover.

First, if we are looking at variability between and within individuals as a possible basis for adaptation and indeed selection, a point worth examining is the variability of rates of protein turnover in man. From our data, within-individual variability, which includes error, is of the order of 10% (Table 1). Between subjects the variability seems to be much greater: in the two studies shown in Table 2 the range between individuals was several-fold. It is greater in study A than in B because in the former the estimates were based on only one end-product, ammonia, whereas in the latter they were derived from the end-product average (Fern *et al.*, 1981). In both sets of paired measurements the rank orders were almost identical.

Table 3. *Allometric relationships with body weight.*

				Reference
Basal metabolic rate (kcal/d)	70.5	×	$W^{0.73}$	(1)
Protein turnover (g/d)	15.8	×	$W^{0.72}$	(2)
Albumin turnover (mg/d)	5.8	×	$W^{0.68}$	(3)
Endogenous N (mg/d)	146	×	$W^{0.72}$	(1)
Creatinine N (mg/d)	12.7	×	$W^{0.9}$	(1)
Liver weight (mammals) (g)	33	×	$W^{0.87}$	(4,5)
Brain weight (mammals) (g)	10	×	$W^{0.70}$	(1,4)
Bone weight (g)	(0.6–2.8)	×	$W^{1.09}$	(6)

References:
(1) Brody (1945)
(2) Waterlow (1984)
(3) Wetterfors (1965)
(4) Stahl (1965)
(5) Prothero (1982)
(6) Günther (1975)

It is worth noting that in study A the group was not homogeneous: it included both sexes and some Asians as well as Caucasians. Unfortunately, BMR was not measured in these subjects.

In two studies BMR and whole body protein turnover have been measured at the same time: by Nair *et al.* (1981a,b) in calorie-restricted obese subjects with and without thyroid hormone therapy; and by Clugston & Garlick (1982) in lean and obese people, both fasting and fed. In both studies there was a significant correlation between protein synthesis rate and BMR.

Next, I thought it might be interesting, since we are concerned in this symposium with comparative nutrition, to look again, over a wide range of animal species, at the inter-relationships between energy metabolism, protein turnover and body weight. Nearly 20 years ago, on the basis of comparisons between rat and man and between infant and adult, I suggested that there might be a rather close relation between whole body protein turnover and BMR (Waterlow, 1968). Later results in different animals showed that this does indeed seem to be the case. Protein turnover, like BMR, varies as approximately the 3/4 power of the body weight (Waterlow, 1984). It has then been calculated that over a range of species, with body weights varying from 0.02 to 500 kg, the energy cost of protein turnover accounts for 15–20% of BMR.* I have tried to find information on this relationship in a wide range of animals, but so far without success except in one rather strange case, the blue mussel. From the data of Hawkins *et al.* (1986), it appears that, just as in mammals, 15–20% of the energy turnover could be accounted for by the energy cost of protein synthesis. It is very interesting that this relation is the same in mussels belonging to fast or slow growing strains, because the rate of protein synthesis is the same; it is the breakdown rate that differs.

In examining energy and protein turnover in animals of different sizes it is necessary to take into account differences in the make-up of the body, as already pointed

*This calculation is based on the assumption that 4–5 moles ATP or GTP are used per mole peptide bond, with no energy cost for protein breakdown. However, it now appears that non-lysosomal protein degradation requires 2 moles ATP per mole peptide bond (Hershko & Ciechanover, 1982; Goldberg *et al.*, 1987), so that the original figure for the cost of protein turnover will be an under-estimate. We cannot tell by how much without more information about the relative contributions of lysosomes and non-lysosomal proteases to protein degradation.

Table 4. *Fractional synthesis rates of mixed tissue proteins of liver and muscle* (% per day).

Animal	*Weight (kg)*	*Method*[a]	*Nutritional state*[b]	*Fractional synthesis rate* *Liver*	*Muscle*	*Liver/muscle*	*Reference*
A. *Mature or nearly mature*[c]							
Rat							
adult	0.75	Inf	PA	54	4.5	12	Waterlow *et al.*, 1978
senescent	0.60	FD	Fed	48	3.7	13	Goldspink *et al.*, 1985
Rabbit	3.6	Inf	Fed	40	2.2	18	Nicholas *et al.*, 1977
Sheep	58	Inf	PA	36	2.2	16	Schaeffer *et al.*, 1986
Man	68	Inf	Fed	—	1.8	—	Halliday *et al.*, 1988
Heifer	220	Inf	Fed	32	1.95	16	Lobley *et al.*, 1980
Steer	250	Inf	?	24.4	2.2	11	Eisemann *et al.*, 1986
B. *Immature, growing*							
Rat							
fetus	0.004	FD	Fed	97.5	20.5	4.8	Goldspink *et al.*, 1985
growing	0.1	Inf	PA	57	15.7	3.7	Garlic *et al.*, 1975
Chick	0.18	FD	Fed	103	19	5.4	Muramatsu *et al.*, 1983; 1985
Lamb							
fetus	?	Inf	Fed	78	26	3.0	Schaeffer & Krishnamurti, 1984
7–8 days	?	FD	?	115	22	5.2	Arnal, M.[d]
Growing	16	Inf	PA	54	4.5	12.0	Davis *et al.*, 1981
Piglet							
20 days	?	FD	?	85	16	5.3	Arnal, M.[d]
Pig	60–90	Inf	?	23	4.2	5.5	Garlick *et al.*, 1976

[a]Inf = constant infusion of isotope; FD = flooding dose.
[b]PA = postabsorptive.
[c]'Nearly mature' = 50% or more of final body weight.
[d]Personal communication.

out in this symposium by Professor Webster (p. 37). There is a huge literature on body scaling, that I am not competent to discuss in detail (see paper by Professor Peters, p. 1). The allometric equations in Table 3 show that liver weight as a fraction of body weight decreases with increasing body weight, but not to the same extent as whole body protein turnover. Between adult rat and man there is a two-fold difference between liver weight per kg body weight, but a five-fold difference in turnover per kg. There are two other large tissues whose mass may be expected to vary with body surface area, both of which are active in protein turnover—the intestinal mucosa (McNurlan & Garlick, 1980) and the skin (Preedy *et al.*, 1983). The brain is an unusual tissue because it has a large oxygen uptake but a rather low rate of protein turnover. If we exclude primates, its mass also seems to vary as the 2/3 power of body weight. Thus the internal organs, as a group, increase in weight more slowly than the body as a whole.

I cannot find direct data for muscle mass. Creatinine excretion varies directly with body weight (Table 3), and this makes sense, since on first principles one would expect muscle mass to vary in this way. However, it may be unwise to suppose that the same factor can be used across the board to derive muscle mass from creatinine production.

If there are large amounts of tissue with exponents of less than 1, and another mass with an exponent of 1, to fill the gap there must be some tissues with an exponent

Table 5. *Plasma concentrations of thyroxine (T_4) and tri-iodothyronine (T_3) in different animals.*

	Body wt (kg)	*Total T_4 (nmol/l)*	*Total T_3 (nmol/l)*	*Reference*
Rat	0.5	63	2.1	Schalch & Cree, 1985
Rabbit	5	22	—	Larsson *et al.*, 1985
Dog	12	29	—	
Piglet	15	30–80	1.0–1.4	Dauncey & Ingram, 1986
Man	70	109	1.8	Larsden, 1986
Sheep	76	60	1.3	Godden & Weeks, 1984
Cattle	500	83	—	Larsson *et al.*, 1985
Horse	1000	22	—	
Chicken	2	20	3.5	Hylka *et al.*, 1986
Salmon		11	—	Larsson *et al.*, 1985
Frog		3	—	

greater than 1. On physical principles one might expect to find such a relationship in those tissues that carry the stresses and strains of weight-bearing and movement—the skeleton, tendons, ligaments, etc. For a series of individual bones, the average exponent relating bone weight to body weight was found to be 1.1 (Günther, 1975).

Fat mass has been found to increase with an exponent of 1.13 (Calder, 1984). (I am indebted to Professor Peters for this information).

My argument therefore is that quite a large part of the difference in whole body protein turnover between large and small animals results from these differences in the make-up of the body rather than from intrinsic differences in the turnover rates of individual proteins. It is unfortunately difficult to find reliable data on protein synthesis rates in different tissues of different animals. The results in Table 4 seem to indicate a smaller span between species than one might expect, with a much greater difference, particularly for muscle, between mature and immature animals.

There is clearly a fascinating field for further enquiry in comparing the turnover rates of individual proteins, such as myofibrillar proteins or liver enzymes, in different species.

Finally, many of us were brought up to believe that the BMR is in some way controlled by thyroid hormones, since measurement of the BMR used to be the standard test of thyroid function. There is also evidence that both the rate of whole body protein turnover (Garrow, 1981; Nair *et al.*, 1981a,b; Wolman *et al.*, 1985) and the number of Na-K-ATPase receptors (Kjeldsen *et al.*, 1984) are responsive to changes in thyroid activity. It might, therefore, be expected that the concentrations of thyroid hormones in the blood might vary inversely with body size. The results in Table 5 show that this idea is totally wrong. It is true that these values represent total T_3 and total T_4, and not the free forms, for which I could not find adequate data. However, for what they are worth they suggest that the differences between animals lie in the number or activity of receptors rather than in the activity of the gland.

My conclusion is that there is plenty of scope for physiological variation in BMR in man. The first component and the most obvious one is variation in body composition. The second component is variation in the amounts or fluxes of what Garby & Larsen (1984) call the dissipative processes. There is a third component resulting from differences in the substrate mixture that is oxidized, carbohydrate producing iso-energetically more ATP than fat or protein. It remains to be seen whether it is necessary to invoke a fourth component, variation in metabolic efficiency, either in the formation of ATP (P/O ratio) or in its utilization (coupling efficiency).

Acknowledgement—I am indebted to Dr David Fleming of the Commonwealth Agriculture Bureaux for the literature search that provided the data for Table 5.

References

Blaxter, K. L. & Waterlow, J. C., eds (1985): *Nutritional adaptation in man.* London: John Libbey.

Brody, S. (1945): *Bioenergetics and growth.* New York: Reinhold Publishing Corp.

Calder, W. A. (1984): *Size, function and life history*. Cambridge, Mass: Bellknap Press.

Clugston, G. A. & Garlick, P. J. (1982): The response of protein and energy metabolism to food intake in lean and obese men. *Hum. Nutr: Clin. Nutr.* **36C**, 57–70.

Dauncey, M. J. & Ingram, D. L. (1986): Influence of a single meal on fractional disappearance and catabolic rates of 3,5,3′-triiodothyronine and thyroxine over 24 hours. *Comp. Biochem. Physiol.* **83A**, 89–92.

Davis, S. R., Barry, T. N. & Hughson, G. A. (1981): Protein synthesis in tissues of growing lambs. *Br. J. Nutr.* **46**, 409–419.

Eisemann, J. H., Hammond, A. C., Rumsey, T. S. & Bauman, D. E. (1986): Tissue protein synthesis rates in beef steers injected with placebo or bovine growth hormone. *J. Animal Sci.* **63**, Suppl. 1, 217.

Fern, E. B., Garlick, P. J., McNurlan, M. A. & Waterlow, J. C. (1981): The excretion of isotope in urea and ammonia for estimating protein turnover in man with (^{15}N) glycine. *Clin. Sci.* **61**, 217–228.

Fern, E. B., Garlick, P. J., Sheppard, H. & Fern, M. (1984): The precision of measuring the rate of whole body nitrogen flux and protein synthesis in man with a single dose of ^{15}N glycine. *Hum. Nutr: Clin. Nutr.* **38C**, 63–73.

Gann, M. (1988): Non-steroid anti-inflammatory agents and protein turnover in the elderly. MSc Thesis, Univ. Aberdeen.

Garby, L. & Larsen, P. S. (1984): Principles and problems of human energy exchange. *Am. J. Physiol.* **247** (Regulatory Integrative Comp. Physiol. 16) R366–R374.

Garlick, P. J., Burk, T. L. & Swick, R. W. (1976): Protein synthesis and RNA in tissues of the pig. *Am. J. Physiol.* **230**, 1108–1112.

Garlick, P. J., Millward, D. J., James, W. P. T. & Waterlow, J. C. (1975): The effect of protein deprivation and starvation on the rate of protein synthesis in tissues of the rat. *Biochim. Biophys. Acta* **414**, 71–84.

Garlick, P. J., McNurlan, M. A., Fern, E. B., Tomkins, A. M. & Waterlow, J. C. (1980): Stimulation of protein synthesis and breakdown by vaccination. *Br. Med. J.* **2**, 263–265.

Garrow, J. S. (1981): Protein turnover and metabolic rate in obesity. In *Nitrogen metabolism in man*, eds J. C. Waterlow and J. M. L. Stephen, pp. 449–456. London: Applied Science Publishers.

Godden, P. M. M. & Weeks, T. E. C. (1984): Influence of chronic thyroxine treatment on plasma hormone and metabolite concentrations and on responses to insulin, glucagon and thyrotrophin releasing hormone in adult sheep. *Hormone Metab. Res.* **16**, 354–358.

Goldberg, A. L., Menon, A. S., Goff, S. & Chin, D. T. (1987): The mechanism and regulation of the ATP-dependent protease La from *Escherichia coli*. *Biochem. Soc. Trans.* **15**, 809–811.

Goldspink, D. F., Lewis, S. E. M. & Kelly, F. J. (1985): Protein turnover and cathepsin B activity in several individual tissues of fetal and senescent rats. *Comp. Biochem. Physiol.* **82B**, 849–853.

Günther, B. (1975): Dimensional analysis and theory of biological similarity. *Physiol. Rev.* **55**, 659–699.

Halliday, D., Pacy, P. J., Cheng, K. N., Dworzak, F., Gibson, J. N. A. & Rennie, M. J. (1988): Rate of protein synthesis in skeletal muscle of normal man and patients with muscular dystrophy: a reassessment. *Clinical Science*, **74**, 237–240.

Hawkins, A. J. S., Bayne, B. L. & Day, A. J. (1986): Protein turnover, physiological energetics and heterozygosity in the blue mussel, *Mytilus edulis*: the basis of variable age-specific growth. *Proc. R. Soc. Lond. B.* **229**, 161–176.

Hershko, A. & Ciechanover, A. (1982): Mechanisms of intracellular protein breakdown. *Ann. Rev. Biochem.* **51**, 335–364.

Hylka, V. W., Tonetta, S. A. & Thommes, R. C. (1986): Plasma iodothyronines in the domestic fowl: newly hatched to early adult stages, with special reference to reverse triiodothyronine (rT3). *Comp. Biochem. Physiol.* **84A**, 275–277.

Kjeldsen, K., Nørgaard, A., Gøtzsche, C. O., Thomassen, A. & Clausen, T. (1984): Effect of thyroid function on number of Na-K pumps in human skeletal muscle. *Lancet* **2**, 8–10.

Larrson, M., Pettersson, T. & Carlstrom, A. (1985): Thyroid hormone binding in serum of 15 vertebrate species: isolation of thyroxine-binding globulin and pre-albumin analogs. *Gen. Comp. Endocrinol.* **58**, 360–363.

Larsden, P. R. (1986): In *The Thyroid*, eds S. H. Ingbar and L. E. Braverman, 5th edition. Chapter 19. Philadelphia: Lippincott.

Lobley, G. E., Milne, V., Lovie, J. M., Reeds, P. J. & Pennie, K. (1980): Whole body and tissue protein synthesis in cattle. *Br. J. Nutr.* **43**, 491–502.

McNurlan, M. A. & Garlick, P. J. (1980): Contribution of rat liver and gastrointestinal tract to whole-body protein synthesis in the rat. *Biochem. J.* **186**, 381–383.

Muramatsu, T., Coates, M. E., Hewitt, D. & Salter, D. N. (1983): The influence of the gut microflora on protein synthesis in liver and jejunal mucosa in chicks. *Br. J. Nutr.* **49**, 453–462.

Muramatsu, T., Salter, D. N. & Coates, M. E. (1985): Protein turnover of breast muscle in germ-free and conventional chicks. *Br. J. Nutr.* **54**, 131–145.

Nair, K. S., Baldwin, I., Halliday, D. & Garrow, J. S. (1981a): Effect of caloric restriction in obese subjects on resting metabolic rate, protein turnover, peripheral T_4 metabolism and glucose oxidation. *Clin. Sci.* **81**, 9P.

Nair, K. S., Halliday, D., Lalloz, M. & Garrow, J. S. (1981b): Rate of protein turnover in obese women on energy restriction and its relationship to extra-thyroidal T_4 metabolism. *Proc. Nutr. Soc.* **40**, 94A.

Nicholas, G. A., Lobley, G. E. & Harris, C. I. (1977): Use of the constant infusion technique for measuring rates of protein synthesis in the New Zealand white rabbit. *Br. J. Nutr.* **38**, 1–17.

Preedy, V. R., McNurlan, M. A. & Garlick, P. J. (1983): Protein synthesis in skin and bone of the young rat. *Brit. J. Nutr.* **49**, 517–523.

Prothero, J. W. (1982): Organ scaling in mammals: the liver. *Comp. Biochem. Physiol.* **71A**, 567–577.

Schaefer, A. L. & Krishnamurti, C. R. (1984): Whole body and tissue fractional protein synthesis in the ovine fetus *in utero*. *Br. J. Nutr.* **52**, 359–369.

Schaefer, A. L., Davis, S. R. & Hughson, G. A. (1986): Estimation of tissue protein synthesis in sheep during sustained elevation of plasma leucine concentration by intravenous infusion. *Br. J. Nutr.* **56**, 281–288.

Schalch, D. S. & Cree, T. C. (1985): Protein utilization in growth: effect of calorie deficiency on serum growth hormone, somatomedins, total thyroxin (T_4) and triiodothyronine, free T_4 index and total corticosterone. *Endocrinology* **117**, 2307–2312.

Stahl, W. R. (1965): Organ weights in primates and other mammals. *Science* **150**, 1039–1042.

Waterlow, J. C. (1968): Observations on the mechanism of adaptation to low protein intakes. *Lancet* **2**, 1091–1097.

Waterlow, J. C. (1984): Protein turnover with special reference to man. *Q. J. Exp. Physiol.* **69**, 409–438.

Waterlow, J. C., Garlick, P. J. & Millward, D. J. (1978): *Protein turnover in mammalian tissues and in the whole body*. Amsterdam: North Holland Publishing Co.

Wetterfors, J. (1965): In *Physiology and pathophysiology of plasma protein metabolism*, eds H. Koblet, P. Vesin, H. Diggelmann and S. Barandum, p. 83. Berne: Huber.

Wolman, S. L., Sheppard, H., Fern, M. & Waterlow, J. C. (1985): The effect of tri-iodothyronine (T_3) on protein turnover and metabolic rate. *Internat. J. Obesity*, **9**, 459–463.

World Health Organization (1985): *Energy and protein requirements*. Report of a joint FAO/WHO/UNU Consultation. WHO Tech. Rep. Ser. 724. Geneva, WHO.

10

Variability in basal metabolic rates of man

P. S. SHETTY and M. J. SOARES*

Introduction

The range of variability in the energy needs of man is based largely on meticulous studies of energy intakes and expenditure which have shown that in any group of 20 or more similar individuals, undertaking much the same activity, the daily energy intake can vary as much as two-fold (Edholm *et al.*, 1955; Rose & Williams, 1961; Widdowson, 1962; Wynn-Jones *et al.*, 1972). Recent reports confirm the wide variation in the daily energy intakes (with coefficients of variation of the order of 15–17% [Rao, 1987] and suggest that a substantial portion (estimated at about 70% in some population groups) of the total variation is largely the result of within-subject or intra-individual variation in intakes (De Boer *et al.*, 1987; Rao, 1987). It is this extraordinary range of variation in energy intakes, both between and within individuals, that has led the recent International Expert Consultation of the FAO/WHO/UNU to state, 'as a matter of principle we believe that estimates of energy requirements should, as far as possible be based on estimates of energy expenditure, whether actual or desirable'.

Energy expenditure is considered as made up of three components, ie basal metabolic rate (BMR), thermogenesis and physical activity; and since BMR constitutes up to 70% of the total energy output, is relatively stable and easily measurable, it is only appropriate that the energy needs of man are based on measures of BMR as a proxy for the total energy output. In this discussion basal metabolic rate (BMR) and resting metabolic rate (RMR) are used synonymously, although conceptual differences exist in the terminology used (Schutz, 1984). Variations in the thermogenic component

*Dr Soares was not present at the symposium.

and the quantum and cost of physical activity can also contribute to variability in energy needs. In this presentation however, we have confined the discussion to variability in BMRs that may result from methodological bias and biological variability in man, both between individuals and within the individual, and the relative importance of each.

Influence of methodology on the variability of BMR

Do the methods used in the measurement of BMR contribute to its variability? This question needs to be tackled at several levels. It is understood that certain stipulated minimal experimental prerequisites such as absence of gross muscular activity, a post-absorptive state, thermo-neutrality, etc are adhered to in order to ensure minimal levels of metabolism and to make comparisons of measurements made elsewhere possible. BMR measurements involve in the first instance an estimation of oxygen consumption of the individual, which is then converted into units of heat or energy output. In general, it is our opinion and that of most groups involved in BMR measurements, that the range of techniques available to measure oxygen consumption provide more or less the same value. We have compared the Douglas bag, Oxylog, HB metabolator, ventilated hood or canopy and whole body calorimeter and found that there are no significant differences between measurements of oxygen consumption obtained by two or more techniques in the same individual at the same time (Shetty *et al.*, 1986). A recent report by Segal (1987) supports these observations.

In the subsequent conversion of oxygen consumption values to energy output many assumptions are made which may influence the final result considered to be the BMR of the subject, expressed in kcals or megajoules per day. The most important of these assumptions are: (1) the value for non-pr tein respiratory quotient (RQ) assumed when the method used does not actually measure the non-protein RQ by not measuring CO_2 production; (2) the equations used in the calculation to convert O_2 consumption and CO_2 production (whether or not nitrogen excretion in the urine is estimated) to energy output; and (3) corrections that are made for differences in the volumes of inspired and expired air when both CO_2 output and O_2 consumption are measured. It is generally believed that these assumptions do not influence the final results over the range of physiological RQs seen. This however, is not correct. The difference between the true non-protein RQ of the subject and the assumed RQ in the calculation (be it 0.82 or 1.0) can introduce a difference of over 5% if the true RQ is as low as 0.77, for the same value of O_2 consumption obtained (Shetty *et al.*, 1986). Garlick *et al.*, (1987) have recently reported a mean RQ of less than 0.8 and if an Oxylog is used, which assumes an RQ of 1 in Weir's equation, the difference in the final value could be as much as 4.6%. Brockway has shown in his recent paper (1987) that the differences due to the various formulae generally used (ie those suggested by Weir [1949], Consolazio *et al.* [1963], Brouwer [1965] and Passmore & Eastwood [1986]) to calculate energy expenditure may cover a range of about 3%. McLean (1984) has also argued that the not uncommon assumption that O_2 consumption is equal to (outlet ventilation × O_2 concentration difference) can produce an error in the estimate of O_2 consumption of the order of ±6%, which emphasizes the importance of correcting for differences in volume flow of inspired and expired air when measuring BMR. McLean states that this error is fortunately cancelled out by an error in the calorific value of O_2 consumed as the RQ varies. However, this is not necessarily correct since calculation of energy output from values for an O_2 deficit of, say, 5%, for a fixed volume of 5 l/min at an assumed RQ of 0.82 using Weir's formula can introduce a net error of between +4.5 and −4.0% for a range of physiological RQs of between 0.71 and 1.0 respectively. One has no option but to state that little credence can be paid to small variations in BMR between individuals or groups of individuals when the differences are less than 5%, unless the methodology and the calculations used to arrive at the value of energy expenditure are comparable.

Inter-individual variability in BMR

It is generally recognized that in a group of apparently comparable individuals there is a considerable inter-individual variation in habitual total energy expenditure. Edholm (1961) reviewed a number of studies in which repeated measurements of total energy expenditure were made. These indicated a coefficient of inter-individual variability of about ±12.5% on a body weight basis. In recent studies where energy intake and physical activity have been controlled and energy output measured by calorimetry, the inter-individual variation in total energy expenditure has been found to have a coefficient of variation (CV) varying between 7.5 and 17.9% (Garby *et al.*, 1984; De Boer, 1985). The larger the variation in body weight among the subjects, the larger the CV of total energy expenditure.

Jéquier & Schutz (1981) compared subjects of similar body weight and body composition and showed that the inter-individual CV of RMR was 13%; other investigators have found inter-individual CVs of RMR between 7.9 and 12.0% in male and female subjects when measured under conditions of controlled intake and activity (Schutz, 1984; De Boer, 1985; Daly *et al.*, 1985); around 9.2% when intake was controlled at two levels of physical activity in males (Dallosso & James, 1984); and of the order of 11.7% in our measurements of 123 male subjects with a CV of body weights of the order of 15.2%. Simultaneous comparisons of the CVs of inter-individual variability of a group of lean male subjects who maintained constant body weight was the order of 10.3% for total energy expenditure and 10.2% for BMR (Dallosso *et al.*, 1982). The last study referred to indicates that the inter-individual variability in total energy output is reflected in the inter-individual variability of BMR in the same subjects, suggesting that the BMR may make a substantial contribution towards the variability of individuals in their habitual energy intakes (James, 1981).

Intra-individual variability in metabolic rate

Sukhatme & Margen (1982) argued that within-individual variations in intakes are more important than between-individual variations, and that the observed inter-individual variations can largely be explained in terms of the intra-individual variations. These investigators consider that the well-documented variation in intakes observed among apparently healthy individuals indulging in similar levels of activity is evidence that different individuals operate at different levels within what they consider to

Table 1. *Intra-individual variations in BMR/RMR.*

		Sex	CV (%)
1.	*Energy intake & physical activity controlled*		
	Jéquier & Schutz, 1981	F	2.0
2.	*Energy intake controlled; physical activity varied*		
	Dallosso & James, 1984	M	2.2
3.	*Energy intake varied; physical activity controlled*		
	Dallosso *et al.*, 1982	M	2.8
4.	*Energy intake & physical activity uncontrolled*		
	Harris & Benedict, 1919	?	4.0
	Berkson & Boothby, 1938	M	3.5
	Berkson & Boothby, 1938	F	4.7
	Soares & Shetty, 1986	M	2.9

Table 2. *Intra-individual variations in 24-hour energy expenditure.*

		Sex	CV %
1.	*Energy intake & physical activity controlled*		
	Dallosso *et al.*, 1982	M	1.5
	Webb & Abrams, 1983	F	3.3
	Webb & Annis, 1983	F	6.0
	Garby *et al.*, 1984	M	2.2
	De Boer, 1985	F	1.9
2.	*Energy intake varied; physical activity controlled*		
	De Boer, 1985	F	2.4
	De Boer, 1985	F	2.6

be the intra-individual range of 'costle s' adaptation. This has resulted in an unsubstantiated claim that intra-individual variations in energy expenditure are also large, with a wide coefficient of variation even in subjects accustomed to similar levels of physical activity every day, and that this wide variation needs to be considered when assessing the energy requirements of an individual (Sukhatme & Narain, 1983). Table 1 summarizes some of the recent data on the within-individual variations in BMR obtained from repeated measurements in the same individual when: (1) energy intake and physical activity have been controlled while in a respiration chamber (Jéquier & Schutz, 1981); (2) energy intake alone was controlled and BMR measurements were made on two levels of physical activity over a 24-hour period (Dallosso & James, 1984); (3) physical activity was kept constant over 24 hours but the energy intake was varied at two different levels (Dallosso *et al.*, 1982); and (4) BMR measurements have been made in free-living subjects in whom neither intake nor activity have been regulated (Harris & Benedict, 1919; Berkson & Boothby, 1938; Soares & Shetty; 1986). The CV of the measured BMR has never exceeded 5% and is frequently below 3%.

Estimation of the CV of 24-hour energy expenditure measurements using whole body calorimetry also leads to similar conclusions (Table 2). Several studies (Dallosso *et al.*, 1982; Webb & Abrams, 1983; Webb & Annis, 1983; Garby *et al.*, 1984; De Boer, 1985) have confirmed the low CV of intra-individual differences in 24-hour energy output when both energy intake and physical activity are tightly regulated as

Table 3. *Intra-individual variations in BMR/RMR with time.*

	Sex	n	Coefficient of variation (%) Days	Weeks	Months
Harris & Benedict, 1919	M	(?)			4.0
Du Bois, 1936	M	(23)		3.5	
	F	(10)		4.7	
Jéquier & Schutz, 1981	F	(14?)	2		
Garby & Lammert, 1984	M	(22)	2.4		
	M	(23)		2.2	
Lammert *et al.*, 1987	M	(7)	3.5	4.3	
	M	(7)		4.8	
Soares & Shetty, 1987	M	(5)		2.9	
	M	(10)			2.5

Table 4. *Intra-individual variations in energy expenditure (EE) and body weight with time.*

	Group	n	Time interval[3] (months)	CV (%) EE	Body weight
BMR[1]					
Males	Entire	(10)	18.2 ± 2.3 (7.0 – 33.0)	2.5	2.5
	Weight stable[4]	(5)	14.4 ± 2.9 (7.0 – 21.0)	3.2	0.6
	Weight change	(5)	22.0 ± 3.0 (15.0 – 33.0)	1.8	4.3
24 hour EE[2]					
Females	Entire	(10)	9.5 ± 2.0 (2.0 – 24.0)	2.4	2.4
	Weight stable[4]	(5)	7.2 ± 2.0 (2.0 – 13.0)	2.0	1.1
	Weight change	(5)	11.8 ± 3.3 (5.0 – 24.0)	2.7	4.1

[1]Soares & Shetty, 1987.
[2]De Boer, 1985 (recalculated).
[3]Mean ± sem; figures in parenthesis = range.
[4]Considered stable if change <2.0% of initial body weight.

is usual in a calorimetry protocol. Even when energy intakes are varied at two different levels, but the activity patterns when inside the calorimeter are maintained constant, the within-individual CVs do not vary by more than 2.4 or 2.6% (De Boer, 1985). When energy intakes are unaltered, but 24-hour energy expenditure is varied at two different levels of activity in the same subject, a large CV (of the order of 9.8%) is seen. This is to be expected since the 24-hour energy output has been deliberately altered in these subjects. However, even in these experimental situations, the CVs of the measured BMR in the same subjects at the two different levels of activity while in the calorimeter is no more than 2.2% (Dallosso & James, 1984).

The overwhelming recent evidence tends to support the view that intra-individual variations in BMR of the same subject are small and probably insignificant even when neither the intakes nor the activity patterns of the individual are controlled.

Reports of BMR measurements made over 50 years ago seem to support the conclusion that the within-subject variations in BMR, even when energy intake and physical activity are uncontrolled, are indeed very small and insignificant. For example Harris & Benedict (1919), in a statistical analysis of subjects observed from 20 to 50 days, reported a CV of 4%. BMR measurements made by Benedict on himself 18 times in 1932 and on 33 consecutive days in 1933 were extraordinarily uniform, being unaffected by variations in the evening meal, or length and depth of sleep during the previous night, or by normal variations in room temperature. Studies reported from the Mayo Clinic in 1936 (Du Bois, 1936) aimed specifically at answering the questions of intra-individual variations concluded that following numerous successive determinations of 10 females aged 18–53 years and 23 males of ages 18–40 years, on each of whom 7 to 15 consecutive morning observations were made, there was a CV of 4.7 and 3.5% respectively (Table 3). More recent measurements of BMRs in 14 subjects (controls & obese), each tested on 5 consecutive days, have confirmed that the CV is low, at around 2% (Jéquier & Schutz, 1981); and 16 male subjects studied on two separate occasions had a CV of less than 3% (Dallosso *et al.*, 1982). Other studies (Garby *et al.*, 1984; Lammert *et al.*, 1987), including our own (Soares & Shetty, 1987), have supported the view that the intra-individual variations in BMR measured over a period of days, weeks or even months, is small and probably not significant.

A critical analysis of the variations seen in BMRs or in 24-hour energy output over a period of up to 36 months when intakes and activity patterns were not controlled over this length of time is represented in Table 4. The BMRs of 10 male subjects measured on a minimum of three occasions over a period of 6 to 36 months showed a mean CV of intra-individual differences (separated from measurement error) of the order of 2.5% (Soares & Shetty, 1987). Five of the 10 individuals who had body weight changes of >2.0% had even smaller CVs (1.8%) as compared to those who had smaller changes in body weight over the period of time. Measurements of 24-hour expenditure by calorimetry in 10 females over a period of 24 months has also shown small CVs of 2.4%; however smaller CVs were seen in those five women who had <2% body weight change over this period (De Boer, 1985). In these females, neither intakes nor activity patterns were controlled, except during the periods when they were strictly on the calorimetry regimes. These recent data support the conclusions that BMRs of individuals are relatively constant over a period of several years despite reasonable fluctuations in body weight, when no attempt is made to regulate either energy intake or physical activity pattern. Earlier reports also verify these observations. Mitchell (1964) mentioned individual cases studied over several years, including measurements made by Eugene Du Bois on himself over a period of 22 years, which permitted him to conclude that the BMRs of adult humans are relatively constant and the range of variation seen within a subject is no greater than that for other physiological data.

Conclusion

In conclusion, it can be stated that the technique and calculations used while estimating BMR can contribute to some extent to differences between groups, which emphasizes the importance of uniformity in methodology if large-scale collection of BMR data worldwide is to help us arrive at energy needs of population groups. Intra-individual variations in energy expenditure and BMRs are small and probably insignificant as compared to a wider range of inter-individual variations. This is in contrast to the wide between-individual variation in energy intake, much of which can be attributed to variation in the intakes of the same individual over a period of time.

Acknowledgements—This study was supported by the Food and Agricultural Organisation, Rome.

References

Berkson, J. & Boothby, W. M. (1938): Studies of the energy metabolism of normal individuals. The interindividual and intraindividual variability of basal metabolism. *Am. J. Physiol.* **121**, 669–683.

Brockway, J. M. (1987): Derivation of formulae used to calculate energy expenditure in man. *Hum. Nutr: Clin. Nutr.* **41C**, 463–472.

Brouwer, E. (1965): Report of subcommittee on constants and factors. In *Third Symposium on energy metabolism*, ed K. L. Blaxter, pp. 441–443. European Association for Animal Production, publ. no. II. London: Academic Press.

Consolazio, C. F., Johnson, R. E. & Pecora, E. (1963): Physiological methods of metabolic functions in man, pp. 313–317. New York: McGraw Hill.

Dallosso, H. M., Murgatroyd, P. R. & James, W. P. T. (1982): Feeding frequency and energy balance in adult males. *Hum. Nutr: Clin. Nutr.* **36C**, 25–39.

Dallosso, H. M. & James, W. P. T. (1984): The effect of fat over-feeding on 24 h energy expenditure. *Br. J. Nutr.* **52**, 49–64.

Daly, J. M., Heymsfield, S. B., Head, C. A., *et al.* (1985): Human energy requirements: overestimation by widely used prediction equation. *Am. J. Clin. Nutr.* **42**, 1170–1174.

De Boer, J. O. (1985): Energy requirements of lean and obese women, assessed by indirect calorimetry. PhD Thesis. Agricultural University, Wageningen, Netherlands.

De Boer, J. O., Knuiman, J. T., West, C. E., *et al.* (1987): Within-person variation in daily dietary intake of boys from Finland, the Netherlands, Italy, the Philippines and Ghana. *Hum. Nutr: Appl. Nutr.* **41A**, 225–232.

Du Bois, E. F. (1936): *Basal metabolism in health and disease*, 3rd edn. Philadelphia: Lea and Febiger.

Edholm, O. G. (1961): Energy expenditure and calorie intake in young men. *Proc. Nutr. Soc.* **20**, 71–76.

Edholm, O. G., Fletcher, J. G., Widdowson, E. M. *et al.* (1955): The energy expenditure and food intake of individual men. *Brit. J. Nutr.* **9**, 286–300.

FAO/WHO/UNU (1985): Energy and protein requirements. Report of a joint FAO/WHO/UNU Expert consultation. *WHO Technical report series* No. 724. Geneva: WHO.

Garby, L. & Lammert, O. (1984): Within-subjects between-days-and-weeks variation in energy expenditure at rest. *Hum. Nutr: Clin. Nutr.* **38C**, 395–397.

Garby, L., Lammert, O. & Nielsen, E. (1984): Between subjects variability in 24 h energy expenditure for a fixed activity programme. In *Human energy metabolism*, ed A. J. H. Van Es. EURO-NUT report 5, p. 209, Wageningen, Netherlands.

Garby, L., Lammert, O. & Nielsen, E. (1984): Within-subjects between weeks variation in 24 h energy expenditure for fixed physical activity *Hum. Nutr: Clin Nutr.* **38C**, 391–394.

Garlick, P. J., McNurlan, M. A., McHardy, K. C., *et al.* (1987): Rates of nutrient utilization in man measured by combined respiratory gas analysis and stable isotopic labelling: effect of food intake. *Hum. Nutr: Clin. Nutr.* **41C**, 177–191.

Harris, J. A. & Benedict, F. G. (1919): *A biometric study of basal metabolism in man*. Carnegie Institution of Washington Publication No. 279.

James, W. P. T. (1981): Individual variability in energy needs. Background paper for joint FAO/WHO/UNU Expert consultation of energy and protein requirements.

Jéquier, E. & Schutz, Y. (1981): The contribution of BMR and physical activity to energy expenditure. In *The body weight regulatory system: normal and disturbed mechanisms*, ed L. A. Cioffi, W. P. T. James and T. B. van Itallie, pp. 89–96. New York: Raven Press.

Lammert, O., Garby, L., Maron, K., *et al.* (1987): Effect of the preceeding days energy intake on the energy cost of rest, arm and leg exercise. *Hum. Nutr: Clin. Nutr.* **41C**, 141–147.

McLean, J. A. (1984): Heat production or oxygen consumption? In *Human energy metabolism*, ed A. J. H. Van Es. EURO-NUT report 5, pp. 187–189. Wageningen, Netherlands.

Mitchell, H. H. (1964): *Comparative nutrition of man and domestic animals* Vol I. New York: Academic Press.
Passmore, R. & Eastwood, M. A. (1986): In *Davidson and Passmore: Human nutrition and dietetics*, 8th edn, pp. 18–19. Edinburgh: Churchill Livingstone.
Rao, S. (1987): Variations in dietary intake in adolescents. *Hum. Nutr: Clin. Nutr.* **41C**, 71–79.
Rose, G. A. & Williams, R. T. (1961): Metabolic studies on large and small eaters. *Brit. J. Nutr.* **15**, 1–9.
Schutz, Y. (1984): Terminology, factors and constants in studies on energy metabolism of humans. In *Human energy metabolism*, ed A. J. H. Van Es. EURO-NUT report 5, pp. 153–168. Wageningen, Netherlands.
Schutz, Y., Bessard, T. & Jéquier, E. (1984): Diet-induced thermogenesis measured over the whole day in obese and non-obese women. *Am. J. Clin. Nutr.* **40**, 542–552.
Segal, K. R. (1987): Comparison of indirect calorimetric measurements of resting energy expenditure with a ventilated hood, face mask and mouth piece. *Amer. J. Clin. Nutr.* **45**, 1420–1423.
Shetty, P. S., Soares, M. J. & Sheela, M. L. (1986): Basal metabolic rate of South Indian males. FAO Report. Rome: FAO.
Soares, M. J. & Shetty, P. S. (1986): Intra-individual variations in resting metabolic rates of human subjects. *Hum. Nutr: Clin. Nutr.* **40C**, 365–369.
Soares, M. J. & Shetty, P. S. (1987): Long term stability of metabolic rates in young adult males. *Hum. Nutr: Clin. Nutr.* **41C**, 287–290.
Sukhatme, P. V. & Margen, S. (1982): In *Newer concepts in nutrition and their implications for policy*, ed P. V. Sukhatme. Pune: MACS.
Sukhatme, P. V. & Narain, P. (1983): Intra-individual variation in energy requirements and its implication. *Ind. J. Med. Res.* **78**, 857–865.
Webb, P. & Abrams, T. (1983): Loss of fat stores and reduction in sedentary energy expenditure from undereating. *Hum. Nutr: Clin. Nutr.* **37C**, 271–282.
Webb, P. & Annis, J. F. (1983): Adaptation to overeating in lean and overweight men and women. *Hum. Nutr: Clin. Nutr.* **37C**, 117–131.
Weir, J. B. (1949): New method for calculating metabolic rate with special reference to protein metabolism. *J. Physiol.* **109**, 1–9.
Widdowson, E. M. (1962): Nutritional individuality. *Proc. Nutr. Soc.* **21**, 121–128.
Wynn-Jones, C., Atkinson, S. J. & Nicholas, P. (1972): Nutrient intake by students over a 3-month period. *Proc. Nutr. Soc.* **31**, 83A–84A.

11

A preliminary analysis of basal metabolic rate and race

C. J. K. HENRY and D. G. REES

Introduction

Almost a century ago, Eijkman (1896), working in Batavia, reported that the basal metabolic rate (BMR) of native Malays was similar to that observed in German subjects. Although his paper was the first to examine the rates of oxygen consumption in two different races, the publication which provoked the greatest controversy was that by Almeida who claimed in 1921 that the BMR of Brazilians was 16–20% below American standards. Since these early and largely conflicting observations, the possible existence of a racial factor influencing BMR has interested both physiologists and nutritionists.

The recent worldwide analysis of BMR in adults by Schofield, Schofield & James (1985) showed that the BMR of Indians was overestimated by 10–11% by the Schofield equations. At the time of this analysis there were insufficient data to determine whether the effect noted in Indians was unique or if it merely reflected a general pattern of metabolism as seen in tropical people. This chapter reviews BMR studies conducted only in the tropics, except for a study of Chippewe Indians (Crile & Quiring, 1939), and attempts to determine whether there is a racial factor in metabolism. It extends the earlier analysis of Quenouille *et al.* (1951) and Schofield *et al.* (1985) and presents data not previously evaluated (Dubois, 1936).

Methods

After careful screening, data were accepted for statistical analysis only if they met the following criteria: (1) BMR measurement was conducted in normal, healthy

Table 1. *List of papers used for analysis.*

Paper no	*Investigators*	*Year*	*Race*	*Location*	*Number*	*Sex*	*Age*	*Technique*
1	Ocampo, Cordero & Conception	1930	Philippino	Manila	104	M/F	14–48	Benedict/Roth respirometer
2	Galvao	1948	Brazilian	Sao Paulo	50	M	20–47	Open circuit
3	Galvao	1950	Brazilian	Sao Paulo	50	M	20–45	Open circuit
4	Orsini	1940	Brazilian	Sao Paulo	242	M	8–18	Benedict spirometer
5	Kise & Ochi	1933	Japanese	Tokyo	94	M/F	50–100	Benedict respiration apparatus
6	Takahira	1925	Japanese	Tokyo	120	M/F	18–58	Closed circuit respiration apparatus
7	Takahira	1925	Japanese	Tokyo	50	M/F	20–49	Closed circuit respiration apparatus
8	Teding Van Berkhout	1929	Malay	Batavia	12	M	19–38	Krough apparatus
9	Goewie & Radsma	1937	Malay	Batavia	58	M	20–50	Knipping apparatus
10	Earle	1928	Chinese	Hongkong	167	M/F	18–32	Benedict apparatus
11	Siddall & Kwok	1937	Chinese	Canton	100	F	15–36	Benedict apparatus
12	Benedict, Kung & Wilson	1937	Chinese	Peiping	120	M/F	15–87	Benedict field apparatus
13	Macgregor & Loh	1940	Chinese Malay Indian Javanese	Singapore	180	M/F	18–26	Benedict recording spirometer
14	Mason & Benedict	1934	Indian	Madras	7	F	19–22	Spirometer
15	Oliveiro	1937	Indian Chinese	Singapore	16	M	21–49	Douglas bag
16	Shattack & Benedict	1931	Mayan	Yucatan	25	M	15–32	Benedict field apparatus
17	Williams & Benedict	1928	Mayan	Yucatan	50	M	16–43	Benedict field apparatus
				Total	1445			

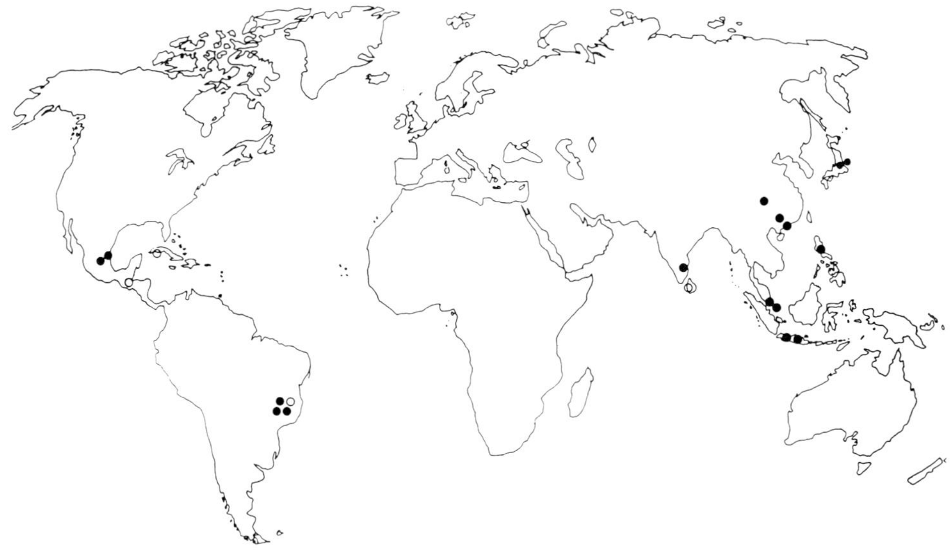

Fig. 1. *Location of BMR studies in various ethnic groups.* ●Studies in present report; ○studies located but not used in present report.

Table 2. *Summary of no. of subjects in each age group.*

	Age group (yrs)					
	3–10	*10–18*	*18–30*	*30–60*	*760*	*All*
Males	39	109	604	220	31	1003
Females	—	4	170	85	42	301
					Total	1304

subjects; (2) BMR was measured under standard conditions, ie post-absorptive, relaxed state; (3) general description of the equipment used for the study was given; and (4) measurements such as weight, height, age, sex were reported.

Results

Applying these strict criteria, 1445 new data points of both sexes and a range of ages were obtained. Several papers were excluded from the analysis as one or more of the criteria were not met. Table 1 summarizes the ethnic groups identified, their source and general description.

Figure 1 shows the location of the various studies. Data from the African continent were conspicuously absent. We excluded 141 cases from further analysis as the sex,

Table 3. *Equations derived for BMR related to body weight in present analysis. BMR MJ/d, weight in kg.*

		n	*R*	*s.e.*
Adults 18 to 30 years				
Males	BMR = 0.0542W + 2.995	604	0.66	0.5376
Females	BMR = 0.0448W + 2.775	170	0.455	0.5030
Adults 30 to 60 years				
Males	BMR = 0.0531W + 2.887	220	0.80	0.5270
Females	BMR = 0.0623W + 1.819	85	0.67	0.6317
	Schofield equation for same age groups			
Adults 18 to 30 years				
Males	BMR = 0.063W + 2.896	2879	0.65	0.6407
Females	BMR = 0.062W + 2.036	829	0.73	0.4967
Adults 30 to 60 years				
Males	BMR = 0.048W + 3.653	646	0.60	0.6997
Females	BMR = 0.034W + 3.538	372	0.68	0.4653

age or weight of the subjects were missing. Repeated measurements made on the same subjects were also deleted. Table 2 presents the data points broken down under each age group.

In keeping with the analyses of Schofield *et al.* (1985) and with Shetty's (1986) comparative study of BMR in adult Indians with predictive equations, the present analysis will be confined to the age group 18–60 years. Linear regression equations of BMR on body weight were obtained and compared with those published by Schofield *et al.* (1985), as shown in Table 3.

Visual inspection of the figures for males in age groups 18–30 and 30–60 (Figs 2 and 3) show that the new regression lines appear to fall below those of Schofield by a significant degree.

This finding is confirmed by hypothesis tests on the difference between BMRs predicted using our regression lines and Schofield's, shown in Figs 2 and 3. The tests were made by calculating approximate t statistics over the range of observed body weights, and using a modification of a method suggested by Steffens (1968), which uses Scheffe's (1959) method of multiple comparisons. These tests indicate that the differences between the predicted BMRs are significant at the 5% level for all weights between 35 and 100 kg in males aged 18–30, and for all weights between 35 and 93 kg in males aged 30–60. In both cases the observed body weight range is 35 to 100 kg. In females the picture is not so clear-cut. In 18–30 year olds (Fig. 4) the lines cross at 43 kg. Clearly differences cannot be significant in this area. However, significant differences were seen in the range 50 to 65 kg.

In 30–60 year old females (Fig. 5), the predicted BMRs were significantly different for body weights between 35 and 53 kg.

Another way to compare the data with Schofield's equation is to calculate for each of our data points the percentage by which the Schofield equation underestimates or overestimates the measured BMR in tropical subjects. This is shown in Table 4.

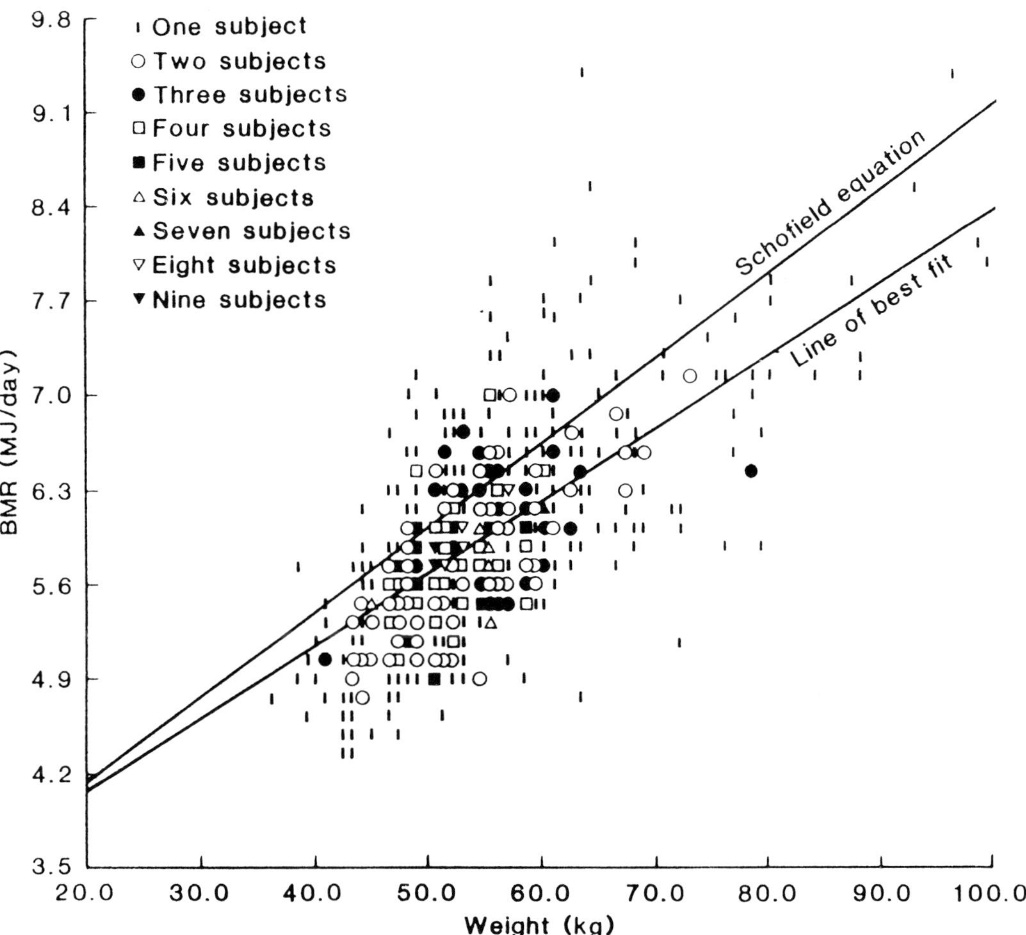

Fig. 2. *Regression of BMR against body weight in 604 males aged 18–30 yrs (see text for explanation).*

In the 18 to 30-year-old males ($n = 604$) the Schofield equation overestimated the group by an average of 7.2%, and in the 30–60-year-old males ($n = 220$) by 8.6%. In the females the overestimate in the 18–30-year-olds ($n = 170$) averaged 2% and in the 30–60-year-olds, 8.9% ($n = 85$). Close examination of the differences for each ethnic group is shown in Table 5.

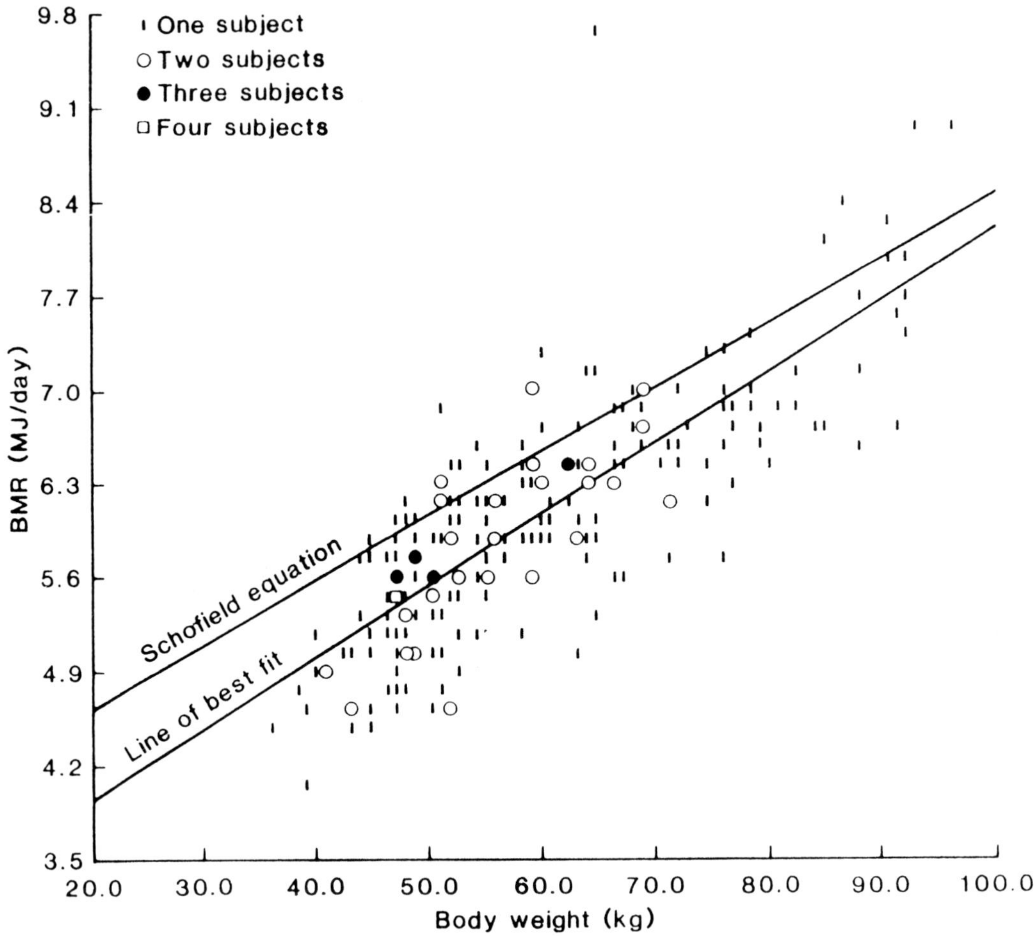

Fig. 3. *Regression of BMR against body weight in 220 males aged 30–60 yrs (see text for explanation).*

In all the S. Asian groups, ie Philippino, Indian, Japanese, Chinese, Malay and Javanese, the differences ranged from 12.7 to 5.1%. It thus appears that the lower BMR reported in Indians is not unique but reflects a phenomenon found in other Asiatic groups as well. Similarly, as first suggested by Almeida in 1921, the Brazilians also had a low BMR compared to the Schofield equations. Exceptions to this general

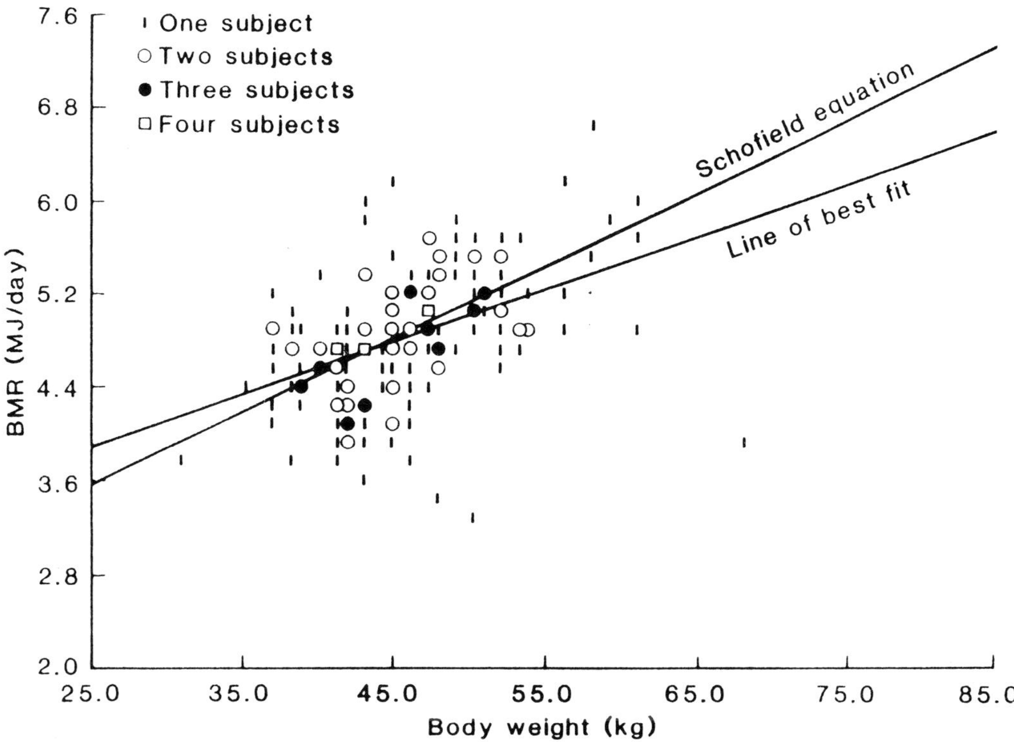

Fig. 4. *Regression of BMR against body weight in 170 females aged 18–30 (see text for explanation).*

Table 4. *The percentages by which Schofield equations overestimate (+) or underestimate (−) the actual BMR in different ethnic groups.*

1. *Males, all ethnicities*

Age group	*Mean %*	*Sample size*
18–30	+7.2	604
30–60	+8.6	220
18–60	+7.6	824

2. *Females, all ethnicities*

Age group	*Mean %*	*Sample size*
18–30	+2.0	170
30–60	+8.9	85
18–60	+4.3	255

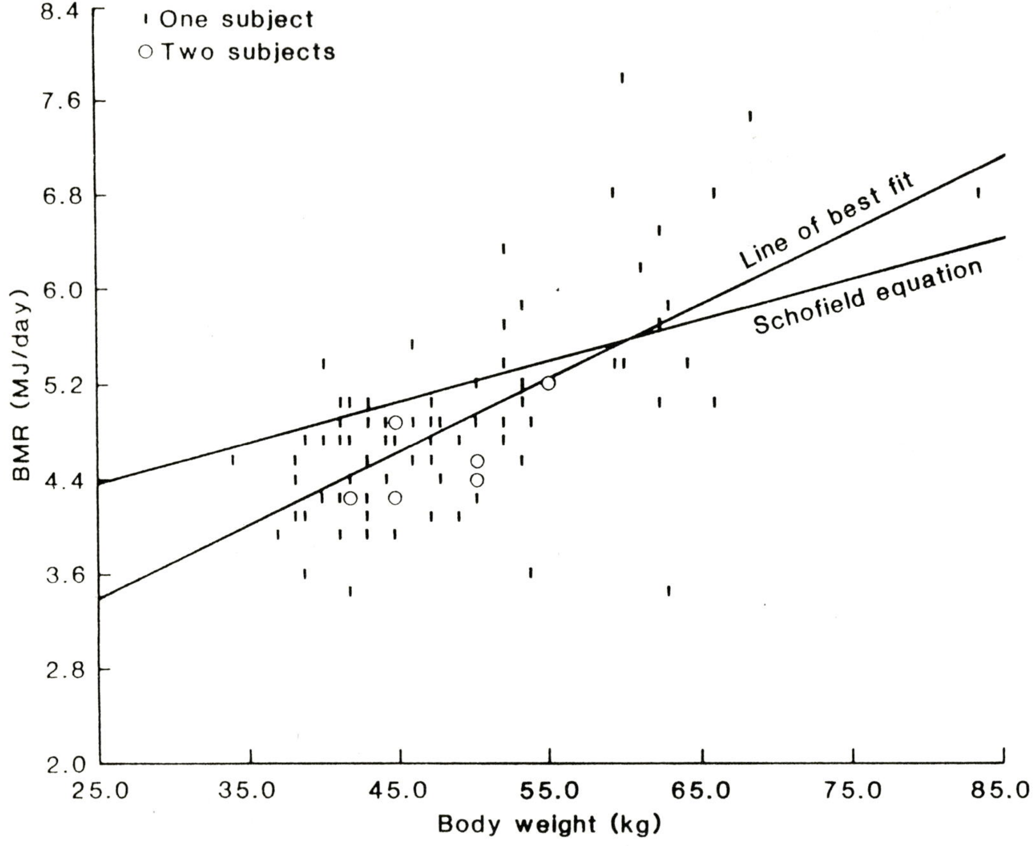

Fig. 5. *Regression of BMR against body weight in 85 females aged 30–60 yrs (see text for explanation).*

rule were the Chippewe Indians, measured in Churchill Bay (N. Canada), who had a higher BMR than predicted by the Schofield equation. Mayans showed no significant difference.

Explanation of this phenomenon is not simple. The study of racial metabolism in the tropics presents unique problems, and the possibility that the racial effect may be complicated by other factors was first suggested by Benedict (1932). Of all the factors that could influence BMR, nutritional status and climate may be the most significant. It is unlikely that the lower BMR observed in the various groups presented here is due to the inclusion of malnourished subjects, since they were reported as normal, healthy individuals. The climatic influence on BMR is more difficult

Table 5. *The percentage by which Schofield equations overestimate (+) or underestimate (−) BMR in different ethnic groups by sex (18–60).*

	Male		*Female*	
Ethnicity	*Mean %*	*Sample size*	*Mean %*	*Sample size*
Philippino	+ 9.6	82	+ 0.3	16
Indian	+ 12.7	48	+ 12.9	7
Japanese	+ 8.3	123	+ 7.9	71
Brazilian	+ 8.1	122	no data	—
Chinese	+ 8.2	232	+ 3.4	156
Malay	+ 9.3	62	no data	—
Javanese	+ 5.1	82	no data	—
Mayan	+ 0.0	68	no data	—
Chippewe Indian	− 18.5	5	− 18.5	5
All	+ 7.6	824	+ 4.3	255

	Male		*Female*	
	Mean %	*Sample size*	*Mean %*	*Sample size*
South Asian	+ 8.4	629	+ 4.7	250
South American and Chippewe Indian	+ 4.6	195	− 18.5	5

to assess and is a problem not yet satisfactorily resolved. Europeans living in the tropics for prolonged periods have been found to have an unchanged (Radsma & Streef, 1932) or lowered BMR (Munro, 1950). Mason & Jacob (1972), who extensively reviewed this topic, concluded that there was considerable variability in the response of BMR to climate. This ranged from no change to a reduction of 24% in BMR on moving to the tropics. Equally significant was the ethnic difference; with a greater proportion of Europeans showing a response to climate than Asians.

Conclusion

In conclusion, a preliminary statistical analysis of various ethnic groups suggests that in peoples living in the tropics (with the exception of Mayans), BMR is lower than predicted by the Schofield equations. Differences were significant for males at all ages from 18 to 60 years. In females the difference was more significant in the 30 to 60-year-old group than in the 18 to 30-year-olds. Although no satisfactory explanation can be offered at this stage for these racial differences, the results are consistent and appear to be genuine. Climate may interact with race to influence metabolism, though it is not clear why in two climatically similar locations, Yucatan and Singapore, the races showed different metabolic responses. Part of the explanation may lie in the varying degrees of muscular relaxation possible in different races, an area that needs closer investigation. Further discussions of energy metabolism in tropical people may need to consider these recorded differences in BMR.

References

Almeida, A. O. (1921): L'emission de chaleur. Le metabolisme basal et le metabolisme minimum de l'homme noir tropical. *J. Physiol. en Path. Gen.* **18**, 958–964.

Benedict, F. G. (1932): The racial elements in human metabolism. *Am. J. Phys. Anthrop.* **16**, 463–473.

Benedict, F. G., Kung, L. & Wilson, S. D. (1937): The basal metabolism and urinary nitrogen excretion of Chinese, Manchus and others of the Mongolian race. *Chinese J. Physiol.* **12**, 67–100.

Crile, G. W. & Quiring, D. P. (1939): Indian and Eskimo metabolism. *J. Nutr.* **18**, 361–368.

Dubois, E. F. (1936): *Basal metabolism in health and disease, 3rd ed.* Philadelphia: Lea and Febiger.

Earle, H. G. (1928): Basal metabolism of Chinese and Westerners. *Chinese J. Physiol.* Report series No. 1, 59–92.

Eijkman, C. (1896): Ueber den Gaswechisel der Tropenbewohner, Speciel mit Bezug auf die frage von der chemischen warmeregulrung. *Arch. f. d. ges. physiol.* **64**, 57–78.

Galvao, P. E. (1948): Human heat production in relation to body weight and surface. II. *J. App. Physiol.* **1**, 395–401.

Galvao, P. E. (1950): Human heat production in relation to body weight and body surface. *J. App. Physiol.* **3**, 21–28.

Goewie, J. B. M. & Radsma, W. (1937): The basal metabolism of different native population groups at Batavia. *Arch. Neerl. de Physiol.* **22**, 297–303.

Kise, Y. & Ochi, T. (1933): Basal metabolism in old people. *J. Lab. Clin. Med.* **19**, 1073–1079.

MacGregor, R. G. S. & Loh, G. L. (1940): The comparison of basal physiological values in racial groups. *J. Malaya Br. Brit. Med. Assoc.* **4**, 449–462.

Mason, E. D. & Benedict, F. G. (1934): The effect of sleep on human basal metabolism, with special reference to South Indian Women. *Am. J. Physiol.* **108**, 377–383.

Mason, E. D. & Jacob, M. (1972): Variations in basal metabolic rate responses to changes between tropical and temperate climates. *Hum. Biol.* **44**, 141–172.

Munro, A. F. (1950): Basal metabolic rates and physical fitness scores of British and Indian males in the tropics. *J. Physiol.* **110**, 356–366.

Ocampo, M., Cordero, N. & Conception, I. (1930): Basal metabolism of Filipinos. *J. Phil. Med. Assoc.* **10**, 357–365.

Oliveiro, C. J. (1937): Basal metabolism in Singapore. *J. Malaya Br. Brit. Med. Assoc.* **1**, 125–133.

Orsini, O. (1940): Metabolismo basal dos Jovens brasileiros. *O. Hospital.* **17**, 59–89.

Quenouille, M. H., Boyne, A. W., Fisher, W. B. & Leitch, I. (1951): Statistical studies of recorded energy expenditure of man. Part I. Basal metabolism related to sex, stature, age, climate and race. Commonwealth Bureau of Animal Nutrition. Tech. Comm. No. 17. Bucksburn, Aberdeen.

Radsma, W. & Streef, G. M. (1932): On metabolism during rest and protein-consumption in Europeans living in the tropics. *Arch. Neerl. de Physiol.* **17**, 97–111.

Schofield, W. M., Schofield, C. & James, W. P. T. (1985): Basal metabolic rate — review and prediction together with an annotated bibliography of source material. *Hum. Nutr: Clin. Nutr.* **39C** (Suppl. 1), 4–96.

Shattack, G. C., Benedict, F. G. (1931): Further studies on the basal metabolism of Maya Indians in Yucatan. *Am. J. Physiol.* **96**, 518–528.

Sheffe, H. (1959): *The analysis of variance.* New York: Wiley.

Shetty, P. S., Soares, M. J. & Sheela, M. L. (1986): Basal metabolic rate of South Indian males. Bangalore: FAO Report.

Siddall, A. C. & Kwok, K. C. (1937): The basal metabolism of Southern Chinese women. *Chinese J. Physiol.* **12**, 389–396.

Steffens, F. E. (1968): On comparing two simple linear regression lines. *S. Afr. Stat. J.* **2**, 33–53.

Takahira, H. (1925): The basal metabolism of normal Japanese men and women. *Rep. Met. Lab. Imperial. Govt. Inst. Nutr.* **1**, 11–36.

Takahira, H., Kitagawa, S., Ishibashi, E. & Kayano, S. (1925): The basal metabolism of common labourers. *Rep. Met. Lab. Imperial Govt. Inst. Nutr.* **1**, 37–42.

Teding van Berkhout, J. P. (1929): Contribution a l'etude du metabolisme basal chez les habitants des tropiques. *Med. deel. v.d. Dienst. d. Volks. in Nederl.-Indie.* **18**, 1–69.

Williams, G. D., Benedect, F. G. (1928): The basal metabolism of Mayans in Yucatan. *Am. J. Physiol.* **85**, 634–649.

Discussion of energy metabolism and basal metabolic rate

Dr Widdowson asked *Dr Prentice* what his experience was in the Gambia as far as energy expenditure was concerned and he replied that research so far supported Dr Widdowson's 1947 observations that there was in fact a two-fold range in the energy expenditure of children in the Gambia, when measured by the doubly-labelled water method.

Dr Dauncey mentioned that their own work had shown basal metabolic rate to be influenced by the previous day's energy intake and asked Dr Henry whether any of the differences in metabolic rate he had reported from the literature could be related to differences in energy intake. *Dr Henry* replied that the information was not provided in many cases.

Professor Waterlow asked how far the lower basal metabolic rate seen in people from tropical regions was related to a low body mass index; and *Dr Henry* again said that no height measurements were available in most cases.

Professor Jackson said that in six normal adults in Jamaica resting energy expenditure was only 88% of that predicted from the Schofield equation, but was the same as predicted in sickle cell disease. He wondered whether chronic disease should be taken into account in tropical climates.

Dr Ingram reported their own study on pigs kept at different temperatures and food intakes. The resting metabolic rate of these pigs measured at thermal neutrality was not affected by the temperature to which they were acclimatized, although it was influenced by food intake.

Professor Garby reported that Dr Dauncey's work suggested there could be approximately a 7% increase in resting metabolic rate when the ambient temperature fell from 28 to 22 degrees centigrade, to which *Dr Henry* replied that the measurements were made at thermal neutrality or on the temperature existing at that day and the room temperatures had in fact varied between 25 and 28 degrees centigrade in most of the papers that he was quoting from.

Professor Garrow wanted to know the coefficient of variation for 24-hour energy expenditure when intake was maintained constant and physical activity was altered.

Dr Shetty replied that a study by Dallosso in lean men showed a coefficient of variation of 9.8% for 24-hour energy output but the intra-individual coefficient of variation was only 2.2% for RMR in the same subjects in whom physical activity had been altered.

Mr Payne commented that an important part of the differences in basal metabolic rate per kilogram body weight between ethnic groups may be artefacts, arising from the use of linear regression equations of BMR on weight, to correct for body size. For example, the study of Indian males by McNeill showed them to have BMR values 12% lower than predicted by the regression equation recommended by FAO (the so-called Schofield equations) for correcting for body weight. However, most of this discrepancy is removed if an exponential equation is used: showing that nearly all the difference in BMR between Indian and Caucasian populations can be accounted for by body size.

This, once again, underlines the points made by *Dr Peters* in his opening talk, regarding the vital importance of properly correcting for allometric factors before drawing conclusions about interspecies or interracial differences.

Dr Henry replied that this needed evaluation.

Professor Waterlow followed this up by saying that from the Schofield equation a 50 kg male would have a 20% lower basal metabolic rate than a 70 kg male, but the rates are the same if they are related to metabolic mass ($wt^{0.7}$). The Schofield equations should be regarded as purely descriptive, without physiological implications.

Professor Webster referred to the work by Koong in which he reported a 40% difference in the basal metabolic rate of pigs by increasing the mass of the intestinal contents, and therefore it was important to consider the prior nutrition immediately before basal metabolic rate was taken if comparisons were going to be made between individuals.

Professor Van Soest backed this up by saying that the variation in transit time in normal subjects which he had studied was very variable and would support the comment made by Webster.

12

Obesity – role of animal models

K. J. McCRACKEN

Introduction

Human obesity, which has been of interest to man for a very long time, has been the subject of intense research effort for most of this century and particularly during the last two decades. Many learned reviews have addressed the complex issues associated with regulation of energy intake and expenditure in human and animal subjects (for example Mayer, 1953; Mayer & Thomas, 1967; Hervey, 1971; McCance, 1972; Garrow, 1974; Bray, 1978; Jeanrenaud, 1978; Himms-Hagen, 1983; Horton, 1983; Le Magnen, 1983; Slattery & Potter, 1985; Bray, 1986; Baile *et al.*, 1986; Sclafani, 1987) and yet many questions remain unanswered or are the subject of intense controversy.

In simple terms, obesity develops when energy intake chronically exceeds energy expenditure and it has frequently been stated that a relatively small imbalance (1%) over a period of years could give rise to the condition. Equally, a 10% excess for one year would give rise to approximately 20% increase in body weight and 50% increase in body energy content. In theory such an imbalance could arise from an increase in energy intake coupled with a smaller increase in expenditure or from a reduction in energy expenditure coupled with no change in energy intake or from a variety of other combinations of these factors. In practice it is probable that a wide range within these combinations can occur. It is of importance to our understanding of the development of obesity, and of relevance to the treatment of pre-obese and obese subjects, that we attempt to clarify this situation. However, despite, or perhaps because of, the proliferation of experimental results, it would appear from an examination of recent reviews (Le Magnen, 1983; Slattery & Potter, 1985) that we are little nearer to finding this particular 'crock of gold' than we were 40 years ago when Newburgh (1944) reviewed the subject.

It is now obvious that the topic is even more complex than Newburgh could have imagined. To provide a synthesis it is necessary to cover such diverse subjects as endocrinology, biochemistry, sensory physiology, neurobiology, psychology and nutrition. Almost all body organs and functions are involved. Much of this complexity has been revealed through the study of animal models.

The purpose of this chapter is to examine the adequacy or otherwise of the models used in the past, the types of question which remain to be answered and the models which may be appropriate in the pursuit of these answers. Even such a limited remit is, to use the words of Le Magnen (1983), 'a daring enterprise' and the present author has already contemplated at length his temerity, not to say foolhardiness, in undertaking such a challenge.

Human obesity

The starting-point for any discussion of the relevance of animal models must be the human and it is assumed that all will agree that the best model is man himself. Therefore, if the question under consideration can be answered by properly-conducted, statistically interpretable, ethical studies on human beings no other approach is valid. For example, studies of methods of weight reduction and their effects on body function and metabolism could come within this definition provided that any drugs, if used, have first undergone pharmacological and toxicological tests on animals. The effects of temperature, exercise and other environmental variables, including short-term overfeeding, all commend themselves for study in man. However, in relation to the development of obesity we are limited, even in nutritional studies, by aesthetic and ethical considerations, by the ability to find 'volunteers' and by the problems of conducting 'controlled' experiments on such devious creatures. It is unlikely that any ethical committee would now permit the Vermont Study (Sims *et al.*, 1968) to be conducted. Equally it would be totally unacceptable to conduct the sort of studies involving specific interference with control systems, which have contributed to our knowledge of the complex interactions which maintain the normal homoeostasis of the intact animal or human. The author will not dwell on the moral, ethical or philosophical aspects of using animals for such purposes but will assume that all scientists adopt a responsible attitude in the use of animals for research and that the techniques employed are justified.

In a subject where controversy and confusion seem to be the key-words it is necessary to start with a statement of what is generally accepted. Human obesity can occur in children but is more frequently manifested in middle-age, is associated with an excess deposition of adipose tissue in combination with a normal or above-normal lean body mass, is defined by an arbitrary cut-off in the distribution curve (eg BMI$>$25; Garrow, 1981) and usually develops insidiously over a period of years (Garrow, 1974). Subjects are frequently hypertensive, hyperinsulinaemic and hypercholesterolaemic and show reduced activity. Resting energy expenditure in absolute terms is normally higher than in lean subjects of comparable height and age (Bray *et al.*, 1970; Irsigler *et al.*, 1979; Ravussin *et al.*, 1982) but is lower when related to body weight or metabolic body size (taken as ${W_{kg}}^{0.75}$ in this paper). Weight reduction can be achieved in most subjects on a strict diet and tends to normalize the clinical parameters. Although the major energy loss is adipose tissue there is a tendency to lose some lean body mass even if protein intake is regarded as adequate. Energy expenditure declines in absolute terms (De Boer, 1985) but remains static or tends to increase per unit body weight. Most subjects have difficulty either in achieving satisfactory reduction or maintaining the new status (Drenick & Johnson, 1978; Dwyer & Berman, 1978).

Controversial aspects

Some of the areas of controversy are: (1) Does the obese subject consume more energy during the static phase of obesity than a comparable lean subject? (2) Is hyperphagia a necessary prerequisite to the development of obesity? (3) What changes occur in energy expenditure during the development of obesity? (4) How do the various neural and endocrine systems interact? (5) What is the potential for treatment of the obese or pre-obese?

One would expect that the answer to the first question would have been established long ago beyond reasonable doubt. However, there are two conflicting schools of thought and even Garrow (1974) avoided reaching a conclusion. Most of the evidence based on assessment of energy intake suggests that obese people eat less than or no more than lean counterparts (Beaudoin & Mayer, 1953; Thomson *et al.*, 1961; Spitzer & Rodin, 1981; Kromhout, 1983; Baecke *et al.*, 1983). This, and the much-quoted studies of Widdowson (1962) and Miller & Payne (1962), have led many research workers to look for a primary alteration in energy expenditure and efficiency of energy utilization as the basis for the development of obesity. On the other hand there is now a firm body of evidence (Irsigler *et al.*, 1979; Ravussin *et al.*, 1982; Blaza & Garrow, 1983; Segal & Gutin, 1983; Webb & Annis, 1983; Schutz *et al.*, 1984; De Boer, 1985) that total energy expenditure is higher in obese subjects in the static phase of obesity. Hence it must be assumed that the values obtained by the normal methods of assessment of energy intake are incorrect. The studies of De Boer (1985) and his colleagues provide an interesting and informative comparison of lean and overweight women. The energy intakes (MJ/d) of the two groups, assessed by the 7 d weighing record method, were respectively 8.61 and 8.78, whereas the measured energy expenditures were 8.62 and 10.70. The conclusion that, as a general rule, the energy intake and expenditure of obese subjects in the static phase is higher than that of lean counterparts at similar levels of activity is supported by the overwhelming bulk of animal studies discussed below even including those relating to hypothalamic lesions or genetic obesity.

In view of the above discussion it is unlikely that the second question 'Is hyperphagia a necessary prerequisite to obesity?' can ever be answered by direct experiment in the human. As discussed by Slattery & Potter (1985) there is a number of situations in animals in which the first signs of the development of obesity appear to precede hyperphagia or occur under pair-fed conditions, eg in genetically obese rodents. It is possible (indeed probable) that in 'metabolic obesity' (Garrow, 1974) or where a subject drastically reduces the normal level of activity, obesity may begin to develop despite a 'normal' intake. A wide range of such situations can be envisaged and modelled in animals and may serve to throw some light on the human situation.

The other three questions are still only partially answered despite the massive research effort on humans and animals, and can be regarded as the major justification for the future use of animal models of obesity.

Animal models

Obesity normally develops over a long time-span and is the result of the integration of adipose tissue storage and loss from conception or, to be more realistic, from birth. Hence any complete understanding of the development of obesity requires consideration of the complete life-span. The normal human is gregarious, omnivorous (with a marked preference for variety), prefers a thermoneutral environment, eats three or four meals per day (at least in affluent societies!) and indulges in a mild degree of exercise. Approximately 40 and 20% of the energy intake are derived from fat and sucrose respectively.

It would seem a reasonable proposition that studies which cannot readily be performed on human subjects should use an animal model as closely related as possible, for example, reasonably large primates. This concept is not new—Garrow (1974) made exactly the same comment in the introduction to his book—yet a survey of the literature reveals that well over 90% of all the published work on animal models of obesity has been, and continues to be, conducted on laboratory rodents. The reasons for this in terms of availability, short life-span, suitability for surgery and for analysis of carcass composition, are obvious. Equally it can be argued that much of what has been achieved in terms of our knowledge of the complexity of the control mechanisms operating in the mammal could not have been achieved without the laboratory rodent. However, it is important that research workers and those providing funds for research should ensure that the right questions are being asked and the most effective means are being applied to obtain the answers. The remainder of this paper will attempt a critical review of the role which animal models have played, particularly in the last ten years, in contributing to our understanding of the development of obesity. Although a number of other animal species could have been included, and are mentioned in passing, the discussion will centre on laboratory rodents and non-human primates.

There are four aspects to any animal model which need to be considered: (1) the timescale of the experimental treatment in terms of age at start and length of period of study; (2) the type and degree of experimental deviation imposed; (3) environmental interactions, and (4) the gender, and in the case of females, the physiological status of the subjects.

Each of these topics is large and, in particular, the subject of sex differences would warrant a review of its own. The author has taken the coward's way out and, apart from the occasional comparison, has excluded it from consideration.

Laboratory rodents

Time-scale of experimental treatments

A number of approaches has been used to modify growth of the rat *in utero* and during early post-natal development. These include increased litter size (Widdowson & McCance, 1960; Stephens, 1980; Oscai, 1982; Harrington & Coscina, 1983; Drenowski *et al.*, 1984), malnutrition of the rat during early pregnancy (Chow & Lee, 1964; Jones *et al.*, 1984, 1986), supplementary feeding during the pre-weaning period (Czajka-Narins & Hirsch, 1974) and chronic intragastric infusion of neonatal rats (West *et al.*, 1982). In some cases these have been coupled with the introduction of high-fat or varied palatable diets at weaning or during the post-pubertal stage (Oscai, 1982; Harrington & Coscina, 1983; Drenowski *et al.*, 1984; Jones *et al.*, 1984, 1986) and with longitudinal studies of behaviour, food intake, growth and body composition.

The studies of Mickelsen and his colleagues (Mickelsen *et al.*, 1955; Schemmel *et al.*, 1969, 1970), employing high-fat or grain diets from weaning, provide longitudinal studies of changes in body weight and composition under conditions of nutritional hyperphagia. Unfortunately the results do not readily lend themselves to detailed investigation of energy utilization. During the last 10 years numerous relatively long-term studies have been conducted on adult rats and mice. These have involved various combinations of experimental deviation which will be discussed in subsequent sections.

Two further categories of time-scale may be defined, namely short-term studies during growth, and short-term studies on adults. Although any generalizations are dangerous it is the author's opinion that such studies, particularly during growth, are less relevant to our understanding of obesity and these have largely been excluded from the subsequent discussion.

Type and degree of experimental deviation

Although it would be possible to create a much longer list of 'experimental deviations' these can be considered under four main headings, (a) nutrition, (b) genetic, (c) hypothalamic lesion, coupled with selective organ removal/interference, (d) combinations of (a)–(c).

(a) Nutrition

Numerous types of dietary model have been studied. These include standard laboratory chows (with or without flavours), diets of altered composition (eg low protein, high fat, high sucrose), varied palatable diets (with or without liquid supplements), physical form of diet (pellets, meal, slurry, liquid), and method of consumption (voluntary *ad libitum*, discrete meals, gastric intubation). The ensuing discussion is not intended to be a comprehensive survey but rather intended to highlight aspects which may contribute to the debate on human obesity and to complement the review of Sclafani (1978).

High-fat diets. These have been used with normal rodents, post-weaning or post-puberty (Mickelsen *et al.*, 1955; Schemmel *et al.*, 1969, 1970; Pitts & Bull, 1977; Oscai, 1982; Oscai *et al.*, 1984; Barr, 1984; Jones *et al.*, 1986; Levin *et al.*, 1986; Corbett *et al.*, 1986), in combination with studies on hypothalamic lesions and as part of studies of genetic obesity (see below). In general, hyperphagia of between 10 and 20% in relation to subjects given low-fat chow was induced and obesity was observed to develop. In some cases it has been claimed that obesity occurred despite a normal energy intake. Study of two recent claims (Oscai *et al.*, 1984; Levin *et al.*, 1986) indicates that these are based on false assumptions with regard to the available (metabolizable) energy content of the diets used. However, one interesting aspect of studies with high-fat diets is the individuality of animal response. For example, Mickelsen *et al.* (1955) reported that only 70% of their rats became obese, ie were clearly above the upper end of the weight range of normal animals. With such variability occurring in a controlled laboratory strain of rat, it is hardly surprising that wide variability exists in the heterogeneous human population.

In many cases the dietary fat contents far exceeded those likely to occur in human diets (eg 85% of energy as fat in the studies of Mickelsen *et al.* [1955], Schemmel *et al.* [1969, 1970] and Pitts & Bull [1977], and 75% as fat in that of Corbett *et al.* [1986]). Hence interpretation of the results must be treated with caution. However, the diet used by Barr (1984) contained only 37% gross energy as fat but induced approximately 15% hyperphagia in three strains of young male rats. A similar level of hyperphagia was observed (Barr & McCracken, unpublished) in adult female rats during a six-week study in which the animals became obese, and by Oscai (1982) in a long-term study on male rats using a diet containing 40% energy as fat. It is therefore possible to produce hyperphagia and obesity in laboratory rodents with a balanced diet of similar composition to that consumed by humans in our affluent society. This provides a useful model for study of diets of different fatty acid composition whilst permitting accurate measurement of energy intake. It may also be possible to identify sub-groups within experimental treatments which do not exhibit obesity and/or hyerphagia and to identify endocrine/metabolic differences which may contribute to our understanding of the development of human obesity.

Varied palatable diets (cafeteria diets). Sclafani & Springer (1976) reported that 'giving an assortment of palatable supermarket foods is a particularly effective way of producing dietary obesity in adult rats'. Since then an avalanche of publications based on studies on 'cafeteria-fed' rats and mice has caused confusion, controversy (Hervey & Tobin, 1983; Rothwell & Stock, 1983) and commentary on the inappropriateness of cafeteria-feeding for studies of thermogenesis (Moore, 1987). There is general agreement, however, that cafeteria-feeding induces hyperphagia and obesity. Although some of the higher estimates of the degree of hyperphagia induced may be due to the problems of accurate measurement of energy intake in a cafeteria system it would seem that hyperphagia of the order of 30 to 40% is common. In a series of 16 experiments with young rats, Barr (1984) obtained values ranging from 16 to 33% and in a 6-week study, hyperphagia in adult virgin females averaged 34%. During this time weight increased by 149 g compared with 55 g for controls. This increase is similar to that observed in adult female rats by Sclafani & Gorman (1977) and would be equivalent to a 60 kg woman gaining 30 kg within a 4-year period. One aspect which was apparent in the Barr (1984) study and which is high-lighted in other studies (Gale *et al.*, 1981; Drenowski *et al.*, 1984) is the large individual variability in weight gain. However, the variability in terms of energy retention versus metabolizable energy intake was no greater than that on the control diet and was similar to that observed in studies on human volunteers (Van Es *et al.*, 1984). Despite the variability, the major conclusion to be drawn from 'cafeteria-fed' rats is that, if humans were like rats , we would all be obese and the abnormal population would be the lean subjects. However there are at least two aspects which have not yet been discussed. First of all, the rat is a nibbler and nocturnal. There is evidence that the introduction of varied palatable foods increases the amount of daylight feeding and meal frequency as well as meal size (Rogers & Blundell, 1984). It is therefore not clear whether the higher sustained degree of hyperphagia observed with cafeteria diets as opposed to high-fat diets is of relevance to the human situation, although it is of interest that similar levels of hyperphagia occur on low-fat varied diets (Barr, 1984; Louis-Sylvestre *et al.*, 1984) and that marked hyperphagia and obesity occurred with a combination of chow and bread (Rogers & Blundell, 1984). Furthermore, Rolls *et al.* (1983) demonstrated that variety in a simple meal enhanced intake and that, over a period of several weeks, simultaneous presentation of several food items results in significantly greater weight gain in male and female rats. The second aspect, activity, is discussed later.

One of the main problems with the use of varied palatable diets is that of definition or control of nutrient intake due to self-selection. This can lead to nutrient deficiencies (Barr & McCracken, 1985) in the diet consumed. For studies where accurate measurement of energy balance is important the use of a small range of foods of different texture/flavour, but of similar nutrient concentration, should improve the accuracy and interpretation of the results obtained.

Despite the criticisms which can be levelled at the cafeteria model, the fact that it simulates an important aspect of the human situation and that variety may play a role in sympathetically-mediated stimulation of energy expenditure would support continued use of well-defined cafeteria diets. One method of presentation which deserves consideration is the provision of five or six discrete meals of 30 minute duration at fixed times. This would more closely mimic the human situation and may induce levels of hyperphagia more in line with those which probably occur in humans.

Sucrose in the diet or as liquid supplement. The role of sucrose and other carbohydrates in relation to the induction of hyperphagia and obesity has recently been thoroughly reviewed (Sclafani, 1987). Two approaches have been adopted in these studies, one involving the incorporation of sucrose or other sugars in the diet (composite diet) and the other the provision of liquid (supplements). In most of the former studies, high-sucrose diets have been found not to alter or even to reduce energy intake but tend to increase body weight and/or body fat. Sclafani (1987) has suggested that this effect may be due to rapid absorption of sucrose leading to hyperinsulinaemia. Others (see Pearce, 1983) have attributed it to a shift in metabolic pathway due to the fructose moiety. Sclafani (1987) has reviewed 19 studies, mainly on adult rats. In 13 of these, food intake was enhanced and in almost all cases body weight and/or body fat were increased. The degree of hyperphagia observed varied from zero to 20% and the contribution of sucrose to total energy was, in some cases, as high as 60%. Careful examination of those studies in which obesity was reported to occur without accompanying hyperphagia (Hill *et al.*, 1980; Rattigan & Clarke, 1984; Sclafani & Xenakis, 1984; Castonguay & Collier, 1986) reveals that energy intakes have apparently been expressed in terms of gross energy or per unit liveweight. Hence the conclusions drawn are not reliable.

In terms of the relevance of these studies to human obesity, two comments are appropriate. First, the levels of sucrose employed in most of the composite diet studies were extremely high, ranging from 30% (Hallfrisch *et al.*, 1981) to 81% (Allen & Leahy, 1966) and it would appear that the contribution of sucrose in liquid-supplemented studies would fall in the same range (Barr, 1984; Sclafani, 1987). Although significant hyperphagia occurs with sucrose supplements it is no greater than that observed with polycose solutions (Sclafani & Xenakis, 1984). Hence, despite the preference expressed by rats for sucrose in two-bottle tests, there is little evidence from the rat data to suggest that the normal levels of sucrose consumed by humans should make a significant contribution to modifying energy intake. The evidence for increased efficiency of energy utilization also seems to be rather tenuous and it is suggested that further studies involving sucrose diets will add little to our understanding of the development of human obesity. However, it would be dangerous to disagree with the statement of Sclafani (1987) that 'the influence of other carbohydrates, rates of carbohydrate digestion and absorption and the post-ingestion modulation of appetite should be considered'.

Gastric intubation. Gastric intubation (Cohn *et al.*, 1955) provides an effective means of control of food intake and meal frequency in the rat. Whereas rats offered a synthetic or chow diet in discrete meals tend to eat less than nibbling counterparts, large excesses of energy can be intubated over long periods (McCracken & McNiven, 1983) and result in extreme obesity. However, the technique may be stressful to the experimental subject as well as to the experimenter and induces metabolic changes which, while they may be partly due to the change in meal pattern, are almost certainly due mainly to the magnitude of the nutrient load (Cohn & Joseph, 1970). In the growing rat there is a marked interference with protein deposition (Cohn & Joseph, 1963; McCracken, 1975; Barr, 1984; Barr & McCracken, 1984) which may be due to increased corticosteroid production (Fletcher, 1986), and there is firm evidence that under pair-feeding conditions energy expenditure is reduced in comparison to 'nibbling' counterparts (Cohn & Joseph, 1959; Barr, 1984). Rothwell & Stock (1979a) have attributed this reduced energy expenditure to inhibition of brown adipose tissue (BAT) thermogenesis. Whether or not this is the whole explanation, the tube-fed adult rat provides an interesting insight into the energy cost of maintenance of obese tissue. McCracken & McNiven (1983), using a synthetic diet containing approximately 20% of energy as sucrose and 35% as fat, force-fed adult female rats for 0, 6, 12, 18, 24 and 30 d so that body weight ranged from 244 to 365 g. Fasting heat production increased from 118 to 160 kJ/d indicating that energy metabolism was closely related to metabolic body size ($W^{0.75}$). During this period, lean body mass (LBM) only increased by 8%. McNiven (1984) demonstrated that the same holds true in the sheep. Since the activity of the obese rats appeared to be lower than for controls, these results strongly suggest that obese tissue makes a major contribution to the maintenance energy requirement. Although there are dangers in drawing analogies from a 300 g rat to a 70 kg human, the fact that resting energy expenditure in many obese humans per unit body weight (or metabolic body size) is lower than in lean counterparts, could indicate an initial low basal energy expenditure as a contributory factor in the development of obesity. Taken with the observation of Leblanc *et al.* (1984) of reduced post-prandial heat production in humans following gastric intubation, the above discussion highlights a potential role for further use of gastric intubation in animals and humans to identify the endocrine implications, particularly in relation to stomach load, gastric emptying and sympathetic stimulation.

(b) Genetic models

Several genetically obese strains of rodent have been identified and studied in considerable detail. These include the yellow strain of mice (Danforth, 1924), the hyperglycaemic (ob/ob) mouse (Ingalls *et al.*, 1950), the Zucker (fa/fa) rat (Zucker and Zucker, 1961), the polygenic obese mouse (Eisen, 1975), the LA/N corpulent rat (Hansen, 1983) bred from the obese, hyperphagic, hypertensive Koletsky strain (Koletsky, 1973), the SHR/N-CP rat (Hansen, 1983), and the db^{Pas} mouse (Aubert *et al.*, 1985). It is not the purpose of this chapter to systematically compare and contrast these models or to provide a synthesis of understanding of the endocrine, biochemical and compositional differences which are observed (see reviews of Mayer, 1953; Coleman, 1978; Himms-Hagen, 1983) and recent papers (Michaelis *et al.*, 1983; Tulp, 1984; Tulp & Buck, 1986; Tulp & McKee, 1986; Tulp *et al.*, 1986; Michaelis *et al.*, 1986). However, some important differences can be highlighted. For example, the onset of obesity in the yellow strain coincided with sexual maturity (Danforth, 1927) and appeared to be associated with hyperphagia and reduced activity (Mayer, 1953), whereas the onset of obesity in the ob/ob mouse and fa/fa rat occurs during the early post-natal period and precedes hyperphagia (Lin *et al.*, 1977; Boissoneault *et al.*, 1978; Thurlby & Trayhurn, 1978). Most of the mutations are single-locus, are associated with extremely high levels of obesity and exhibit low body temperatures and increased cold sensitivity (Himms-Hagen, 1983). However, it would appear that the LA/N corpulent rats differ from the ob/ob mouse and fa/fa rat in that, although obesity is observed around 5 weeks of age, hyperphagia precedes the onset of obesity (Tulp & McKee, 1986) and lean body mass is increased, whereas the reverse is true for the latter strains. Since it would appear that the genetically related aspects of human obesity are not associated with single-locus defects (DHSS/MRC, 1976; Foch & McClean, 1980) it can be argued that the polygenic obese mouse (Eisen, 1975; Robeson *et al.*, 1981) represents a potentially better model than the ob/ob mouse and fa/fa rat upon which a vast amount of research has been lavished.

One area in which the genetic models can be particularly effective relates to the development of therapeutic drugs. This is well illustrated by the effect of the β-adrenergic agonist BRL 26830A on the ob/ob mouse and Zucker (fa/fa) rat (Arch & Ainsworth, 1983). Another example is the recent publication on the anti-obesity action of S-(+)-1-(4-chlorophenylthiomethyl)-N-methylethylamine fumarate (AO-124) which suppressed food intake in a dose-dependent manner in normal, Zucker (fa/fa), and VMH-obese rats (Ikeda *et al.*, 1986).

One further aspect of most studies using genetic mutations merits comment and criticism. Because obese strains exhibit spontaneous hyperphagia on low-fat chow, most research has been conducted without giving due attention to the role of diet composition. For example, elegant studies were conducted which demonstrated the important role of the adrenal in correcting the hyperphagia, obesity and reduced skeletal muscle gain in obese mice given chow (Saito & Bray, 1984; Smith & Romsos, 1985) and the importance of corticosteroids in stimulating hyperphagia in adrenalectomized animals (Bruce *et al.*, 1982), but Smith & Romsos (1985) and Grogan *et al.* (1987) have shown that adrenalectomy fails to exert these effects in ob/ob mice fed purified high-fat or high-glucose diets as opposed to a non-purified diet. This illustrates the difficulty of interpretation of responses even within a species when dealing with a problem of multifactorial origin.

Despite these criticisms, it is obvious that the study of genetic models has contributed enormously to our knowledge of the complexity of the factors which affect energy intake and expenditure within the mammalian system. It is to be hoped that future studies will take more account of the interactions with diet and other factors relevant to the human.

(c) Hypothalamic obesity

Since the report by Hetherington & Ranson (1940) that large electrolytic lesions in the hypothalamus of rats resulted in obesity, a considerable amount of research has been conducted using this model. Various other types of lesion have been produced by peripheral injection of, eg, gold thioglucose (GTG) (Waxler & Brecher, 1950), monosodium glutamate (Olney, 1969) and bipiperidyl-mustard (Jagot *et al.*, 1980), by knife cuts (Sclafani & Berner, 1977), and by local administration of a variety of chemical substances including GTG (Smith & Britt, 1971), 6-hydroxydopamine (Kapatos & Gold, 1973), norepinephrine (Shizamu *et al.*, 1986) and neuropeptide Y (Stanley *et al.*, 1985). These studies have been extended to a wide range of species (Bell, 1971) and numerous reviews have been published (for example, Mayer, 1953; Kennedy, 1961; Mayer & Thomas, 1967; Frohman, 1978; Bray & York, 1979; Bray *et al.*, 1981; Le Magnen, 1983; Bray, 1986). Many elegant experiments have been conducted in which VMH-lesioned animals have been subjected to adrenalectomy (Bruce *et al.*, 1982; Debons *et al.*, 1986), vagotomy (Powley & Opsahl, 1974; Sclafani, 1981), sympathecomy (Bray *et al.*, 1981), hypophysectomy (York & Bray, 1972), jejunoileal bypass (Sclafani *et al.*, 1980), and pancreatic transplant (Bray *et al.*, 1981). In some cases the timing of these events in relation to production of the VMH lesion has been shown to modify the course of development of hyperphagia and obesity (York & Bray, 1972; Sclafani *et al.*, 1980).

The recent reviews of Le Magnen (1983) and Bray (1986) provide a marvellous synthesis of the current situation and Bray (1986) has developed a fascinating model for the hypothalamic control of feeding and provided a succinct summary which is reproduced as follows: 'the levels of hormones such as insulin, adrenal steroids, gonadal steroids and growth hormone play an important role in predicting energy balance. The two limbs of the autonomic nervous system also modify energy expenditure. Hypothalamic obesity and genetic obesity are associated with lower sympathetic activity whereas the weight reduction associated with lateral hypothalamic lesions is accompanied by increased sympathetic activity. This suggests that the activity of the sympathetic nervous system is inversely related to energy stores . . . and that both hormonal factors and the autonomic nervous system seem to be able to independently modulate energy stores'.

In the face of such elegant studies and hypotheses it may seem hypercritical to ask if the studies are as relevant to the human situation as they could be. However, it is of interest to note that out of twenty important papers published in the last 7 years, twelve employed chow only and seven used high-fat diets (most of them supplying 60% energy from fat). Only one (Sclafani *et al.*, 1981) compared different dietary regimens and this paper demonstrated that although vagotomy blocks hyperphagia and obesity on chow diets or even with supplemented sucrose it fails to normalize intake and weight gain when a varied palatable diet is offered. As with the genetic model therefore, diet composition and physical form play an important role which appears to have been underestimated or overlooked in studies involving hypothalamic obesity. This aspect, and other environmental considerations which will be discussed below, should be given higher priority in future studies using this interesting model.

(d) Combination of factors

Relatively few of the studies discussed above involved combinations of the different models of obesity but the results obtained indicate the importance of a multifactorial approach to the problem of obesity. In particular those of Smith & Romsos (1985) and Grogan *et al.* (1987) in the ob/ob mouse and that of Sclafani *et al.* (1981) with VMH rats demonstrate the roles of nutrient content and variety in altering the response to other experimental deviations. Similarly the papers by Gale *et al.* (1981) and Tulp & Shields (1984) suggest that the introduction of a varied palatable diet to adult Zucker (fa/fa) rats or LA/N-cp rats in the static phase of obesity induces a greater degree of hyperphagia than in lean counterparts. Unfortunately, no measurements of food intake or energy expenditure are available from these studies. Whilst the problems inherent in the design and interpretation of multifactorial studies should not be taken lightly it would appear that useful insights into the control of metabolism would be obtained if this approach were adopted more widely. Furthermore, it has been amply demonstrated that the problem of obesity requires a multidisciplinary approach and that interpretation of many studies has been hampered by insufficient simultaneous measurements or in some cases failure to interpret nutritional data correctly by those whose expertise lies in other directions. If effective use is to be made of animal models in the future it would seem that larger teams or increased inter-laboratory collaboration must be considered.

Environmental interactions

Earlier in this chapter the human model was discussed in terms of a number of social and environmental factors; man is gregarious, prefers thermoneutral zone, eats three or four meals per day, indulges in some degree of exercise. For sound experimental reasons we normally separate our laboratory rodents into individual cages, especially if we wish to measure food intake. We weigh them frequently and subject them to a daily routine which is convenient for us. These are all factors which may vary from one laboratory to another and probably within laboratories and yet may have profound effects on behaviour and food intake of our experimental subjects. For example, we are all aware that food intake of rats is increased by frequent weighing, ie handling. If all animals are treated alike within an experiment this may not be a matter for great concern. However, two other features of most studies on laboratory rodents are of the utmost importance but have been overlooked or ignored in the vast majority of studies. These are (a) room temperature and (b) the role of exercise.

(a) Temperature

Although it has been known for the last 40 years (Swift, 1944) that the lower critical temperature of the rat is around 27°C, almost all studies have been conducted at between 21° and 24°C. In view of the numerous reports indicating the importance of the sympathetic nervous system in the regulation of food intake and energy expenditure it is remarkable that so little attention has been paid to the effects of temperature and that so many studies have been conducted at temperatures which may be comfortable for the investigator but do nothing for the usefulness of the experimental model. The few studies which have been undertaken underline the importance of this variable.

Vander Tuig *et al.* (1980) measured the maintenance energy requirements of young obese ob/ob and lean mice at 33°C. In the ob/ob mice expenditure was similar at 33°C to that reported by Lin *et al.* (1979) but in the lean mice the maintenance requirement was reduced by 25%. Fletcher (1986) studied lean and obese (fa/fa) rats at 22 or 30°C. At 30°C rectal temperature was normalized in the fatty Zucker, and both food intake and the degree of hyperphagia relative to the controls were lower. Plasma corticosteroid levels were higher in obese rats at both temperatures but the phenotypic difference was greater at 30°C. Probably correlated with this, protein deposition was significantly reduced in the fatty Zucker at 30°C whereas no significant difference was observed at 22°C.

There do not appear to be any direct comparisons of temperature above and below the thermoneutral zone in adult models of obesity. However, Rowe & Rolls (1981) compared 18°C and 25°C in both cafeteria-fed and control rats. At the lower temperature, as would be expected, rats ate more irrespective of diet, but gained less weight. When the varied palatable foods were withdrawn and replaced by chow the rats at the lower temperature tended to lose weight whereas body weight increased at 25°C. The persistent obesity observed after withdrawal of cafeteria foods (Rolls *et al.*, 1980) is in contrast to the rapid weight normalization in the studies of Sclafani & Gorman (1977) and may be related to the lower temperatures employed by the latter (Rolls *et al.*, 1980).

Barr & McCracken (1984) observed high efficiency of utilization of cafeteria diets and no increase in heat production per unit metabolic body size relative to controls in studies at 29°C. This observation was in marked contrast to the results of Rothwell & Stock (1979b) using rats of similar origin and weight but an environmental temperature of 24°C. Recently Rothwell & Stock (1986) have reported a comparison at 24°C and 29°C. The results at 29°C were in line with those of Barr & McCracken (1984), whereas those at 24° broadly agreed with those of Rothwell & Stock (1979b). This study suggests that the role of brown adipose tissue in 'diet-induced' thermogenesis may have been grossly overestimated because of the experimental models used.

The evidence cited above is regarded by the author as a major indictment of most of the studies which have been conducted on laboratory rodents.

(b) Exercise

Although a number of reports have demonstrated the effect of exercise on food intake and body composition of rats fed laboratory chow (Mayer *et al.*, 1954; Stevenson *et al.*, 1966; Crews *et al.*, 1969; Ring *et al.*, 1970; Applegate *et al.*, 1982) relatively little attention has been paid to the role of activity during the development of hyperphagic obesity.

However, Pitts & Bull (1977) studied the effects of forced exercise on male rats given chow or a high-fat diet. In both cases there was a marked reduction in weight gain but the effect was greater on the high-fat diet.

Rolls & Rowe (1979) observed a marked reduction in the body-weight gain of males given a palatable diet when allowed spontaneous exercise in a running wheel. Voluntary activity tended to be higher on the palatable diet than on chow. In contrast they noted that exercising females increased intake and showed little difference in body weight on either diet compared with non-exercising counterparts.

Recently Tulp & Jones (1987) reported that forced exercise early in the lifespan of LA/N corpulent female rats reduced the degree of obesity which occurred on a chow diet but did not normalize body composition. However, the reduction in weight gain compared to sedentary animals was greater than for their lean counterparts.

The paper of Pitts (1984) should be compulsory reading for every student of nutrition and anyone contemplating experimental studies on energy balance. This paper examined changes in weight and body composition from weaning to 260 d of age in males and 130 d in females in relation to diet, age and activity. The diets were chow or high-fat and in the case of the males three activity regimens were compared (spontaneous running, adequate cage size, restricted cage size). The results for males showed up highly significant activity/diet interactions on body fat, with restricted activity rats given chow showing a reduction in intake, body weight and fat, those on the high-fat diet having the highest weight and body fat. The spontaneously-exercising high-fat rats had similar body composition at 260 d to those given chow in adequate cages. As in the study of Rolls & Rowe (1979) the spontaneously-exercising females increased food intake and maintained similar body weight and composition to non-exercising females. As Pitts (1984) states in his discussion 'if we had achieved the usual objective of letting only one parameter vary at a time . . . we would have been left in ignorance of the multiple existing interactions. However, such interactions are a fundamental characteristic of living organisms largely avoided by investigators, perhaps because they can be nearly overwhelming'.

Non-human primates

Compared with the enormous literature on laboratory rodents, that on non-human primates (mainly the rhesus monkey, *Macaca mulatta*) is relatively small. The studies can be divided into three broad categories: (a) those which studied the normal pattern of intake and growth and the development of spontaneous obesity; (b) those where obesity was induced by dietary means; and (c) those where obesity resulted from lesions in the ventromedial hypothalamus.

Spontaneous obesity

Although studies on adolescent rhesus monkeys (McHugh & Moran, 1978) have demonstrated a remarkable degree of accuracy in the regulation of food intake on a chow diet following intragastric preloads, and Hansen *et al.* (1981) have shown that monkeys regulate intake on liquid feeds with considerable precision over a wide range of dilution, there are reports of spontaneous obesity in older animals given laboratory chow. Hamilton *et al.* (1972) classified obesity as animals above 15 kg and observed hyperinsulinaemia, reduced glucose tolerance, hyperlipidaemia and high plasma cholesterol in the majority of animals, and overt diabetes in two. They subsequently reported on the stages of development of diabetes mellitus (Hamilton & Ciaccia, 1978). The syndrome of spontaneous obesity in rhesus monkeys has since been studied by Jen *et al.* (1985) and Kemnitz & Francken (1986). Spontaneous obesity has also been reported in several other species of macaques (Kemnitz, 1984). According to Hamilton *et al.* (1976) animals that develop obesity tend to eat more earlier in life than those which remain lean in adulthood, but the data for food intake over a 28-week period (Hamilton, 1972) showed quite large differences in intake of animals of similar weight and weight gain.

These animals obviously represent an interesting model of one type of human obesity and the painstaking long-term studies which have been, and no doubt will continue to be, conducted provide an unique opportunity to study the development of the disease in conjunction with accurate measurements of food intake and various metabolic parameters.

Diet-induced obesity

Three recent papers have described the induction of obesity in three different species of monkey by different dietary means. Ausman *et al.* (1981) fed semipurified diets containing 20–30% of energy as fat and 25–35% energy as sucrose to squirrel monkeys (*Saimiri sciureus*) and cebus monkeys (*Cebus albifrons*). Infants were hand-reared on liquid semipurified diets and transferred to the experimental diets at between 5 and 12 months of age. No differences in body weight were observed between experimental and normal animals until around 3 years of age. Those changed from the high-fat/sucrose diet to chow at 2 years of age maintained adult weights similar to control animals in the breeding colony whilst those maintained on the experimental diets continued to gain weight. Those which survived to six years of age were almost double the weight of controls. Carcass analysis revealed that lean body mass was increased by 35 and 50% respectively in obese males and females and that the weight of fat was increased six-fold in males and nine-fold in females. Calculations based on the regression of weight change on energy intake suggest that the efficiency of utilization of energy for gain was at least 75%. During static obesity the energy intake of animals, 80% overweight, was approximately 20% higher than for controls, but maintenance requirement per unit metabolic body size was only 76% of that in lean animals.

In contrast, neither males nor females of the *C. albifrons* spp. showed any tendency for excess weight gain during similar longitudinal studies.

Wene *et al.* (1982) identified flavour preferences in baboons (*Papio sp*) and when preferred flavours were offered over a nine-week period, intake was increased by up to 30% over base-line values. The weight increases recorded suggested a high efficiency of conversion of the excess intake to body tissue.

The report of Jen & Hansen (1984) is of interest in terms of the role of the stomach and gastrointestinal system in satiety. Rhesus monkeys fitted with intragastric cannulae were fed between 100 and 165% of base-line oral intake for periods between 50 and 130 d. Excess voluntary consumption averaged 19% with 100% infusion and 5% with 125% infusion and it took subjects up to one week to reduce voluntary intake to these levels following a change in gastric load. Gross obesity was induced, with one animal reaching 67% overweight in 100 d. After withdrawal of intragastric infusion, low intakes and rapid weight loss occurred. There was considerable individual variation but the stabilized post-obese weight averaged 14% above that of the pre-experimental period. In one animal infusion was gradually reduced and weight stability coupled with initiation of oral consumption occurred at approximately 110% of the pre-experimental intake.

All of these results indicate the potential value of non-human primates as models of diet-induced obesity. There is obviously scope for further application of the variety of systems which have been applied to laboratory rodents. In particular there would seem to be a case for studies using varied palatable diets.

Hypothalamic obesity

Hamilton & Brobeck (1964) produced lesions in the VMH of rhesus monkeys. Within 36 h of the operation, marked hyperphagia and behavioural changes occurred and rapid weight gain was observed over a period of months or years. Based on subjective assessment the animals were judged to have become less active. In contrast to the rat model, lesioned monkeys were highly motivated to obtain food in difficult situations. Food intake during static obesity was lower than during the dynamic phase but was well above the pre-operation levels. Hamilton *et al.* (1972) observed similar metabolic changes in lesioned rhesus monkeys to those seen in animals with spontaneous obesity.

Conclusions

Whilst this chapter falls far short of a comprehensive study of animal models of obesity, it is the author's hope that some of the objectives established in the introduction have been achieved. There can be no doubt that animal models have contributed immensely to our understanding of the complexities of mammalian metabolism in relation to energy balance and obesity no less than in many other aspects of physiological control of body functions. However, it is important to remember, in the immortal words of Edholm (1973), that 'man is not a rat' and it is the responsibility of those who use animal models to ensure that differences between the model and the man should be minimized, and, if recognized, the implications understood. The important interactions of diet, gender, age, temperature and activity have been high-lighted and the main theme of this paper is encapsulated in the statement of Adolph (1982): 'An organism is an integrated system by virtue of the fact that none of its properties is entirely uncorrelated, but that most are demonstrably interlinked; not just by single chains, but by a greater number of criss-crossed linkages'; and that of Pitts (1984): 'The simultaneous study of multiple interacting variables is the next appropriate step in this field of research'.

The results obtained with non-human primates suggest that despite the obvious experimental difficulties involved, relative to laboratory rodents, these offer potential for fruitful multifactorial studies provided that appropriate multidisciplinary teams can be developed to fully exploit the opportunities presented. Although models other than rodents and monkeys have largely been ignored in this paper there may well be a role for these. In particular the miniature pig, which has been widely used as a model of other diseases in man, may, by virtue of its similar size and similarities in digestive function, prove to be a useful model of obesity. The normally high appetite and predisposition to obesity of the pig may be of use in tests of drugs to prevent or reduce obesity. It is concluded that animal models may, with careful management, make a major contribution to our further understanding of obesity.

References

Adolph, E. F. (1982): Physiological integrations in action. *Physiologist* **25**, Suppl., 1–67.
Allen, R. J. L. & Leahy, J. S. (1966): Some effects of dietary dextrose, fructose, liquid glucose and sucrose in the adult male rat. *Br. J. Nutr.* **20**, 339–347.
Applegate, E. A., Upton, D. E. & Stern, J. S. (1982): Food intake, body composition and blood lipids following treadmill exercise in male and female rats. *Physiol. Behav.* **28**, 917–920.
Arch, J. R. S. & Ainsworth, A. T. (1983). Thermogenic and anti-obesity activity of a novel β-adrenoreceptor agonist (BRL 26830A) in mice and rats. *Am. J. Clin. Nutr.* **38**, 549–558.
Aubert, R., Herzog, J., Camus, M. C., Guenet, J. L. & Lemmonier, D. (1985): Description of a new model of genetic obesity: the db^{Pas} mouse. *J. Nutr.* **115**, 327–333.
Ausman, L. M., Rasmussen, K. M. & Gallina, D. L. (1981): Spontaneous obesity in maturing squirrel monkeys fed semipurified diets. *Am. J. Physiol.* **241**, R316–R321.
Baecke, J. A. H., Van Staveren, W. A., Burema, J. (1983): Food consumption, habitual physical activity and body fatness in young Dutch adults. *Am. J. Chem. Nutr.* **37**, 278–286.
Baile, C. A., McLaughlin, C. L. & Della-Fera, M. A. (1986): Role of cholecystokinin and opioid peptides in control of food intake. *Physiol. Rev.* **66**, 172–234.
Barr, H. G. (1984): Factors influencing food intake and energy balance in the laboratory rat. PhD thesis, The Queen's University of Belfast.
Barr, H. G. & McCracken, K. J. (1985): High efficiency of energy utilization in 'cafeteria'- and force-fed rats kept at 29°C. *Br. J. Nutr.* **51**, 379–387.
Bell, F. R. (1971): Hypothalamic control of food intake. *Proc. Nutr. Soc.* **30**, 103–109.
Beaudoin, R. & Mayer, J. (1953): Food intake of obese and non-obese women. *J. Am. Diet. Ass.* **29**, 29–33.
Blaza, S. & Garrow, J. S. (1983): Thermogenic response to temperature, exercise and food stimulae in lean and obese women, studied by 24-hour direct calorimetry. *Br. J. Nutr.* **49**, 171–180.
Boissoneault, G. A., Hornshuh, M. J., Simons, J. W., Romsos, D. R. & Leveille, G. A. (1978): Oxygen consumption and body fat content of young, lean and obese (ob/ob) mice. *Proc. Soc. Exptl. Biol. Med.* **157**, 402–406.
Bray, G. A. (1978): Endocrine factors in the modulation of food intake. *Proc. Nutr. Soc.* **37**, 301–309.
Bray, G. A. (1986): Autonomic and endocrine factors in the regulation of energy balance. *Fed. Proc.* **45**, 1404–1410.
Bray, G. A., Inoue, S. & Nishizawa, Y. (1981): Hypothalamic obesity: the autonomic hypothesis and the lateral hypothalamus. *Diabetol.* **20**, 366–377.
Bray, G. A., Schwartz, M., Rozin, R. & Lister, J. (1970): Relationship between oxygen consumption and body composition of obese patients. *Metabolism* **19**, 418–429.
Bray, G. A. & York, D. A. (1979): Hypothalamic and genetic obesity in experimental animals: an autonomic and endocrine hypothesis. *Physiol. Rev.* **59**, 719–809.
Bruce, B. K., King, B. M., Phelps, G. R. & Veitia, M. C. (1982): Effects of adrenalectomy and corticosterone administration on hypothalamic obesity in rats. *Am. J. Physiol.* **243**, E152–157.
Castonguay, T. W. & Collier, G. H. (1986): Diet balancing: some limitations. *Nutr. Behav.* **3**, 43–55.
Chow, B. F. & Lee, C. J. (1964): Effect of dietary restriction of pregnant rats on body weight gain of the offspring. *J. Nutr.* **82**, 10–18.
Cohn, C. & Joseph, D. (1959): Changes in body composition attendant on force-feeding. *Am. J. Physiol.* **196**, 965–968.
Cohn, C. & Joseph, D. (1963): Feeding frequency and protein metabolism. *Am. J. Physiol.* **205**, 71–78.
Cohn, C. & Joseph, D. (1970): Effects of caloric intake and feeding frequency on carbohydrate metabolism of the rat. *J. Nutr.* **100**, 78–84.
Cohn, C., Schrago, E. & Joseph, D. (1955): Effect of food administration on weight gains and body composition of normal and adrenalectomised rats. *Am. J. Physiol.* **180**, 503–507.
Coleman, D. L. (1978): Genetics of obesity in rodents. In *Recent advances in obesity research* II., ed G. A. Bray, pp. 142–152. London: Newman Publishing.
Corbett, S. W., Stern, J. S. & Keesey, R. E. (1986): Energy expenditure in rats with diet-induced obesity. *Am. J. Clin. Nutr.* **44**, 173–180.
Crews, E. L., Fuge, K. W., Oscai, L. B., Holloszy, J. O. & Shank, R. E. (1969): Weight, food intake and body composition: effect of exercise and of protein deficiency. *Am. J. Physiol.* **216**, 359–363.

Czajka-Narins, D. M. & Hirsch, J. (1974): Supplementary feeding during the preweaning period. *Biol. Neonate.* **25**, 176–185.
Danforth, C. H. (1924): Adiposity and doubling as constituent traits in the mouse. *Anat. Record.* **29**, 354.
Danforth, C. H. (1927): Hereditary adiposity in mice. *J. Hered.* **18**, 153–162.
De Boer, J. O. (1985): Energy requirements of lean and overweight women assessed by indirect calorimetry. PhD thesis, Wageningen.
Debons, A. F., Tse, C. S., Zurek, L. D., Abrahamsen, S. & Maayan, L. A. (1986): Adrenalectomy-induced anorexia in gold thioglucose-induced obese mice: metabolic and hormonal changes. *Physiol. Behav.* **38**, 111–117.
DHSS/MRC (1976): *Research on obesity*, ed W. P. T. James. London: HMSO.
Drenick, E. J. & Johnson, D. (1978): Weight reduction by fasting and semi-starvation in morbid obesity: long-term follow-up. *Int. J. Obesity* **2**, 123–132.
Drenowski, A., Cohen, A. E., Faust, J. M. & Grinker, J. A. (1984): Meal-taking behaviour is related to pre-disposition to dietary obesity in the rat. *Physiol. Behav.* **32**, 61–67.
Dwyer, J. T. & Berman, E. M. (1978): Battling the bulge: a continuing struggle. Two year follow-up of successful losers in a commercial dieting concern. In *Recent advances in obesity research* II, ed G. A. Bray, pp. 227–294. London: Newman Publishing.
Edholm, O. G. (1973): Energy expenditure and food intake. In *Regulation de l'equilibre energetique chez l'homme*, ed M. Apfebaum, pp. 51–60. Paris: Masson.
Eisen, E. J. (1975): Population size and selection intensity effects on long-term selection response in mice. *Genetics* **79**, 305–323.
Fletcher, J. M. (1986): Effects on growth and endocrine status of maintaining obese and lean Zucker rats at 22°C and 30°C from weaning. *Physiol. Behav.* **37**, 597–602.
Foch, T. T. & McClean, G. E. (1980): Genetics, body weight and obesity. In *Obesity*, ed A. J. Stunkard, pp. 48–71. Philadelphia: W. B. Saunders.
Frohman, L. A. (1978): The syndrome of hypothalamic obesity. In *Recent advances in obesity research II* ed G. A. Bray, pp. 133–141. London: Newman Publishing.
Gale, S. K., Van Itallie, T. B. & Faust, I. M. (1981): Effects of palatable diets on body weight and adipose tissue cellularity in the adult obese female Zucker rat (fa/fa). *Metabolism* **30**, 105–110.
Garrow, J. S. (1974): *Energy balance and obesity in man*. New York: North Holland/American Elsevier.
Garrow, J. S. (1981): *Treat obesity seriously*. Edinburgh: Churchill Livingstone.
Grogan, C. K., Kim, H. K. & Romsos, D. R. (1987): Effects of adrenalectomy on energy balance in obese (ob/ob) mice fed high carbohydrate or high fat diets. *J. Nutr.* **117**, 1115–1120.
Hallfrisch, J., Cohen, L. & Reiser, S. (1981): Effects of feeding rats sucrose in a high fat diet. *J. Nutr.* **111**, 531–536.
Hamilton, C. L. (1972): Long term control of food intake in the monkey. *Physiol. Behav.* **9**, 1–6.
Hamilton, C. L. & Brobeck, J. R. (1964): Hypothalamic hyperphagia in the monkey. *J. Comp. Physiol. Psychol.* **57**, 271–278.
Hamilton, C. L. & Ciaccia, P. J. (1978): The course of development of glucose intolerance in the monkey (*Macaca mulatta*). *J. Med. Primatol.* **7**, 165–173.
Hamilton, C. L., Ciaccia, P. J. & Lewis, D. O. (1976): Feeding behaviour in monkeys with and without lesions of the hypothalamus. *Am. J. Physiol.* **230**, 818–830.
Hamilton, C. L., Kuo, P. T. & Feng, L. Y. (1972): Experimental production of syndrome of obesity, hyperinsulinaemia and hyperlipidemia in monkeys. *Proc. Soc. Expt. Biol. Med.* **140**, 1005–1008.
Hansen, B. C., Jen, K. L. & Kribbs, P. (1981): Regulation of food intake in monkeys: response to caloric dilution. *Physiol. Behav.* **26**, 479–486.
Hansen, C. T. (1983): Two new congenic rat strains for nutrition and obesity research. *Fed. Proc.* **42**, 537.
Harrington, M. E. & Coscina, D. V. (1983): Early weight gain and behavioural responsibility as predictors of dietary obesity in rats. *Physiol. Behav.* **30**, 763–770.
Hervey, G. R. (1971): Physiological mechanisms for the regulation of energy balance. *Proc. Nutr. Soc.* **30**, 109–116.
Hervey, G. R. & Tobin, G. (1983): Luxuskonsumption, diet-induced thermogenesis and brown fat: a critical review. *Clin. Sci.* **64**, 7–18.
Hetherington, A. W. and Ranson, S. W. (1940): Hypothalamic lesions and adiposity in the rat. *Anat. Rec.* **78**, 149–172.
Hill, W., Castonguay, T. W. & Collier, G. H. (1980): Taste or diet balancing? *Physiol. Behav.* **24**, 765–767.

Himms-Hagen, J. (1983): Brown adipose tissue thermogenesis in obese animals. *Nutr. Revs.* **41**, 261–267.

Horton, E. S. (1983): Introduction: an overview of the assessment and regulation of energy balance in humans. *Am. J. Clin. Nutr.* **38**, 972–977.

Ikeda, H., Shimakawa, K., Kito, G., Meguro, K., & Matsuo, T. (1986): The anti-obesity action of (S)-(+)-1-(4-chlorophenylthiomethyl)-N-methylethylamine fumarate (AO-124): *Eur. J. Pharmacol.* **125**, 201–210.

Ingalls, A. M., Dickie, M. M. & Snell, G. D. (1950): Obese, a new mutation in the house mouse. *J. Hered.* **41**, 317–318.

Irsigler, K., Veitl, V., Sigmund, A., Tschegg, E. & Kunz, K. (1979): Calorimetric results in man: energy output in normal and overweight subjects. *Metabolism* **28**, 1127–1132.

Jagot, S. A., Webb, G. P., Rogers, P. D. & Dickerson, J. W. T. (1980): The induction of obesity in the rat with bipiperidyl mustard. *Br. J. Nutr.* **44**, 253–255.

Jeanrenaud, B. (1978): An overview of experimental models of obesity. In *Recent advances in obesity research II*, ed G. A. Bray, pp. 111–122. London: Newman Publishers.

Jen, K. L. C. & Hansen, B. C. (1984): Feeding behaviour during experimentally induced obesity in monkeys. *Physiol. Behav.* **33**, 863–869.

Jen, K. L. C., Hansen, B. C. & Metzger, B. L. (1985): Adiposity, anthropometric measures and plasma insulin levels of rhesus monkeys. *Int. J. Obesity* **9**, 213–224.

Jones, A. P., Assimon, S. A. & Friedman, M. J. (1986): The effect of diet on food intake and adiposity in rats made obese by gestational undernutrition. *Physiol. Behav.* **37**, 381–386.

Jones, A. P., Simpson, E. & Friedman, M. I. (1984): Gestational undernutrition and the development of obesity in rats. *J. Nutr.* **114**, 1484–1492.

Kapatos, G. & Gold, M. R. (1973): Evidence for ascending noradrenergic mediation of hypothalamic hyperphagia. *Pharmacol. Biochem. Behav.* **1**, 81–88.

Kemnitz, J. W. (1984): Obesity in macaques: Spontaneous and induced. In *Advances in veterinary science and comparative medicine*, ed A. G. Hendrickx, C. E. Cornelius and C. F. Simpson, pp. 81–114. Academic Press: Orlando, Florida.

Kemnitz, J. W. & Francken, G. A. (1986): Characteristics of spontaneous obesity in male rhesus monkeys. *Physiol. Behav.* **38**, 477–483.

Kennedy, G. C. (1961): The central nervous regulation of caloric balance. *Proc. Nutr. Soc.* **20**, 58–64.

Koletsky, S. (1973): Obese spontaneously hypertensive rats — a model for study of atherosclerosis. *Expt. Mol. Pathol.* **19**, 53–60.

Kromhout, D. (1983): Energy and macronutrient intake in lean and obese middle-aged men (the Zutphen Study): *Am. J. Clin. Nutr.* **37**, 295–299.

Leblanc, T., Cabanac, M. & Samson, P. (1984): Reduced post-prandial heat production with gavage as compared with meal-feeding in human subjects. *Am. J. Physiol.* **246**, E95–E101.

Le Magnen, J. (1983): Body energy balance and food intake: a neuroendocrine regulatory mechanism. *Physiol. Rev.* **63**, 314–385.

Levin, B. E., Triscari, J. & Sullivan, A. C. (1986): Metabolic features of diet-induced obesity without hyperphagia in young rats. *Am. J. Physiol.* **251**, R433–R440.

Lin, P. Y., Romsos, D. R. & Leveille, G. A. (1977): Food intake, bodyweight gain and body composition of the young obese (ob/ob) mouse. *J. Nutr.* **107**, 1715–1723.

Louis-Sylvestre, J., Giachetti, J. & Le Magnen, J. (1984): Sensory versus dietary factors in cafeteria-induced overweight. *Physiol. Behav.* **32**, 901–905.

McCance, R. A. (1972): The composition of the body: its maintenance and regulation. *Nutr. Revs.* **42**, 1269–1279.

McCracken, K. J. (1975): The effect of feeding pattern and protein intake on energy metabolism of rats. *Br. J. Nutr.* **33**, 277–289.

McCracken, K. J. & McNiven, M. A. (1983): Effects of overfeeding by gastric intubation on body composition of adult female rats and on heat production during feeding and fasting. *Br. J. Nutr.* **49**, 193–202.

McHugh, P. R. & Moran, T. H. (1978): Accuracy of the regulation of caloric ingestion in the rhesus monkey. *Am. J. Physiol.* **235**, R29–R34.

McNiven, M. A. (1984): The effect of body fatness on energetic efficiency and fasting heat production in adult sheep. *Br. J. Nutr.* **51**, 297–304.

Mayer, J. (1953): Genetic, traumatic and environmental factors in the etiology of obesity. *Physiol. Rev.* **33**, 472–508.

Mayer, J., Marshall, N. B., Vitale, J. J., Christensen, J. H., Mashayekhi, M. B. & Store, F. J. (1954): Exercise, food intake and body weight in normal rats and genetically obese mice. *Am. J. Physiol.* **177**, 544–548.

Mayer, J. & Thomas, D. W. (1967): Regulation of food intake and obesity. *Science*, **156**, 328–337.

Michaelis, D. E., Ellwood, K. C., Hallfrisch, J. & Hansen, C. T. (1983): Effect of dietary sucrose and genotype on metabolic parameters on a new strain of genetically obese rat: LA/N-corpulent. *Nutr. Res.* **3**, 217–228.

Michaelis, D. E., Ellwood, K. C., Tulp, O. L. & Greenwood, M. R. C. (1986): Effect of feeding sucrose or starch diets on parameters of glucose tolerance in the LA/N corpulent rat. *Nutr. Res.* **6**, 95–99.

Michelsen, O., Takahashi, S. & Craig, C. (1955): Experimental obesity 1. Production of obesity in rats by feeding a high fat diet. *J. Nutr.* **57**, 541–554.

Miller, D. S. & Payne, P. R. (1962): Weight maintenance and food intake. *J. Nutr.* **78**, 255–262.

Moore, B. J. (1987): The cafeteria diet—an inappropriate tool for studies of thermogenesis. *J. Nutr.* **117**, 227–231.

Newburgh, L. H. (1944): Obesity 1. Energy metabolism. *Physiol. Rev.* **24**, 18–31.

Olney, J. W. (1969): Brain lesions, obesity and other disturbances in mice treated with monosodium glutamate. *Science* **16**, 719–721.

Oscai, L. B. (1982): Dietary-induced severe obesity: a rat model. *Am. J. Physiol.* **242**, R212–R215.

Oscai, L. B., Brown, M. M. & Miller, W. C. (1984): Effect of dietary fat on food intake, growth and body composition in rats. *Growth* **48**, 415–424.

Pearce, J. (1983): Fatty acid synthesis in liver and adipose tissue. *Proc. Nutr. Soc.* **42**, 263–271.

Pitts, G. C. (1984): Body composition in the rat: interactions of exercise, age, sex and diet. *Am. J. Physiol.* **246**, R495–R501.

Pitts, G. C. & Bull, L. S. (1977): Exercise, dietary obesity and growth in the rat. *Am. J. Physiol.* **232**, R38–R44.

Powley, T. L. & Opsahl, C. A. (1974): Ventromedial hypothalamic obesity abolished by subdiaphragmatic vagotomy. *Am. J. Physiol.* **226**, 25–33.

Rattigan, S. & Clark, M. G. (1984): Effect of sucrose solution drinking option on the development of obesity in rats. *J. Nutr.* **114**, 1971–1977.

Ravussin, E., Burnand, B., Schutz, Y. & Jéquier, E. (1982): Twenty-four-hour energy expenditure and resting metabolic rate in obese, moderately obese and control subjects. *Am. J. Clin. Nutr.* **35**, 566–573.

Ring, G. C., Bosch, M. & Lo, C. S. (1970): Effects of exercise on growth, resting metabolism and body composition of Fischer rats. *Proc. Soc. Exp. Biol. Med.* **133**, 1162–1165.

Robeson, B. C., Eisen, E. J. & Leatherwood, J. M. (1981): Adipose cellularity, serum glucose, insulin and cholesterol in polygenic obese mice fed high-fat or high-carbohydrate diets. *Growth* **45**, 198–215.

Rogers, P. J. & Blundell, J. E. (1984): Meal patterns and food selection during the development of obesity in rats fed cafeteria diets. *Neurosci. Behav. Rev.* **8**, 441–453.

Rolls, B. J. & Rowe, E. A. (1979): Exercise and the development and persistence of dietary obesity in male and female rats. *Physiol. Behav.* **23**, 241–247.

Rolls, B. J., Rowe, E. A. & Turner, R. C. (1980): Persistent obesity in rats following a period of consumption of a mixed, high energy diet, *J. Physiol.* **298**, 15–427.

Rolls, B. J., van Duijvenvorde, P. M. & Rowe, E. A. (1983): Variety in the diet enhances intake in a meal and contributes to the development of obesity in the rat. *Physiol. Behav.* **31**, 21–27.

Rothwell, N. J. & Stock, M. J. (1979a): Regulation of energy balance in two models of reversible obesity in the rat. *J. Comp. Physiol. Psychol.* **93**, 1024–1034.

Rothwell, N. J. & Stock, M. J. (1979b): A role for brown adipose tissue in diet-induced thermogenesis. *Nature* **281**, 31–35.

Rothwell, N. J. & Stock, M. J. (1983): Luxuskonsumption, diet-induced thermogenesis and brown fat: the case in favour. *Clin. Sci.* **64**, 19–23.

Rothwell, N. J. & Stock, M. J. (1986): Influence of environmental temperature on energy balance, diet-induced thermogenesis and brown fat activity in 'cafeteria'-fed rats. *Br. J. Nutr.* **56**, 123–129.

Rowe, E. A. & Rolls, B. J. (1981): Effects of environmental temperature on dietary obesity and growth in rats. *Physiol. Behav.* **28**, 218–226.

Saito, M. & Bray, G. A. (1984): Adrenalectomy and food restriction in the genetically obese (ob/ob) mouse. *Am. J. Physiol.* **246**, R20–R25.

Schemmel, R., Mickelsen, O. & Tolgay, Z. (1969): Dietary obesity in rats: influence of diet, weight, age and sex on body composition. *Am. J. Physiol.* **216**, 373–379.

Schemmel, R., Mickelsen, O. & Gill, J. L. (1970): Dietary obesity in rats: body weight and body fat accretion in seven strains of rats. *J. Nutr.* **100**, 1041–1048.

Schutz, Y., Bessard, T. & Jéquier, E. (1984): Diet-induced thermogenesis measured over a whole day in obese and non-obese women. *Am. J. Clin. Nutr.* **40**, 542–552.

Sclafani, A. (1978): Dietary obesity. In *Recent advances in obesity research II* ed G. A. Bray, pp. 123–132. London: Newman Publishing.

Sclafani, A. (1981): The role of hyperinsulinaemia and the vagus nerve in hypothalamic hyperphagia re-examined. *Diabetol.* **20**, 402–410.

Sclafani, A. (1987): Carbohydrate, taste, appetite and obesity: an overview. *Neurosci. Behav. Rev.* **11**, 131–153.

Sclafani, A., Aravich, P. F. & Landmann, M. (1981): Vagotomy blocks hypothalamic hyperphagia in rats on a chow diet and sucrose solutions but not on a palatable mixed diet. *J. Comp. Physiol. Psychol.* **95**, 720–734.

Sclafani, A. & Berner, C. N. (1977): Hyperphagia and obesity produced by parasagittal and coronal hypothalamic knife-cuts: further evidence for a longitudinal feeding inhibitory pathway. *J. Comp. Physiol. Psychol.* **91**, 1000–1018.

Sclafani, A. & Gorman, A. N. (1977): Effects of age, sex and prior body weight on the development of dietary obesity in adult rats. *Physiol. Behav.* **18**, 1021–1026.

Sclafani, A., Koopmans, H. S. & Appelbaum, K. A. (1980): Hypothalamic hyperphagia and obesity in rats with jejunoileal bypass. *Am. J. Physiol.* **239**, G387–G394.

Sclafani, A. & Springer, D. (1976): Dietary obesity in adult rats. Similarities to hypothalamic and human obesity syndromes. *Physiol. Behav.* **17**, 461–471.

Sclafani, A. & Xenakis, S. (1984): Sucrose and polysaccharide induced obesity in the rat. *Physiol. Behav.* **32**, 169–174.

Segal, K. R. & Gutin, B. (1983): Thermic effects of food and exercise in lean and obese women. *Metabolism* **32**, 581–589.

Shizamu, T., Noma, M. & Saito, M. (1986): Chronic infusions of norepinephrine into the ventromedial hypothalamus induce obesity in rats. *Brain. Res.* **369**, 215–223.

Sims, E. A. H., Goldman, R. F., Glick, C. M., Horton, E. S., Kelleher, P. C. & Rowe, D. W. (1968): Experimental obesity in man. *Trans. Assoc. Am. Phycns.* **81**, 153–170.

Slattery, J. M. & Potter, R. M. (1985): Hyperphagia: a necessary precondition to obesity? *Appetite* **6**, 133–142.

Smith, C. J. V. & Britt, D. C. (1971): Obesity in the rat induced by hypothalamic implants of gold thioglucose. *Physiol. Behav.* **7**, 7–10.

Smith, C. K. & Romsos, D. R. (1985): Effects of adrenalectomy on energy balance of obese mice are diet dependent. *Am. J. Physiol.* **249**, R13–R22.

Spitzer, L. & Rodin, J. (1981): Human eating behaviour: a critical review of studies in normal weight and overweight individuals. *Appetite* **2**, 293–329.

Stanley, B. G., Kyrkouli, S. E., Lampert, S. & Leibowitz, S. F. (1986): Neuropeptide Y chronically injected into the hypothalmus: a powerful neurochemical inducer of hyperphagia and obesity. *Peptides* **7**, 1189–1192.

Stephens, D. N. (1980): Growth and development of dietary obesity in adulthood of rats which have been undernourished during development. *Br. J. Nutr.* **44**, 215–227.

Stevenson, J. A. F., Box, B. M., Feleki, V. & Beaton, J. R. (1966): Bouts of exercise and food intake in the rat. *J. Appl. Physiol.* **21**, 118–122.

Swift, R. W. (1944): The effect of feed on the critical temperature of the albino rat. *J. Nutr.* **28**, 359–364.

Thomson, A. M., Billewicz, W. Z. & Passmore, R. (1961): The relation between caloric intake and body weight in man. *Lancet* **1**, 1027–1028.

Thurlby, P. L. & Trayhurn, P. (1978): The development of obesity in preweanling obob mice. *Br. J. Nutr.* **39**, 397–402.

Tulp, O. L. (1984): Impaired activation of thermogenesis in the corpulent rat. *Life Sci.* **35**, 1699–1704.

Tulp, O. L. & Buck, C. L. (1986): Caffeine and ephedrine stimulated thermogenesis in LA-corpulent rats. *Comp. Biochem. Physiol.* **85C**, 17–19.

Tulp, O. L., Hansen, C. T. & Michaelis, O. E. (1986): Nonshivering thermogenesis in the diabetic SHR/N-cp (corpulent) rat. *Physiol. Behav.* **36**, 127–131.
Tulp, O. L. & Jones, C. T. (1987): Effects of increased energy expenditure on weight gain and adiposity in the LA-corpulent rat. *Comp. Biochem. Physiol.* **86A**, 67–72.
Tulp, O. L. & McKee, T. D. (1986): Triiodothyronine (T3) neogenesis in lean and obese LA/N-cp rats. *Biochem. Biophys. Res. Comm.* **1440**, 134–142.
Tulp, O. L. & Shields, S. J. (1984): Thermogenesis in cafeteria-fed LA/N-cp (corpulent) rats. *Nutr. Res.* **4**, 325–332.
Van Es, A. J. H., Vogt, J. E., Niessen, C. H., Veth, J., Rodenburg, L., Teeuwse, V., Dhyvetter, J., Deurenberg, P., Hautvast, J. G. A. J. & Van der Beek, E. (1984): Human energy metabolism below, near and above energy equilibrium. *Br. J. Nutr.* **52**, 429–442.
Vander Tuig, T. G., Romsos, D. R. & Leveille, G. A. (1980): Changes in body composition of adult obese (ob/ob) and lean mice fed restricted levels of diets high in carbohydrate, fat or protein. *Int. J. Obesity* **4**, 79–85.
Waxler, H. & Brecher, G. (1950): Obesity and food requirements in albino mice following administration of goldthioglucose. *Am. J. Physiol.* **162**, 428–433.
Webb, P. & Annis, J. F. (1983): Adaptation of overeating in lean and overweight men and women. *Hum. Nutr: Clin. Nutr.* **37C**, 117–131.
Wene, J. D., Barnwell, G. M. & Mitchell, D. S. (1982): Flavour preferences, food intake, and weight gain in baboons (*Papio sp.*). *Physiol. Behav.* **28**, 569–573.
West, D. B., Diaz, J. & Woods, S. C. (1982): Infant gastrostomy and chronic formula infusion as a technique to overfeed and accelerate weight gain of neonatal rats. *J. Nutr.* **112**, 1339–1343.
Widdowson, E. M. (1962): Nutritional individuality. *Proc. Nutr. Soc.* **21**, 121–128.
Widdowson, E. M. & McCance, R. A. (1960): Some effects of accelerating growth. 1. General somatic development. *Proc. Roy. Soc.* **B152**, 188–206.
York, D. A. & Bray, G. A. (1972): Dependence of hypothalamic obesity on insulin, the pituitary and the adrenal gland. *Endocrinol.* **90**, 885–894.
Zucker, L. M. & Zucker, T. F. (1961): Fatty, a new mutation in the rat. *J. Hered.* **52**, 275–278.

* * * * *

Discussion

Dr York felt that the speaker had not sufficiently emphasized the advantages of the animal model. These models could be used to identify the causes of obesity and to describe the metabolic and physiological changes which are secondary to the developing obesity. Virtually all our understanding of these aspects of obesity has come initially from studies on animal obesities. An example of this has been our understanding of insulin resistance. In obesity it has been shown to be secondary to the hypersecretion of insulin and the mechanisms through which insulin resistance develop have been demonstrated. In addition, these animal models have made a great contribution to our understanding of the central mechanisms regulating energy balance and have shown the close integration between the regulation of food intake and the regulation of the metabolic responses to feeding through the autonomic nervous system. Criticism of the animal models on the basis of their normal high carbohydrate diet, as opposed to the high fat diet of man, seems unwarranted since virtually all the studies have shown the obesities to be exaggerated by feeding high fat diets. Certainly without the animal models, our understanding of obesity would be extremely limited.

Professor Kritchevsky suggested that the laboratory rat was in fact an 'obese' rat. He drew attention to the different effects of restriction of energy intake on body composition of the normal and LA/N corpulent rat. Whereas the lean body mass was conserved at the expense of fat in the normal rat this did not happen in the LA/N corpulent. *McCracken* agreed that compared with animals in the wild the sedentary laboratory rat could be regarded as 'obese' but drew attention to the effects of exercise in the paper of Pitts (1984).

Professor Webster raised the question of whether the study of energy metabolism in rats should be made only at thermoneutrality. He felt that at 30°C the rats were close to the upper limit at which they could control their body temperature and he suggested that, contrary to the recommendation that studies be conducted at temperatures only within the narrow thermoneutral zone, temperature should be included as an experimental variable. *McCracken* responded to this by pointing out that the thermoneutral zone for the rat was approximately 28–33°C [Swift (1944)] rather similar to that of naked man consuming a maintenance intake. Hence studies at 29 or 30° were well within the comfort zone and therefore equivalent to the conditions man prefers for himself. However he agreed that useful information could be obtained from the factorial approach, as had been demonstrated in the study of Fletcher (1986).

Dr Prentice questioned the suitability of the arboreal species of monkeys as a model since he understood that the excess fat is enteroabdominal and not subcutaneous. *McCracken* replied that as far as he was aware the distribution of fat in the rhesus and squirrel monkeys was similar to that observed in the obese human.

Mr Payne commented that one of Dr McCracken's objections to the rat as a model for obesity in the human was that the rat is a 'nibbler' rather than a meal eater. He asked if Dr McCracken could suggest what would be an appropriate pattern of feeding in an animal as small as a rat, which could be accepted as equivalent to man. The allometric principles outlined earlier by *Dr Peters* suggest that meal frequency should be inversely proportional to the fourth root of body weight, which would imply a meal frequency for a rat-sized meal eater of between 20 and 30 meals per day.

13

Atherosclerosis

DAVID KRITCHEVSKY

Introduction

Atherosclerosis is a disease of multiple aetiology. It is a disease for which there is no certain ante-mortem medical diagnosis and thus instead we have statistical diagnosis in the form of risk factors. The three generally accepted major risk factors are elevated blood pressure, elevated plasma cholesterol and cigarette smoking. Recently obesity and diabetes have also been cited as important risk factors. Hopkins & Williams (1981) identified over 200 risks related to atherosclerosis, classifying them as initiators, promoters, potentiators and precipitators.

Adams (1964) presented a flow sheet of the various metabolic relationships possible in human atherosclerosis. In his scheme, intimal thickening held a central position and was shown to interact with mural thrombi, lipid overloading and mechanical stress. Lipid overloading was, in turn, related to lipid synthesis and absorption, which affect plasma lipid levels. Although most discussions of atherosclerosis center on lipidaemia and lipoproteinaemia, it should be noted that there is a number of conditions which can be classified as non-atheromatous ischaemic heart disease (Harrison & Reeves, 1968).

Davignon (1978) has also devised a graphic scheme aimed at explaining all of the interacting factors in atherosclerosis. He divides the scheme into three areas: *ecology* which includes the known risk factors, genetics and other factors including dietary components, stress and viruses; *the circulating blood* which contains hormones, lipoproteins and platelets; and *the arterial wall* itself with its own biochemical, metabolic and structural properties.

The 'natural history' of atherosclerosis has been discussed by Adams (1964) and by Vastesaeger & Delcourt (1962). Adams (1964) reviewed the reports of spontaneous

Table 1. *Characteristics of atheromata*. After Adams (1964).

Distal aorta	*Proximal aorta*	*Fibro fatty lesions*	*Fibrous lesion*
Man	Rabbit	Man	Young rat
Buzzard	Chicken	Reptiles	Old rabbit
Turkey	Pigeon	Chicken	Dog
Dog	Cow	Buzzard	Cat
Cat	Young pig	Turkey	Elephant
Elephant		Pigeon	
Old pig		Young pig	
		Old rat	
		Pig	
		Cow	
		Baboon	
		Monkey	

Table 2. *Characteristics of atherosclerosis in animal species commonly used in atherosclerosis research** (0–4 scale). After Wissler & Vesselinovitch (1974).

Species	*Spontaneous disease*	*Sensitivity to diet*	*Distribution of lesions**	*Small artery involvement*
Rabbit	0.5	4	1	4
Chicken	2	4	0.5	4
Rat	0	1	0.5	3
Pig	1	2	2	2
Squirrel monkey	2	4	3.5	2
Rhesus monkey	0	4	3.5	1

*Compared to men.

atherosclerosis in animals, including snakes, lizards, rats, rabbits, cats, pigs, dogs, sheep, bears, cattle, horses, elephants, primates and wild and domestic fowl. He has also listed the dissimilarities between location and type of human and animal lesions (Table 1). Adams (1964) concluded that intimal thickening of the artery is the initiating factor in human atherosclerosis. Vastesaeger & Delcourt (1962) personally examined the coronary arteries of 146 wild and 403 captive vertebrates and in 134 they also examined the aortas. In their examination they found that atherosclerosis always developed in arteries already showing intimal sclerosis, which they took to be a basic condition for spontaneous atherosclerosis. They concluded: 'spontaneous atherosclerosis may develop in fishes living in their natural habitat, feeding on a diet rich in unsaturated fats; in captive birds whose dietary fats are mostly unsaturated (crane, tree duck, pelican); and in wild mammals whose diet is free of animal fats, in freedom as well as in captivity (deer, camel, tapir).

Wissler & Vesselinovitch (1974) reviewed the characteristics of atherosclerosis in animal species commonly used in atherosclerosis research (Table 2) and found none to be ideal.

The ensuing discussion will be related to atherosclerosis in those species most often used in experimental atherosclerosis research.

Experimental atherosclerosis research

1. Rabbit

The rabbit was the first animal used for the study of atherosclerosis. In the first decade of this century Ignatowski (1908, 1909) was able to induce lesions in weanling rabbits by feeding them milk and eggs, and in adult rabbits by feeding them meat. Ignatowski's hypothesis was that a toxic metabolite of animal protein was the causal agent. Since Ignatowski fed milk, eggs and meat it has often been concluded that their cholesterol content was the real cause of the observed lesions. However, Knack (1915) compared the effects of 0.5–4.5 g of crystalline cholesterol per day with those of a diet containing milk and eggs and providing 300 mg of cholesterol daily. All of the rabbits fed the milk-egg diet exhibited atherosclerosis whereas only one-third (4/12) of those fed the crystalline cholesterol were atherosclerotic. Newburgh and his colleagues (1920, 1922, 1923) showed that rabbits fed meat or casein developed atherosclerosis. The diets used provided only 28–36 mg cholesterol daily. In a later study (Clarkson & Newburgh, 1926) rabbits were fed 25, 113, 253 or 507 mg cholesterol daily and atherosclerosis was found to develop only in those groups fed considerably more cholesterol than was provided by the meat diet.

Anitschkow & Chalatow (1913) and Wacker & Hueck (1913) independently showed that rabbits fed cholesterol developed atherosclerosis and fatty livers. Anitschkow and Chalatow were convinced that a cholesterol-rich diet was sufficient to reproduce the human process, whereas Wacker and Hueck pointed out that the severity of lesions was not correlated with either the duration of feeding or the total amount of ingested cholesterol. These two studies set the stage for decades of research in atherosclerosis and have still eclipsed research on the atherogenic effects of other dietary components.

Normal cholesterol levels of rabbits vary by breed and sex (Wang *et al.*, 1954; Fillios & Mann, 1956; Roberts *et al.*, 1974; De Hoff-Sparks & Kritchevsky, 1982). Rabbits may be hyper- or hypo-responders and the trait may be heritable. Cholesterol-fed rabbits become hypercholesterolaemic within a week or two. Rabbits fed cholesterol with no added fat develop severe atherosclerosis but exhibit relatively low plasma cholesterol levels (Kritchevsky *et al.*, 1961). When saturated fat is present in the diet, it is more cholesterolaemic and atherogenic than unsaturated fat. Thus rabbits fed 2% cholesterol and 6% coconut oil for 8 weeks exhibit serum cholesterol levels and atherosclerosis grade (0–4 severity) of 73.2 mMol/l and 2.70 respectively, whereas the cholesterol level is 49.4 mMol/l and severity of atherosclerosis is 1.45 when 6% corn oil is fed (Kritchevsky, 1970). There are exceptions to the generalization concerning fat saturation and atherosclerosis, however. Peanut oil which has an iodine value of about 90–95 is unexpectedly atherogenic for rats (Gresham & Howard, 1960), rabbits (Kritchevsky *et al.*, 1971), and monkeys (Vesselinovitch *et al.*, 1974; Kritchevsky *et al.*, 1982a). Cocoa butter, on the other hand, with an iodine value of 35, is significantly less atherogenic than either palm kernel oil (iodine value 25), palm oil (iodine value 50) or coconut oil (iodine value 10) (Kritchevsky & Tepper, 1965a; Kritchevsky *et al.*, 1982b). The anamolous behavior of these two fats may be due to the structure of peanut oil and the stearic acid content of cocoa butter, respectively.

The cholesterol-fed rabbit model has been criticized as being an example of a cholesterol storage disease in a herbivore. It is possible to render rabbits hyperlipoproteinaemic and atherogenic by feeding a cholesterol-free, semipurified diet containing saturated fat (Lambert *et al.*, 1958; Malmros & Wigand 1959; Kritchevsky & Tepper, 1965b).

Using the semipurified diet it has been possible to compare effects of other nutrients on atherosclerosis and to show that fructose is more cholesterolemic and atherogenic than other carbohydrates (Kritchevsky *et al.*, 1973b) and that animal protein is more atherogenic than vegetable protein (Kritchevsky *et al.*, 1983). The different effects of animal and vegetable proteins may be due to the ratio of lysine to arginine (Kritchevsky, 1979).

The principal objection to the use of the rabbit as a model for atherosclerosis is its unusual susceptibility to cholesterol feeding, which results in lipid storage in many organs. Even the cholesterol-free model can yield rather high levels of serum cholesterol. Furthermore, the rabbit lesion is an uncomplicated one and hence unlike that of man. Constantinides (1965) reported that he could produce rabbit aortic lesions similar to those of man by a regimen of cholesterol feeding alternating with administration of viosterol and sex hormones. The process takes several years. Wilson *et al.* (1982) produced aortic lesions similar to those seen in man by feeding rabbits one of two semipurified diets in which the major source of fat was either 20% corn oil or 19% butter fat plus 1% corn oil. The diet contained 19.8% of energy as protein (casein), 35.8% as carbohydrate (sucrose) and 44.4% as fat. The feeding period was five years, which places this modality beyond the time scale of the usual grant-supported experiment!

2. *Rat*

The rat, because of its low cost and easy handling would be an ideal model for atherosclerosis research were it not resistant to most standard dietary manipulations. The methods used to promote atherosclerosis in rats involve feeding cholesterol, saturated fat and sodium cholate (Wissler *et al.*, 1954; O'Neal *et al.*, 1961), or saturated fat, cholesterol, cholic acid and thiouracil (Hartroft *et al.*, 1952). Feeding of cholesterol to hypophysectomized rats will produce lesions (Patek *et al.*, 1963), as will feeding saturated fat to rats with essential fatty acid deficiency (Morin *et al.*, 1964). Cholesterol plus high doses of vitamin D_2 has also been found to produce lesions (Aubert *et al.*, 1974).

The requirement for some factor in addition to cholesterol (thiouracil, vitamin D_2 etc) renders these models even less physiological than the cholesterol-fed rabbit. The spontaneously obese, hypertensive rat described by Koletsky (1973) would seem to be an ideal model since it exhibits spontaneous atherosclerosis and a lesion containing some characteristics akin to those of the human lesion, but not much work has been reported since this rat was introduced. One drawback to the use of rats is their small body and artery size.

3. *Dog*

The dog is not a popular model for atherosclerosis research. The dogs' naturally-occurring lesions are sclerotic rather than atheromatous (Lugenbuhl *et al.*, 1965). Dogs can be rendered atherosclerotic by feeding cholesterol, saturated fat and thiouracil

(Steiner & Kendall, 1946; DiLuzio & O'Neal, 1962). When using this regimen it is possible to identify hypo- and hyper-responders (DePalma *et al.*, 1972). When dogs are fed a semipurified diet containing 5% cholesterol and 15–20% coconut oil for about a year they become atherosclerotic (Malmros & Sternby, 1968). The difficulty of establishing lesions in the dog and the expense of maintenance militate against widespread use of this model.

4. *Swine*

The pig would appear to be an ideal model for atherosclerosis research, being omnivorous, having large vessels, being available in purebred lineage, and possessing cardiorespiratory physiology and coronary anatomy similar to those of man. Spontaneous atherosclerosis is seen in pigs and it becomes more severe with age (Gottlieb & Lalich, 1954; Skold & Getty, 1961). Lesions occur in the aorta and in the coronary, iliac and intracranial arteries (Ratcliffe & Luginbuhl, 1971). Atherogenic diets will enhance atherosclerosis in swine (Downie *et al.*, 1963) and if fed long enough will produce myocardial infarction (Lee *et al.*, 1971).

One drawback to using the pig is its large size, unpleasant disposition and the cost of handling. Minipigs are small compared to normal pigs but are still a handful. Atherogenic diets will lead to aortic lesions in minipigs (Mahley *et al.*, 1975) and intimal thickening has also been observed (Stout, 1982). The Yucatan pig is said to be considerably smaller and more docile than other pigs (Reitman *et al.*, 1982) and may become a useful model, but there is virtually no recorded experience with this particular strain.

5. *Avian models*

The principal disadvantage of working with any avian model is that it is not a mammal. Still they have been used to provide data which have been helpful to our understanding of atherosclerosis.

(a) Chickens. Chickens exhibit aortic and coronary artery lesions. Atherosclerosis can be induced or exacerbated in chickens by dietary cholesterol, hypertension or undernutrition. Saturated fat enhances cholesterol-induced atherosclerosis. In a book written in 1953, Katz & Stamler summarized the data relating to experimental atherosclerosis in chickens.

When normocholesterolaemic chickens are infected with a herpes virus (Marek's disease) they develop atherosclerosis (Fabricant *et al.*, 1983). The effects of the virus are magnified when the chickens are fed an atherogenic regimen.

(b) Pigeons. The White Carneau pigeon develops spontaneous atherosclerosis which is similar to that seen in man (Clarkson *et al.*, 1959; Prichard *et al.*, 1962). When fed cholesterol, these pigeons develop more severe and fattier lesions (St. Clair, 1983). Show Racer pigeons have little atherosclerosis and provide a good comparison to the White Carneau for special studies. Wagner *et al.*, (1973) bred a strain of White Carneau pigeon with severe aortic atherosclerosis and a Show Racer with very little atherosclerosis. There are biochemical differences between aortic composition and

aortic metabolism of these two strains (Kritchevsky & Kothari, 1973; Wagner & Nohlgren, 1981). Pigeons are easy and inexpensive to maintain and are long-lived (10–15 years) but their value as a model diminishes because they are not mammals.

(c) Japanese quail. Japanese quail are very susceptible to cholesterol feeding and there has been a report of myocardial infarction in this bird (Ojerio *et al.*, 1972; Shih, 1983). These birds are very small so working with them may be difficult.

6. *Primates*

Non-human primates would seem to be animals of choice for the study of atherosclerosis. They are omnivorous, resemble man in many aspects of cardiovascular and pulmonary physiology and their lesions resemble those of man histologically and in distribution. The disadvantages are difficulty in procurement, expense, and the need for special housing and special handling.

The rhesus monkey (*Macaca mulatta*) has been used most extensively in atherosclerosis research. Although the incidence of spontaneous atherosclerosis is low (Chawla *et al.*, 1967) this strain of monkey can be rendered arteriosclerotic by a pyridoxine-deficient diet (Rinehart & Greenberg, 1951) and atherosclerotic by feeding cholesterol (Mann & Andrus, 1956). The lesions have been described by Taylor *et al.* (1962, 1963a,b), who also described one case of myocardial infarction. In general the severity of atherosclerosis is related to degree of hypercholesterolaemia.

The stumptail macaque (*Macaca arctoides*) is more susceptible to cholesterol-feeding than most other primates (Bullock *et al.*, 1975). They also develop the most severe atherosclerosis and highest tissue cholesterol levels. They tend to become obese with age which adds to their similarity to man, and are also very susceptible to hypertension (Pick *et al.*, 1974). However, there are relatively few of these monkeys in the wild and importation has been banned.

Pigtail macaques (*Macaca nemestrina*) have not been studied extensively as models for atherosclerosis although they do respond to a high cholesterol diet (McMahan *et al.*, 1980).

The squirrel monkey (*Saimiri sciureus*) is a New World monkey which exhibits spontaneous atherosclerosis despite relatively low serum cholesterol levels (Lofland *et al.*, 1967; Middleton *et al.*, 1967; Malinow *et al.*, 1966; McCombs *et al.*, 1969). Clarkson *et al.* (1971) described hyper- and hypo-responding squirrel monkeys and this difference appears to be under genetic control. The disadvantages of using this monkey lie in its small size and an endemic arteritis found in many monkeys caught in the wild (Hayes *et al.*, 1972). Presently, they cannot be imported.

The African green monkey (*Cercopithecus aethiops*) is coming into greater use. On an atherogenic regimen they develop aortic lesions similar to those seen in man (Bullock *et al.*, 1975; Wagner & Clarkson, 1975). When fed cholesterol they exhibit elevated levels of LDL and a lipoprotein profile similar to that seen in humans with Type II A familial hypercholesterolaemia (Rudel, 1980). They are susceptible to hypercholesterolaemia and atherosclerosis when fed semipurified, cholesterol-free diets (Kritchevsky *et al.*, 1977).

Fincham *et al.* (1987) have reported on a long term (47 month) study in which female vervet monkeys were fed a ‘Western’ diet, a ‘prudent’ diet (Table 3),

Table 3. *Characteristics of Chow (HCD), prudent diet (PD) and Western diet (WD).* After Fincham *et al.* (1987).

	Diet		
	HCD	PD	WD
Energy (kcal)	345	245	361
% energy from:			
Saturated fat	1.7	6.4	20.2
Monoene	3.3	7.5	14.9
Polyene	3.3	11.3	6.2
Total lipid	12	29	47
CHO	75	57	39
Protein	14	14	14
Cholesterol (mg/kcal)	Tr	0.8	0.33
Sugar/complex CHO	0/100	0.35	0.35
Animal/vegetable protein	0.3	1.08	2.57
Crude fibre (g)	5.4	5.4	3.0
Ca (mg)	345	82	78
P (mg)	259	140	164

Table 4. *Aortic atherosclerosis in vervet monkeys fed prudent diet (PD), Western diet (WD), or WD then PD.* After Fincham *et al.* (1987).

	Diet		
	PD	WD/PD	WD
Total surface lesion (%)	27.8	22.3	53.2
Surface lipid area (%)	27.4	21.0	43.8
Non-lipid area (%)	0.4	1.3	9.4
Surface lesion score	51.5	37.6	142.8
Lipid staining (score)	80.0	112.0	125.0

PD or WD fed 47 months. WD/PD = WD fed for 20 months then PD for 27 months.

or commercial ration. One group of monkeys were fed the Western diet for 20 months and then placed on the prudent diet for the next 27 months. The data (Table 4) show that switching from Western diet to prudent diet yielded atheromata which were generally similar in nature to those seen in monkeys subsisting on the prudent diet for the duration of the study. A surprising finding was that the prudent diet, which contained virtually no cholesterol, had a polyunsaturated to saturated fatty acid ratio of 1.77 compared to 0.31 for the Western diet, and contained 38% less fat than the Western diet, still led to appreciable atherosclerosis. These data reflect the susceptibility of the vervet monkey and suggest it might be a good model for atherosclerosis in work involving fats and other dietary constituents.

Diets high in cholesterol raise cholesterol levels in spider monkeys (*Ateles geoffroyi*) (Srinivasan *et al.*, 1972) and marmosets (Dreizen *et al.*, 1973).

Jokinen *et al.* (1985) consider the cynomolgus macaque (*Macaca fasicularis*) to be the best monkey model for human atherosclerosis. Their lesions are morphologically similar to those of man, they exhibit a male-female difference in susceptibility and have a relatively high rate of myocardial infarction. Diet-induced lesions have been described by a number of investigators including Kramsch & Hollander (1968); Prathap (1975); Armstrong (1976); and Wagner *et al.*, (1978). Their lipoprotein patterns resemble those of humans (Hamm *et al.*, 1983; Rudel & Pitts, 1978).

Table 5. *Diet and atherosclerosis in baboons*. After Kritchevsky *et al.* (1980).

Regimen	*Parameter* Serum cholesterol (mM/l)	Aortic sudanophilia (%)	Plaques
Fructose	4.24 ± 0.26	11.3 ± 4.2	3/6
Sucrose	4.24 ± 0.31	10.4 ± 5.4	2/6
Starch	4.61 ± 0.60	21.3 ± 8.9	1/6
Glucose	4.48 ± 0.62	17.2 ± 10.3	0/6
Lactose	4.92 ± 0.41	65.8 ± 13.6	5/6
Control	2.62 ± 0.10	1.4 ± 0.4	0/6

Diet contained: 40% carbohydrate; 25% casein; 13.9% coconut oil; 15% cellulose; 5% salt mix; 1% vitamin mix; and 0.1% cholesterol. Three male, three female baboons per group.

Although baboons exhibit considerable aortic fatty streaking in the wild (McGill *et al.*, 1960), when fed a diet containing fat and cholesterol under laboratory conditions for four years (Strong & McGill 1967) they develop only moderate cholesterolaemia and not much more than fatty streaking. Gresham *et al.* (1965) fed baboons butter plus cholesterol for 18 months and only saw fatty streaking.

Kritchevsky *et al.* (1974) fed baboons semipurified diets containing different carbohydrates for one year. They observed moderate increases in serum cholesterol and triglycerides and some sudanophilia, which was most severe in the animals fed fructose and least severe in those fed glucose. In a later study (Kritchevsky *et al.*, 1980) they added 0.1% cholesterol to the diet and after 17 months they observed atherosclerosis (Kritchevsky *et al.*, 1982c) in several of the groups. The results are detailed in Table 5. The severity of sudanophilia was greater in the female aortas in every case except that of the lactose-fed group. Since lactose had not been fed in the earlier study another experiment was carried out involving only lactose, lactose + 0.1% cholesterol and control groups. After 9 months serum cholesterol levels (mM/l) were: lactose 3.86 ± 0.10; lactose-cholesterol 4.43 ± 0.23, and control 2.54 ± 0.05. The percentage of aortic sudanophilia was: lactose 2.2 ± 0.7 (0/6 plaques); lactose-cholesterol 20.8 ± 7.4 (1/6 plaques); and control 0.3 ± 0.2 (0/6 plaques). In this experiment aortic sudanophilia was more severe in the females fed the lactose-cholesterol diet. The baboon is a species which is readily available but its relative resistance to atherosclerosis makes it unsuitable for most studies. In addition it is difficult to handle because of its strength, size and disposition.

Conclusion

Stehbens (1986) has reviewed the vascular complications in experimental atherosclerosis. He concludes that the vast differences between the human and experimental lesions preclude the conclusion that the two have the same aetiology, and that it is not wise to extrapolate from the cholesterol-fed animal to man. Stehbens admits that hyperlipoproteinemia can contribute to atherosclerosis but believes that more effort should be placed on detailed comparison of atherosclerosis in normal and hyperlipoproteinaemic individuals. As Pope said in his Essay on Man, 'The proper study of mankind is man.'

References

Adams, C. W. M. (1964): Arteriosclerosis in man, other mammals and birds. *Biol. Rev.* **39**, 372–423.

Anitschkow, N. & Chalatow, S. (1913): Uber experimentelle cholesterinsteatose und ihre bedeutung fur die entstehung pathologischer prozess. *Z. Allg. Pathol. Patholog. Anat.* **24**, 1–9.

Armstrong, M. L. (1976): Atherosclerosis in rhesus and cynomolgus monkeys. *Primates Med.* **9**, 16–40.

Aubert, D., Ferrand, J. C., Lacaze, B., Pepin, O., Panak, E. & Podesta, M. (1974): Atherogenese experimentale chez le rat Wistar. *Atherosclerosis* **20**, 263–280.

Bullock, B. C., Lehner, N. D., Clarkson, T. B., Feldner, M. A., Wagner, W. D. & Lofland, H. B. (1975): Comparative primate atherosclerosis. I. Tissue cholesterol concentrations and pathologic anatomy. *Exp. Molec. Pathol.* **22**, 151–175.

Chawla, K. K., Murthy, C. D. S., Chakravarti, R. N. & Chuttani, P. N. (1967): Arteriosclerosis and thrombosis in wild rhesus monkeys. *Am. Heart J.* **73**, 85–91.

Clarkson, S. & Newburgh, L. N. (1926): The relation between atherosclerosis and ingested cholesterol in the rabbit. *J. Exp. Med.* **45**, 595–612.

Clarkson, T. B., Lofland, H. B. Jr., Bullock, B. C. & Goodman, H. O. (1971): Genetic control of plasma cholesterol. Studies on squirrel monkeys. *Archs Pathol.* **92**, 37–45.

Clarkson, T. B., Prichard, R. W., Netsky, M. G. & Lofland, H. B. (1959): Atherosclerosis in pigeons: its spontaneous occurrence and resemblence to human atherosclerosis. *Archs Pathol.* **68**, 143–147.

Constantinides, P. (1965): *Experimental atherosclerosis*. Amsterdam: Elsevier Publ. Co.

Davignon, J. (1978): The lipid hypothesis: pathophysiological basis. *Archs Surg.* **113**, 28–34.

De Hoff-Sparks, J. L. & Kritchevsky, D. (1982): Distribution of plasma lipids and glucose in two breeds of rabbit. *Artery* **11**, 136–144.

DePalma, R. G., Insull, W., Bellon, E. M., Roth, W. T. & Robinson, A. V. (1972): Animal models for the study of progression and regression of atherosclerosis. *Surgery* **72**, 268–278.

DiLuzio, N. R. & O'Neal, R. M. (1962): The rapid development of arterial lesions in dogs fed an "infarct-producing" diet. *Exp. Molec. Pathol.* **1**, 122–132.

Downie, H. G., Mustard, J. F. & Rowsell, H. C. (1963): Swine atherosclerosis: the relationship of lipids and blood coagulation to its development. *Ann. NY Acad. Sci.* **104**, 539–562.

Dreizen, S., Levy, B. M. & Bernick, S. (1973): Diet-induced atherosclerosis in the marmoset. *Proc. Soc. Exp. Biol. Med.* **143**, 1218–1223.

Fabricant, C. G., Fabricant, J., Minick, C. R. & Litrenta, M. M. (1983): Herpesvirus-induced atherosclerosis in chickens. *Fed. Proc.* **42**, 2476–2479.

Fillios, L. C. & Mann, G. V. (1956): The importance of sex in the variability of the cholesterolemic response of rabbits fed cholesterol. *Circulation Res.* **4**, 406–412.

Fincham, J. E., Woodroof, C. W., van Wyk, M. J., Capatos, D., Weight, M. J., Kritchevsky, D. & Rossouw, J. E. (1987): Promotion and regression of atherosclerosis in Vervet monkeys by diets realistic for Westernised people. *Atherosclerosis* **66**, 205–213.

Gottlieb, H. & Lalich, J. J. (1954): The occurrence of arteriosclerosis in the aorta of swine. *Am. J. Pathol.* **30**, 851–855.

Gresham, G. A. & Howard, A. N. (1960): The independent production of atherosclerosis and thrombosis in the rat. *Br. J. Exp. Pathol.* **41**, 395–402.

Gresham, G. A., Howard, A. N., McQueen, J. & Bowyer, D. E. (1965): Atherosclerosis in primates. *Br. J. Exp. Pathol.* **46**, 94–103.

Hamm, T. E. Jr., Kaplan, J., Clarkson, T. B. & Bullock, B. C. (1983): Effects of gender and social behavior on the development of coronary artery atherosclerosis in cynomolgus macaques. *Atherosclerosis* **48**, 221–223.

Harrison, T. R. & Reeves, T. J. (1968): *Principles and problems of ischemic heart disease* pp. 42–54. Chicago: Year Book Medical Publishers.

Hartroft, W. S., Ridout, J. H., Sellars, E. A. & Best, C. H. (1952): Atheromatous changes in aorta, carotid and coronary arteries of choline-deficient rats. *Proc. Soc. Exp. Biol. Med.* **81**, 384–393.

Hayes, K. C., Westmoreland, N. P. & Faherty, J. P. (1972): An aortitis in the squirrel monkey and its effect on atherosclerosis. *Exp. Molec. Pathol.* **17**, 334–347.

Hopkins, P. N. & Williams, R. R. (1981): A survey of 246 suggested coronary risk factors. *Atherosclerosis* **40**, 1–52.

Ignatowski, A. (1908): Influence de la nourriture animale sur l'organisme des lapins. *Arch. Med. Exp. Anat. Pathol.* **20**, 1–20.

Ignatowski, A. (1909): Uber die wirkung des tierischen eiweisses auf die aorta und die parenchymatosen organe der kaninchen. *Virchow's Arch. Pathol. Anat. Physiol. Klin. Med.* **198**, 248–270.

Jokinen, M. P., Clarkson, T. B. & Prichard, R. W. (1985): Animal models in atherosclerosis research. *Exp. Molec. Pathol.* **42**, 1–28.

Katz, L. N. & Stamler, J. (1953): *Experimental atherosclerosis*. Springfield, Ill: C. C. Thomas.

Knack, A. V. (1915): Uber cholesterinsklerose. *Virchow's Arch. Pathol. Anat. Physiol. Klin. Med.* **220**, 36–52.

Koletsky, S. (1973): Obese spontaneously hypertensive rats — a model for study of atherosclerosis. *Exp. Molec. Pathol.* **19**, 53–60.

Kramsch, D. M. & Hollander, W. (1968): Occlusive atherosclerotic disease of the coronary arteries in monkeys (*Macaca irus*) induced by diet. *Exp. Molec. Pathol.* **9**, 1–22.

Kritchevsky, D. (1970): Role of cholesterol vehicle in experimental atherosclerosis. *Am. J. Clin. Nutr.* **23**, 1105–1110.

Kritchevsky, D. (1979): Vegetable protein and atherosclerosis. *J. Am. Oil Chem. Soc.* **56**, 135–146.

Kritchevsky, D., Davidson, L. M., Kim, H. K., Krendel, D. A., Malhotra, S., Mendelsohn, D., vanderWatt, J. J., duPlessis, J. P. & Winter, P. A. D. (1980): Influence of type of carbohydrate on atherosclerosis in baboons fed semipurified diets plus 0.1% cholesterol. *Am. J. Clin. Nutr.* **33**, 1869–1887.

Kritchevsky, D., Davidson, L. M., Kim, H. K., Krendel, D. A., Malhotra, S., vanderWatt, J. J., duPlessis, J. P., Winter, P. A. D., Ipp, T., Mendelsohn, D. & Bersohn, I. (1977): Influence of semipurified diets on atherosclerosis in African green monkeys. *Exp. Molec. Pathol.* **26**, 28–51.

Kritchevsky, D., Davidson, L. M., Shapiro, I. L., Kim, H. K., Kitagawa, M., Malhotra, S., Naer, P. P., Clarkson, T. B., Bersohn, I. & Winter, P. A. D. (1974): Lipid metabolism and experimental atherosclerosis in baboons: influence of cholesterol-free, semi-synthetic diets. *Am. J. Clin. Nutr.* **27**, 29–50.

Kritchevsky, D., Davidson, L. M. & vanderWatt, J. J. (1982c): The influence of carbohydrates on atherosclerosis in primates. In *Metabolic effects of utilizable dietary carbohydrate*, ed S. Reiser, pp. 141–174. New York: Marcel Dekker, Inc.

Kritchevsky, D., Davidson, L. M., Weight, M., Kriek, N. P. J. & duPlessis, J. P. (1982a): Influence of native and randomized peanut oil on lipid metabolism and aortic sudanophilia in the Vervet monkey. *Atherosclerosis* **42**, 53–58.

Kritchevsky, D. & Kothari, H. (1973): Aortic cholesterol esterase: studies in white Carneau and Show Racer pigeons. *Biochim. Biophys. Acta* **326**, 489–491.

Kritchevsky, D., Langan, J., Markowitz, J., Berry, J. F. & Turner, D. A. (1961): Cholesterol vehicle in experimental atherosclerosis. III. Effect of absence or presence of fatty vehicle. *J. Am. Oil Chem. Soc.* **38**, 74–76.

Kritchevsky, D. & Tepper, S. A. (1965a): Cholesterol vehicle in experimental atherosclerosis. VII. Influence of naturally occurring saturated fats. *Med. Pharmacol. Exp.* **12**, 315–320.

Kritchevsky, D. & Tepper, S. A. (1965b): Factors affecting atherosclerosis in rabbits fed cholesterol-free diets. *Life Sci.* **4**, 1467–1471.

Kritchevsky, D., Tepper, S. A., Bises, G. & Klurfeld, D. M. (1982b): Experimental atherosclerosis in rabbits fed cholesterol-free diets. X. Cocoa butter and palm oil. *Atherosclerosis* **41**, 279–284.

Kritchevsky, D., Tepper, S. A., Czarnecki, S. K., Klurfeld, D. M. & Story, J. A. (1983): Effects of animal and vegetable protein in experimental atherosclerosis. In *Animal and vegetable proteins in lipid metabolism and atherosclerosis*, eds M. J. Gibney and D. Kritchevsky, pp. 85–100. New York: Alan R. Liss, Inc.

Kritchevsky, D., Tepper, S. A. & Kitagawa, M. (1973b): Experimental atherosclerosis in rabbits fed cholesterol-free diets. 3. Comparison of fructose and lactose with other carbohydrates. *Nutr. Rep. Int.* **7**, 192–202.

Kritchevsky, D., Tepper, S. A., Vesselinovitch, D. & Wissler, R. W. (1971): Cholesterol vehicle in experimental atherosclerosis. 11. Peanut oil. *Atherosclerosis* **14**, 53–64.

Lambert, G. F., Miller, J. P., Olsen, R. T. & Frost, D. V. (1958): Hypercholesterolemia and atherosclerosis induced in rabbits by purified high fat rations devoid of cholesterol. *Proc. Soc. Exp. Biol. Med.* **97**, 544–549.

Lee, K. T., Jarmolych, J., Kim, D. N., Grant, C., Krasney, J. A., Thomas, W. A. & Bruno, A. M. (1971): Production of advanced atherosclerosis myocardial infarction and 'sudden death' in swine. *Exp. Molec. Pathol.* **15**, 170–190.

Lofland, H. B., St. Clair, R. W., MacNintch, J. E. & Prichard, R. W. (1967): Atherosclerosis in new world primates: biochemical studies. *Archs Pathol.* **83**, 211–214.

Lugenbuhl, H., Jones, J. E. T. & Detweiler, D. K. (1965): The morphology of spontaneous atherosclerotic lesions in the dog. In *Comparative atherosclerosis*, eds J. C. Roberts, Jr. and R. Straus, pp. 161–169. New York: Harper and Row.

Mahley, R. W., Weisgraber, K. H., Innerarity, T., Brewer, H. B., Jr. & Assmann, G. (1975): Swine lipoproteins and atherosclerosis changes in the plasma lipoproteins and apoproteins induced by cholesterol feeding. *Biochemistry* **14**, 2817–2823.

Malinow, M. R., Maruffo, C. A. & Perley, A. M. (1966): Experimental atherosclerosis in squirrel monkeys (*Saimiri sciurea*). *J. Path. Bact.* **92**, 491–510.

Malmros, H. & Sternby, N. H. (1968): Induction of atherosclerosis in dogs by a thiouracil-free semi-synthetic diet containing cholesterol and hydrogenated coconut oil. *Prog. Biochem. Pharmacol.* **4**, 482–487.

Malmros, H. & Wigand, G. (1959): Atherosclerosis and deficiency of essential fatty acids. *Lancet* **2**, 749–751.

Mann, G. V. & Andrus, S. B. (1956): Xanthomatosis and atherosclerosis produced by diet in an adult rhesus monkey. *J. Lab. Clin. Med.* **48**, 533–550.

McCombs, H. L., Zook, B. C. & McGandy, R. B. (1969): Fine structure of spontaneous atherosclerosis of the aorta in the squirrel monkey. *Am. J. Pathol.* **55**, 235–252.

McGill, H. C., Jr., Strong, J. P., Holman, R. L. & Werthessen, N. T. (1960): Arterial lesions in the Kenya baboon. *Circulation Res.* **8**, 670–679.

McMahan, M. R., Rhyne, A. L., Lofland, H. B. & Sackett, G. P. (1980): Effects of sex, age and dietary modification on plasma lipids and lipoproteins of *Macaca nemestrina*. *Proc. Soc. Exp. Biol. Med.* **164**, 27–34.

Middleton, C. C., Clarkson, T. B., Lofland, H. B. & Prichard, R. W. (1967): Diet and atherosclerosis of squirrel monkeys. *Archs Pathol.* **83**, 145–153.

Morin, R. J., Bernick, S. & Alfin-Slater, R. B. (1964): Effects of essential fatty acid deficiency and supplementation on atheroma formation and regression. *J. Atheroscler. Res.* **4**, 387–396.

Newburgh, L. H. & Clarkson, S. (1922): Production of arteriosclerosis in rabbits by diets rich in animal protein. *J. Am. Med. Ass.* **79**, 1106–1108.

Newburgh, L. H. & Clarkson, S. (1923): The production of arteriosclerosis in rabbits by diets containing meat. *Archs Intern. Med.* **31**, 653–676.

Newburgh, L. H. & Squier, T. L. (1920): High protein diets and arteriosclerosis in rabbits: a preliminary report. *Archs Intern. Med.* **26**, 38–40.

Ojerio, A. D., Pucak, G. J., Clarkson, T. B. & Bullock, B. C. (1972): Diet-induced atherosclerosis and myocardial infarction in Japanese quail. *Lab. Anim. Sci.* **22**, 33–39.

O'Neal, R. M., Still, W. J. S. & Hartroft, W. S. (1961): Experimental atherosclerosis in the rat. *J. Path. Bact.* **82**, 183–188.

Patek, P. R., Bernick, S., Ershoff, B. H. & Wells, A. (1963): Induction of atherosclerosis by cholesterol feeding in the hypophysectomized rat. *Am. J. Pathol.* **42**, 137–150.

Pick, R., Johnson, P. J. & Glick, G. (1974): Deleterious effects of hypertension on the development of aortic and coronary atherosclerosis in stumptail macaques (*Macaca speciosa*) on an atherogenic diet. *Circulation Res.* **35**, 472–482.

Prathap, K. (1975): Diet-induced aortic atherosclerosis in Malaysian long-tailed monkeys (*Macaca irus*). *J. Pathol.* **115**, 163–174.

Prichard, R. W., Clarkson, T. B., Lofland, H. B., Jr., Goodman, H. O., Herndon, C. N. & Netsky, M. G. (1962): Studies on the atherosclerotic pigeon. *J. Am. Med. Ass.* **179**, 49–52.

Ratcliffe, H. L. & Luginbuhl, H. (1971): The domestic pig: a model for experimental atherosclerosis. *Atherosclerosis* **13**, 133–136.

Reitman, J. S., Mahley, R. W. & Fry, D. L. (1982): Yucatan miniature swine as a model for diet-induced atherosclerosis. *Atherosclerosis* **43**, 119–132.

Rinehart, J. F. & Greenberg, L. D. (1951): Pathogenesis of experimental arteriosclerosis in pyridoxine deficiency: with notes on similarities to human arteriosclerosis. *Archs Pathol.* **51**, 12–18.

Roberts, D. C. K., West, C. E., Redgrave, T. G. & Smith, J. B. (1974): Plasma cholesterol concentration in normal and cholesterol-fed rabbits. Its variation and heritability. *Atherosclerosis* **19**, 369–380.

Rudel, L. L. (1980): Plasma lipoproteins in atherogenesis in nonhuman primates. In *The use of nonhuman primates in cardiovascular diseases*, ed S. S. Kalter, pp. 37–57. Austin, Texas: University of Texas Press.
Rudel, L. L. & Pitts, L. L. II (1978): Male-female variability in the dietary cholesterol-induced hyperlipoproteinemia of cynomolgus monkeys (*Macaca fasicularis*). *J. Lipid Res.* **19**, 992–1003.
St. Clair, R. W. (1983): Metabolic changes in the arterial wall associated with atherosclerosis in the pigeon. *Fed. Proc.* **42**, 2480–2485.
Shih, J. C. (1983): Atherosclerosis in Japanese quail and effect of lipoic acid. *Fed. Proc.* **42**, 2494–2497.
Skold, B. H. & Getty, R. (1961): Spontaneous atherosclerosis in swine. *J. Am. Vet. Med. Ass.* **139**, 655–660.
Srinivasan, S. R., Dalferes, E. R., Jr., Ruiz, H., Pargaonkar, P. S., Rhadakrishnamurthy, B. & Berenson, G. S. (1972): Rapid serum lipoprotein changes in spider monkeys on short-term feeding of high cholesterol-high saturated fat diet. *Proc. Soc. Exp. Biol. Med.* **141**, 154–160.
Stehbens, W. E. (1986): Vascular complications in experimental atherosclerosis. *Prog. Cardiovasc. Dis.* **29**, 221–237.
Steiner, A. & Kendall, F. E. (1946): Atherosclerosis and arteriosclerosis in dogs following ingestion of cholesterol and thiouracil. *Archs Pathol.* **42**, 433–444.
Stout, L. C. (1982): Pathogenesis and diffuse intimal thickening (DIT) in aortas and coronary arteries of 2½-year-old miniature pigs. *Exp. Molec. Pathol.* **37**, 427–432.
Strong, J. P. & McGill, H. C. Jr. (1967): Diet and experimental atherosclerosis in baboons. *Am. J. Pathol.* **50**, 669–690.
Taylor, C. B., Cox, G. E., Manalo-Estrella, P. & Southworth, J. (1962): Atherosclerosis in rhesus monkeys. II. Arterial lesions associated with hypercholesterolemia induced by dietary fat and cholesterol. *Archs Pathol.* **74**, 16–34.
Taylor, C. B., Manalo-Estrella, P. & Cox, G. E. (1963a): Atherosclerosis in rhesus monkeys. V. Marked diet-induced hypercholesterolemia with xanthomatosis and severe atherosclerosis. *Archs Pathol.* **76**, 239–249.
Taylor, C. B., Patton, D. E. & Cox, G. E. (1963b): Atherosclerosis in rhesus monkeys. VI. Fatal myocardial infarction in a monkey fed fat and cholesterol. *Archs Pathol.* **76**, 404–412.
Vastesaeger, M. M. & Delcourt, R. (1962): The natural history of atherosclerosis. *Circulation* **26**, 841–855.
Vesselinovitch, D., Getz, G. S., Hughes, R. H. & Wissler, R. W. (1974): Atherosclerosis in monkeys fed three food fats. *Atherosclerosis* **20**, 303–321.
Wacker, L. & Hueck, W. (1913): Uber experimentelle atherosklerose und cholesterinamie. *Muenchner Med. Wochenschr.* **60**, 2097–2100.
Wagner, W. D. & Clarkson, T. B. (1975): Comparative primate atherosclerosis. II. A biochemical study of lipids, calcium and collagen in atherosclerotic arteries. *Exp. Molec. Pathol.* **23**, 96–121.
Wagner, W. D., Clarkson, T. B., Feldner, M. A. & Prichard, R. W. (1973): The development of pigeon strains with selected atherosclerosis characteristics. *Exp. Molec. Pathol.* **19**, 304–319.
Wagner, W. D. & Nohlgren, S. R. (1981): Aortic glycosaminoglycans in genetically selected WC-2 pigeons with increased atherosclerosis susceptibility. *Arteriosclerosis* **1**, 192–201.
Wagner, W. D., St. Clair, R. W. & Clarkson, T. B. (1978): Angiochemical and tissue cholesterol changes in *Macaca fasicularis* fed an atherogenic diet for three years. *Exp. Molec. Pathol.* **28**, 140–153.
Wang, C. J., Schaefer, L. E., Drackman, S. R. & Adlersberg, D. (1954): Plasma partition of the normal and cholesterol-fed rabbit. *J. Mt. Sinai Hosp.* **21**, 19–25.
Wilson, R. B., Miller, R. A., Middleton, C. C. & Kinden, D. (1982): Atherosclerosis in rabbits fed a low cholesterol diet for five years. *Arteriosclerosis* **2**, 228–241.
Wissler, R. W., Eilert, M. L., Schroeder, M. A. & Cohen, L. (1954): Production of lipomatous and atheromatous arterial lesions in the albino rat. *Archs Pathol.* **57**, 333–351.
Wissler, R. W. & Vesselinovitch, D. (1974): Comparative pathogenic patterns in atherosclerosis. *Adv. Lipid Res.* **6**, 181–206.

* * * * *

Discussion

Professor Gurr suggested that few animals show comparable atheroma to man, and *Professor Kritchevsky* admitted that in most experimental animals the pathology resembled early human atheroma rather than the complex lesions seen in human vascular disease. *Professor Gurr* also wished to know about familial hypercholesterolaemia and whether the atheroma in this condition was the same as in naturally occurring atheroma in older people. Nobody was able to answer this.

Dr Sanders suggested that the effect of fish oil in inhibiting atherosclerosis was independent of its effects on serum cholesterol. *Kritchevsky* said that fish protein itself also reduces atheroma and therefore perhaps it would be more advisable to eat whole fish rather than the oil of fish by itself.

Dr Widdowson recommended using the elephant as an experimental animal for atherosclerosis based on work by McCulloch.

Dr Eastwood wondered whether the resistance to atheroma was due to variation in the composition of bile acids. *Kritchevsky* said there was no evidence so far but he did wonder whether the speed of inhibiting cholesterol synthesis may play a part.

Professor Garrow asked if the mechanisms which resulted in increased coronary heart disease during stress were known. *Kritchevsky* said that this was speculative but that it could operate via the adrenals or catecholamines. He cited a study where cholesterol was measured in 177 U.S. generals over a period of five years, and of these individuals 16 had a coronary thrombosis during the period. These 16 individuals showed a fluctuation in cholesterol of over 50% during the course of the study leading up to their coronary event, thereby suggesting that it might have been cholesterol fluctuation rather than the absolute value which was associated with coronary heart disease.

Dr Stevens wondered whether reptilian species with a long life span showed atheroma and whether their arteries would provide reasonable models but there did not seem to be any evidence to substantiate this.

Sir Christopher Booth wondered whether the hypercholesterolaemic agents which are on the market affected the atheroma as well as lowering the serum cholesterol. *Kritchevsky* said that this was not at the moment known but there were some modern ultrasonic techniques which were now looking at this. He also suggested that regression of atheroma was unlikely in his view and in any event there have been very few studies in this field. *Booth* also asked about the value of plasmaphoresis, but *Kritchevsky* did not know whether a trial had been done; he had not seen any report of this.

Professor Waterlow asked whether the sex difference that occurs in man is also found in experimental models and *Kritchevsky* noted that female vervets seem to have more atheromatous lesions than males, but in most studies it is only the males that have been used because of the knowledge that *homo sapiens* males tend to be the ones to have increased coronary heart disease.

Professor MacDonald asked whether stearic acid was a non-cholesterolaemic saturated fatty acid as implied by a remark made by Kritchevsky at the beginning of his talk. *Kritchevsky* said that stearic acid certainly looks interesting because in the early studies oils rich in stearic (such as cocoa butter) were not very cholesterolaemic or atherogenic—certainly less than one would expect from their level of saturation.

Sir Christopher Booth asked what were the causes of reduced ischaemic heart disease found in recent years in the United States. *Kritchevsky* thought that it might be due to reduced incidence of smoking, better treatment of high blood pressure, and lower cholesterol in the diet leading to lower plasma cholesterol, but it was difficult to single out any of these factors. Cardio-pulmonary resuscitation had also improved considerably, which might be influencing mortality.

Dr Sanders commented that ischaemic heart disease rates had declined in women in 26 countries between 1950–1978 in contrast to the marked increase in rates in men in most of the countries. *Kritchevsky* was not aware of these data.

14

Comparative infant nutrition in man and other animals

R. G. WHITEHEAD and A. A. PAUL

Introduction

When one compares what is known about the nutritional aspects of animal husbandry and the nutritional health care of the young human being, one cannot escape the conclusion that feeding strategies for the young animal are often on a much firmer scientific basis. Why should this be so? Partly it must be that with animals one usually has a relatively clear cut and *simple* objective. Precisely what this objective is, of course, varies depending on the animal in question and the use to which it is to be put, but there is rarely such a multiplicity of potentially conflicting objectives as one finds in man.

In cows or pigs reared for meat one usually needs to achieve a given carcass composition and animal size as quickly and cheaply as possible. One is not concerned about whether this rate of growth or body composition is going to be deleterious to the animal's long-term quality of life because there is going to be no long term! Even with non-food animals such as the racehorse, the prime objective is still clear cut and well defined: the athletic performance of the young adult. There has to be little or no concern for how he is going to fare in middle or old age. In man, on the other hand, our concept of what constitutes the best infant diet has to take into account ultimate health and well-being throughout the whole age-range with the later stages of life being of particular importance. Most sets of dietary guidelines, for example the British NACNE ones (Health Education Council, 1983), are mainly concerned with health issues which only become clinical problems over the age of 40 years.

There is increasing discussion nowadays in paediatric circles about the long-term importance of dietary patterns set in very early life. Infant feeding cannot be considered just in terms of the best diet whilst that individual is still a young baby. Possible

Comparative Nutrition, ed K. Blaxter & I. Macdonald. ©John Libbey 1988.

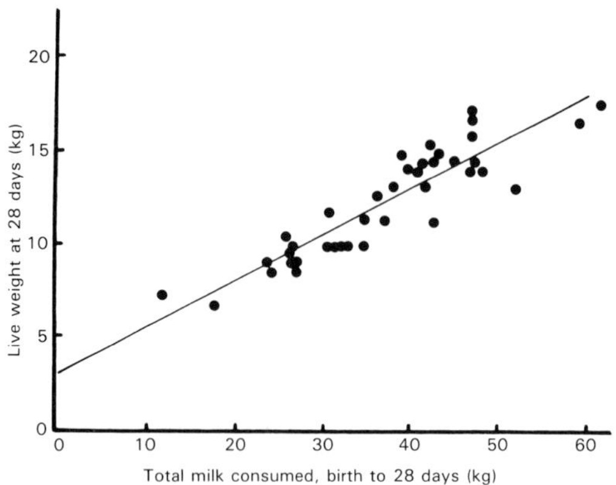

Fig. 1. *Relationship between weight of suckling lambs at 1 month and total amount of milk consumed.* Each point represents either a singleton lamb or the mean of twin or triplet sets. (From Wallace, 1948).

long-term biochemical 'programming' that might occur in early life, or behavioural characteristics and habits that might become set, have also to be taken into account. It has to be admitted that such discussions can be rather academic, however, for a variety of reasons, not least the virtual lack of really relevant basic, scientific information. What is becoming apparent, nevertheless, is that there is probably no such thing as an infant dietary practice which is likely to be optimal for all subsequent physiological requirements and desired lifestyles right throughout life into old age. Very precise prescriptions for infant feeding could very well have to involve 'physiological trade-offs'.

Although the situation in animals might be more simple than in man, comparative evaluations can provide valuable clues of clinical importance, as this short review will try to demonstrate. It will be shown that different attitudes towards infant feeding practices can produce variations in the growth of babies which parallel similar differences that have long been known in animals. These will be examined in terms of their potential long-term sequelae.

Postnatal animal growth and maternal lactational performance

One objective which seems to dominate much of the husbandry of the young animal is achieving the maximum rate of growth from the earliest possible age. This is usually for economic reasons, as in the beef, pork and sheep industries for example, but in a number of other species it is widely believed that the size of the animal at the end of the weaning period tends to determine how well he is going to keep on growing and hence his final adult stature.

In this regard, the lactational capacity of the mother can be a prime consideration (Blaxter, 1961) and female breeding animals are frequently selected because of their individual abilities to produce large amounts of milk. A good example of the importance of lactational capacity in animals was published by Wallace (1948) who studied the growth of lambs up to 28 days in relation to their total milk intake over this period as a whole (Fig. 1). Ewes which were able to produce the most milk quite clearly had the biggest offspring by one month. Exactly the same has been shown in beef calves (Yates *et al.*, 1971) and in foals (Doreau *et al.*, 1986). In many of the multi-littered

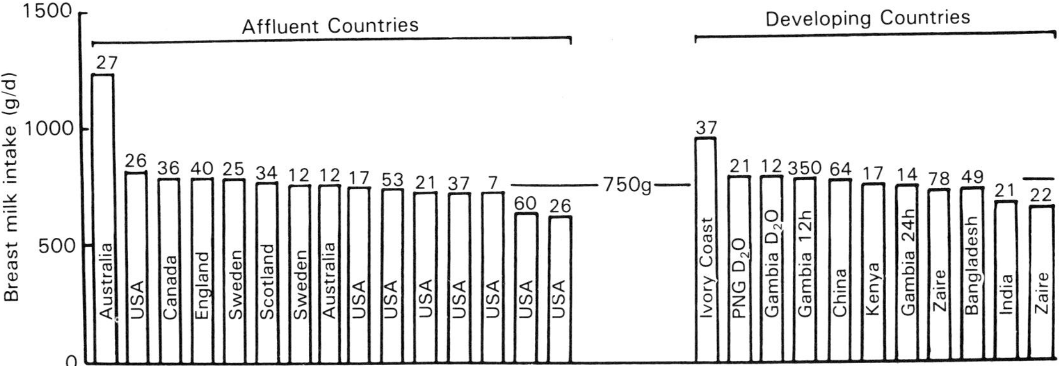

Fig. 2. *Breast-milk intake at 3 months of age from measurements made after 1975 in affluent and developing countries.* Numbers of subjects are shown at the top of each column. (From Prentice *et al.*, 1986).

species, it is well known that the young of smaller litters grow much more quickly than when there are a larger number of animals in a litter, again because of the greater amount of milk each individual receives. This is a well-known phenomenon both in farm animals (Wallace 1948; Blaxter 1961), and in laboratory animals such as rats and mice (Widdowson & McCance, 1960; Knight *et al.*, 1986).

Whilst the lactational capacity of the female of all mammalian species is clearly of critical importance and factors which might impair lactation, such as genetics or maternal diet, can greatly influence the growth of offspring, one needs to bear in mind that the human baby grows much more slowly in relative terms than the great majority of other animals (Payne & Wheeler, 1968; Oftedahl, 1984).

The practical consequence is that the nutritional stress of lactation on the human mother is less than it is in most other animals and she has to be very undernourished before her milk yield is likely to be severely affected. Primates such as the baboon behave similarly to man, and Roberts *et al.* (1985) showed that reducing maternal dietary energy intake by 20% had little or no effect on milk output. It was not until energy intake was reduced by 40% that a significant difference could be detected. Even so, at 9–10 weeks such mothers were still producing as much as 75% of the milk of well-nourished controls.

There has been much discussion about the ability of Third World women living on marginal food intakes to lactate adequately. Our conclusion (Prentice *et al.*, 1986) is that human milk output in most Third World countries is very similar to that of healthy, well-motivated mothers in the UK (Fig. 2). In The Gambia, for example, only during the annual 6 to 12-week hungry season is the milk intake of young babies demonstrably lower. It is because human lactational performance is well protected even in quite deprived mothers that this mode of feeding is so important in terms of the survival of babies in the Third World.

Whilst the genetic component in determining relative lactational performance is well established in farm animals, this topic is a much more controversial issue in the human. This is because of the difficulty in distinguishing between true biological variations in lactational capacity and the adverse effects of various behavioural and sociological factors which may have a negative influence on the opportunities or the

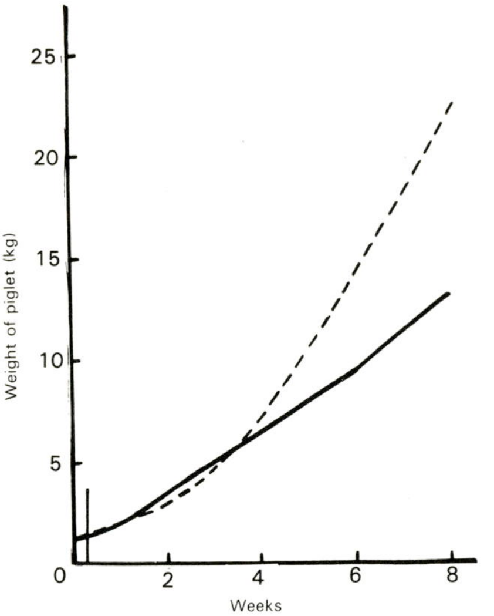

Fig. 3. *Weight growth of littermate piglets reared artificially (broken line) compared with those reared on a sow (full line).* Both lots received the same creep feed. From Braude (1954).

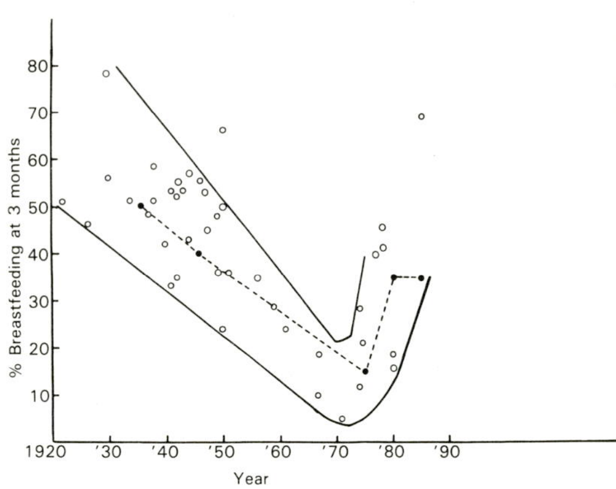

Fig. 4. *Proportions of mothers breastfeeding at 3 months in England and Wales from 1920 to 1985.* Closed symbols refer to national surveys. Open symbols refer to individual cities and towns from 29 different studies. (Whitehead & Paul, 1987).

willingness of the mother to breast-feed. We believe, however, that there is also true biological variation in the human. Our studies in Cambridge and in The Gambia have shown that part of this variation can be accounted for by differences in the size of babies at birth and their subsequent rates of growth, but there is more to it than that. In The Gambia, where our colleagues have been able to observe the same mothers through a number of successive pregnancy/lactation cycles, they have had the quite unusual opportunity of being able to compare these women's lactational performances with those of their own mothers who became pregnant at the same time (Prentice *et al.*, 1986). Not only was there a close association between the measured milk outputs from reproductive cycle to reproductive cycle in the same woman, but a good correlation was also found between the lactational performances of the two generations. Although this does not prove a genetic factor, it makes one likely.

Artificial milks and animal growth

Nowadays the whole question of using infant milk formulas in human feeding is so full of emotional controversy that one often hesitates to raise the topic, even in a rational discussion. An analysis of data in the literature, however, would indicate that in man as well as in animals, the young offspring can be made to grow more quickly if 'artificial' milks are introduced early into the diet either as a substitute or as a complement. This has been dramatically demonstrated by Braude (1954) in pigs (Fig. 3) and it is now common practice to wean piglets completely from the mother at around 3 weeks (Fowler, 1981). This is partly to restore the mothers' fertility as quickly as possible but also to encourage faster infant growth. By 8 weeks the artificially-fed animal can be twice as heavy as the one fed by the sow. Non-human primates also show greater weight gains when artificially-fed from birth than when reared on their mothers' milk (Kerr, 1972).

Human lactation and approved infant milk formulas

It is not always appreciated how much the way we feed our babies has fluctuated throughout this century. Until about 1970 there was a steady decline in the proportion being breastfed. Fig. 4 shows this for the United Kingdom at 3 months of age (Whitehead & Paul, 1987). Whilst there did appear to be some improvement between 1975 (Martin, 1978) and 1980 (Martin & Monk 1982) the OPCS 1985 National Survey (Martin, private communication) showed no further improvement, which would be in accord with our own observations. Importantly, all studies on this subject have demonstrated a marked social class influence, with the wives of professional workers breastfeeding in much larger numbers and for considerably longer than those of semi-skilled or unskilled workers.

But the trends in human infant feeding patterns were not just confined to breastfeeding. The composition of infant milk formulas has also been changed considerably in an attempt to mimic as closely as possible the composition of human milk. Up to 1940 diluted cow's milk with added sugar was the main type of milk used and even when full-cream milk powders became more common, sugar still had to be added, in variable amounts, by mother to meet the changing needs of baby as he grew older.

Really major compositional changes were initiated around 1975 and now, in most formulas, the butter fat has been completely replaced by vegetable oils and there have also been changes in the casein to whey ratio. Significantly, sucrose no longer has to be added by the mother. Another important observation around the early 1970s was that British mothers were tending to make up liquid milks from the powder in too concentrated a manner and this led to concern about the incidence of hypernatraemia (Davies, 1973). This latter problem has largely been solved, partly as a result of the changes in the infant milk powder composition, but mainly via more precise mixing instructions and improved 'scoop' designs (DHSS, 1980). All these changes have contributed to alterations in the dietary energy content of the made-up formulas and also to the consequent energy intake of the baby. The total energy consumption of the bottle-fed child is now much closer to that of the breast-fed one during the period of exclusive milk feeding.

Replacement of milk by more solid foods in animals

Sooner or later, in all species, solid foods begin to be consumed as well as milk. The effect of the timing of this introduction of solids to the growth of calves is well demonstrated in Fig. 5 (Richardson *et al.*, 1978). Those calves which did not receive solids until 26 weeks were some 20 kg lighter than those which had been given moderate amounts of solids from an earlier age, and about 35 kg less than the ones for which liberal solids were made available.

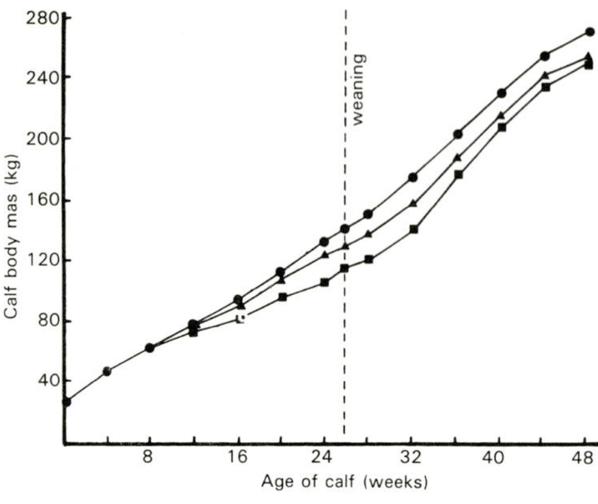

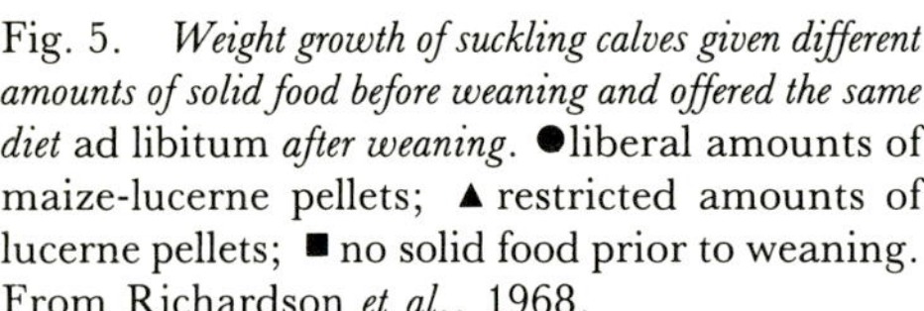
Fig. 5. *Weight growth of suckling calves given different amounts of solid food before weaning and offered the same diet* ad libitum *after weaning.* ●liberal amounts of maize-lucerne pellets; ▲ restricted amounts of lucerne pellets; ■ no solid food prior to weaning. From Richardson *et al.*, 1968.

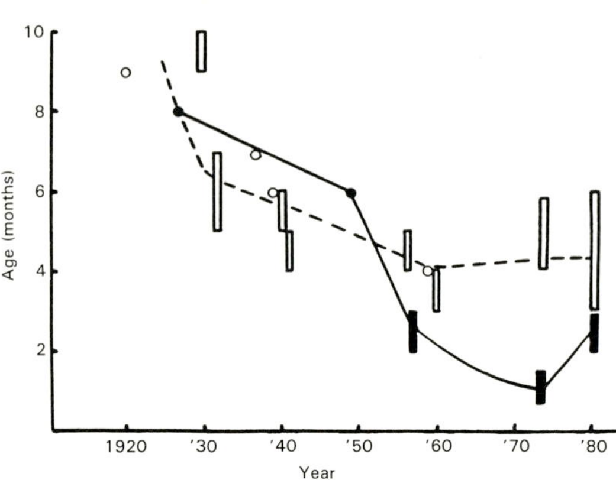

Fig. 6. *Age of introduction of solid foods in the UK from 1920 to 1980* (Whitehead & Paul, 1987). Solid symbols are means or ranges of reported age of introduction. Open symbols are the mean or range of recommendations given by various authors advising on infant feeding.

The data in Fig. 5 are a good example of the long-term effect of maintaining a high *initial* rate of growth. Even though all the groups of calves were given solid food *ad lib.* after 26 weeks, even by 1 year complete weight catch-up had not been achieved and the differences at 26 weeks tended to be maintained. McCance and Widdowson (Widdowson & McCance, 1960; Widdowson, 1970) have demonstrated a similar persistence of growth 'retardation' in a variety of other species including rats and pigs.

As we will show, these animal experiences have their direct parallels in the human infant and his responses to the way he is being fed.

The weaning process in the human infant

When solids should be introduced into the human baby's diet, like virtually every other facet of infant feeding, is again a matter of considerable controversy. Mainly because of the relative biochemical and physiological immaturity of the infant's gut, most paediatric authorities have recommended that babies should not be given non-milk solids until at least 4 months. As Fig. 6 shows, however, there have been major differences during this century between what experts have been advising and what has been done in practice. The 1960s and early 1970s was a period when solids were being given especially early and in 1974 the official Department of Health and Social Security's guide to infant feeding (DHSS, 1974) reported that '. . . in general babies are offered solids when between 3 and 4 *weeks* of age, although it is not unusual to find babies being fed solids in the first fortnight of life' Again, although the national OPCS survey conducted in 1980 (Martin & Monk, 1982) showed some improvement, the 1985 follow-up (Martin, 1987 personal communication) was as discouraging about the introduction of solids as it had been

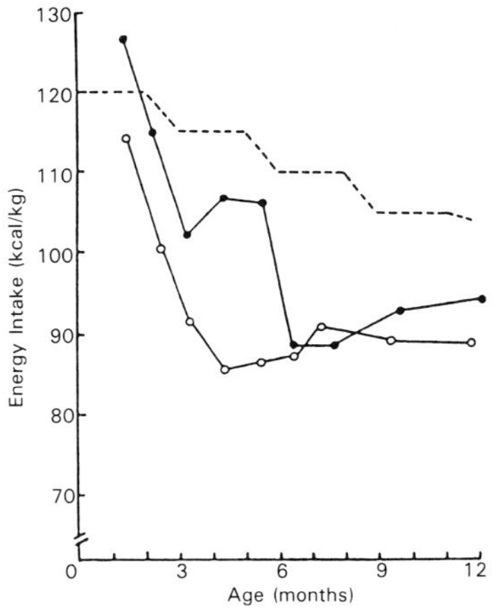

Fig. 7. *Measured metabolizable energy intakes (kcal/kg body weight) of Cambridge babies in 1980,* ○ *breast-fed to at least 4 months (n = 48),* ● *bottle-fed (n = 9), compared to the WHO/FAO (1973) estimated requirements (dotted lines).*

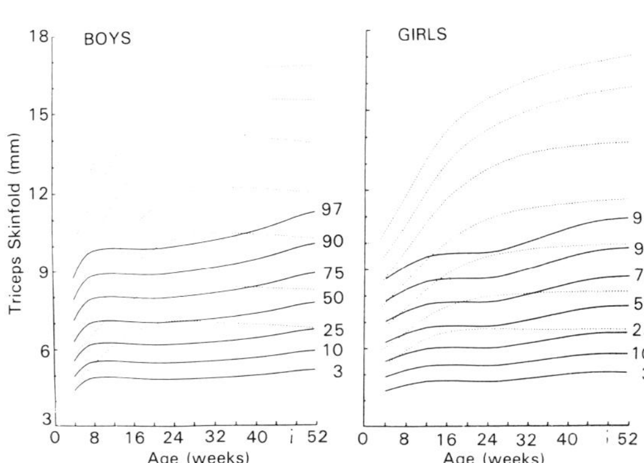

Fig. 8. *3rd to 97th centiles of triceps skinfold thickness of Cambridge babies in 1984–5 (72 boys and 60 girls), solid lines, compared to Tanner centiles (Tanner and Whitehouse, 1975), dotted lines.*

about the incidence of breastfeeding: the improvement of the late 1970s had not continued into the 1980s.

Nutritional significance of fluctuations in infant feeding patterns

It is not easy to ascertain with complete certainty what the nutritional consequences of all these fluctuations in human infant feeding patterns have been. Such data are difficult to collect and unfortunately the subject has not been pursued in a systematic way through the decades. Nevertheless, it is possible to speculate that the swing towards the consumption of over-concentrated infant formula milks instead of breast-milk, plus the increasingly early introduction of non-milk solids, as was occurring during the 1950s and 1960s, would have tended to boost the total energy intake as similar practices did in the animals we have been discussing. Likewise one might predict that babies whose mothers have in recent years been trying to follow more closely the DHSS advice about infant feeding would receive somewhat less dietary energy than must have been typical of the 1960s.

This certainly seems to have been the case in Britain. Figure 7 shows the measured energy intakes of the breast- and bottle-fed babies whom we have studied in Cambridge (Whitehead & Paul 1984) and for comparison the WHO/FAO (1973) safe levels of dietary energy intake. These latter values were based on typical food energy intakes during the 1950s and 1960s. Our values are some 20% down on the older ones. Findings similar to these have been observed by a number of other investigators in recent years in Sweden and the USA (Kylberg *et al.*, 1986; Kohler *et al.*, 1984; Dewey & Lonnerdahl, 1983) although these contrast with French infants, where intakes are still reported to be as high as those found in the 1960s (Boggio *et al.*, 1984).

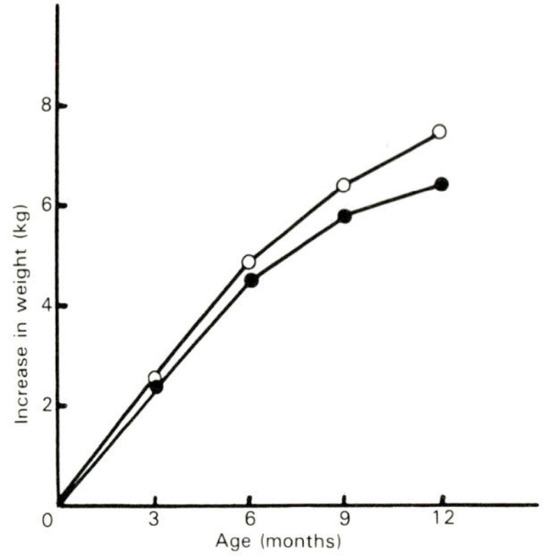

Fig. 9. *Gain in weight during the first year of life of artificially-fed boys (○) compared to boys breast-fed to at least 4 months (●) in the UK in 1949–50.* (Ministry of Health, 1959).

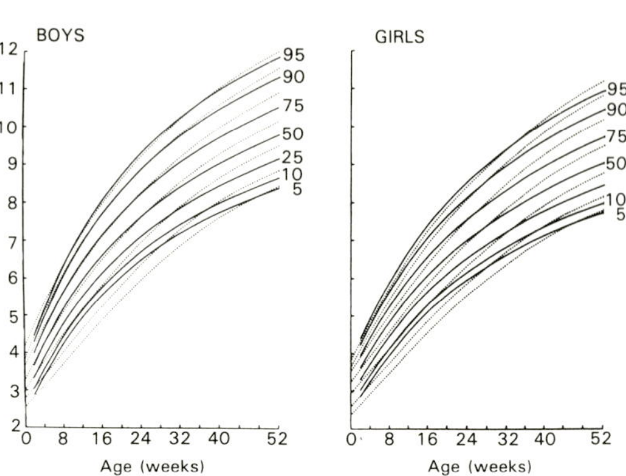

Fig. 10. *5th to 95th centiles of weight of Cambridge babies in 1984–5 (72 boys and 60 girls), solid lines, compared to NCHS centiles (Hamill, 1977), dotted lines.*

Growth and human infant feeding patterns

If the energy intake of the human infant really has changed in Cambridge in the way postulated, one might expect that the adipose tissue stores would have been affected. This does indeed seem to have been the case. Figure 8 shows our Cambridge 3rd to 97th centile values for triceps skinfolds together with the Tanner Revised Standards (Tanner & Whitehouse, 1975) for comparative purposes. These were published in 1975 but were based on data collected by Hutchinson-Smith (1973) in Derbyshire between 1966 and 1967. This was at about the trough of breastfeeding and the peak of early weaning practices (Figs. 4 and 6). The differences between the two sets of reference data are remarkable. Although the Tanner 50th centile values averaged around 11.5–12.0 mm between 6 and 18 months, the same values for the Cambridge boys were only 8 mm, a figure close to the old 10th centile.

The fact that average skinfold thickness values are often significantly smaller now than the Tanner reference values has been reported by a number of investigators including Schluter *et al.* (1976) from Germany, Boulton (1981) from Australia, and Yeung (1983) from Canada. It is of course not possible to be sure that these differences are due to diet but it would seem an obvious explanation. The main difference between the two sets of UK data is that while the Tanner values showed a steady rise from 2–6 months, this did not occur in the Cambridge cohort nor in the other data sets we have cited. If the cause is a dietary one, a likely explanation would thus seem to be the timing of the introduction of weaning foods and the amounts given.

The fact that weight growth in healthy young infants is influenced by how they are fed has been observed by a number of other investigators. One of the best early examples is that published by the old British Ministry of Health (1959) and based on children studied as part of a national survey in 1950. Figure 9 shows the relative rates of growth of initially breast- and bottle-fed boys of that day after standardizing for factors such as social class and geographical area of the country. Quite clearly the breast-fed babies grew more slowly. We can only speculate as to why the difference

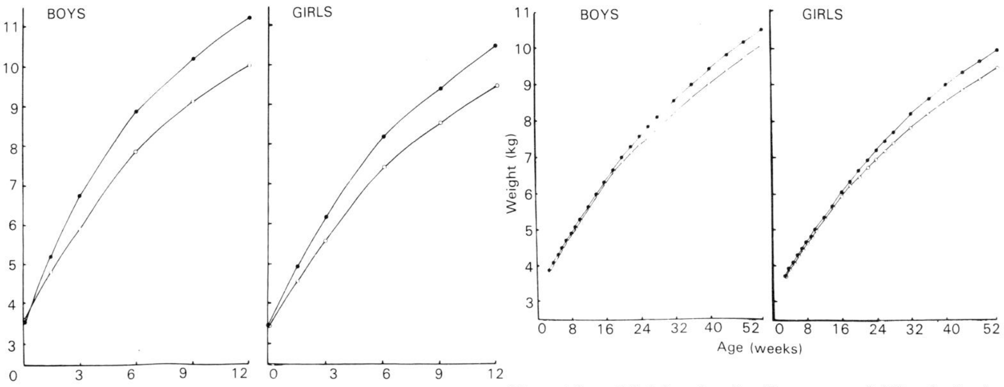

Fig. 11. *Weights of Australian infants in the first year of life in 1964 (●) and 1979 (○).* (Gracey 1987).

Fig. 12. *Weights in the first year of life obtained nationally in The Netherlands in 1965 (●) and 1980 (○).* (Roede & van Wieringen, 1985).

in growth trajectories was maintained long after solids must have been introduced. It is known, however, that bottle-fed children tend, even in present-day Cambridge, to receive solids earlier and in greater amounts than breast-fed ones. Whatever the explanation there is a remarkable similarity between the data in Fig. 9 and those already described in farm animals (Fig. 3) fed in similar ways.

The weight growth curves for our Cambridge cohorts relative to the Tanner & Whitehouse (1973) UK reference values and the internationally adopted NCHS standards (Hamill, 1977) are published elsewhere in detail (Whitehead *et al.*, 1988) but in brief the weight gain of the Cambridge children, which initially showed a somewhat accelerated velocity, started to slow after 3–4 months, such that by 10 months the 50th centile for weight in our Cambridge cohort of boys lay close to the NCHS 25th centile, although it had been on the 60th centile at 3 months. This difference in pattern of growth is summarized in Fig. 10.

These growth patterns are not confined to Cambridge. In recent years there has been an increasing number of publications showing the same findings, from many parts of the industrialized world. It is quite clear that the detailed shapes of the growth curves for infancy can be quite different now from what they used to be.

Figure 11 shows contrasting 50th centile values for growth in Australian infants collected in 1964 and 1980 (Bell & Lay, 1968; Hitchcock *et al.*, 1982). Interestingly the generally lighter 1980 data are almost identical with other Australian values collected in 1932. This indicates a peak in infant body-mass around the 1960s (Gracey, 1987). The Netherlands is a country with an excellent record of producing high quality national data on growth at regular intervals. Figure 12 compares growth data in infants in 1965 and 1980 (Roede & Van Wieringen, 1985). The similarities between the Australian and Dutch data, in terms of change over the same time period, is very apparent.

It must be emphasized that we cannot say for certain that these different patterns in weight growth are related to diet. In neither the Dutch nor the Australian growth studies were quantitative dietary assessments performed. In the Cambridge data contained in Fig. 10, it did seem that the rate of deceleration of growth relative to

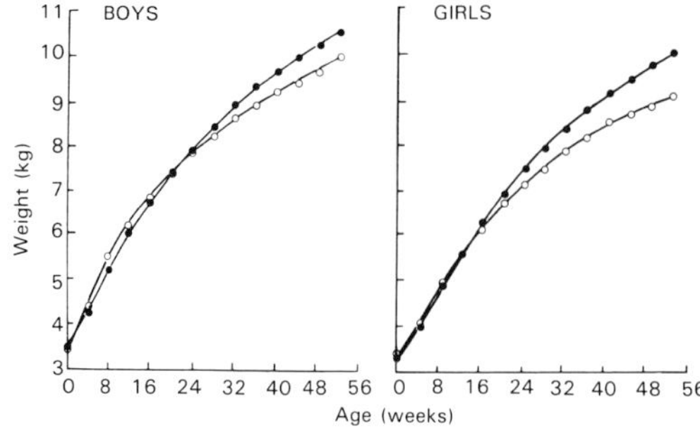

Fig. 13. *Weights of first born infants breast-fed to at least 5.5 months in the present Cambridge growth study (○), 1984–5, compared to Cambridge first-born infants breast-fed to at least 3 months measured by Smith and Widdowson (●) in 1960–64.* (Widdowson 1983).

the NCHS reference centiles was related to the time of weaning (Whitehead *et al.*, 1986) and it is interesting that a further cohort of children, studied by Owen *et al.* (1984) in New Mexico, who received no solids until 6 months had virtually the same rate of growth deceleration as the sub-group of Cambridge children who were not weaned until after 4 months.

In further support of the data in Figs 11 and 12, we compare in Fig. 13 the weight growth of a group of Cambridge children studied by Widdowson in the 1960s (Widdowson, 1983) with our own from the 1980s. Growth progress, once the weaning process had been initiated, was again quite clearly different. Is the faster rate of growth of the 1960s' Cambridge children due to a less severe attitude towards weaning? We shall probably never know for certain.

Long-term significance of differences in human infant growth

Important long-term considerations in man must be the secular trends in height growth and more especially, in growth in head circumference (because of the close relationship between this measurement and brain size).

In our Cambridge cohorts height growth exhibited somewhat similar trends to weight but the difference from NCHS reference values was less extreme. In the Dutch studies, the difference in height between the 1960s and 1980s was even less. For Australia no differences in height between 1964 and 1980 were observed (Gracey, 1987). The extent to which there is a change in the pattern of height growth will only be answered with certainty by further more detailed studies.

With head circumference the situation appears to be more clear-cut. This measurement is dramatically different from virtually all the other developmental trends we have studied, in that it shows no crossing of the standard reference centile lines. Indeed, all the centiles are higher, at all stages of infancy, than the corresponding Tanner reference values (Whitehead *et al.*, 1988), the 50th centile of the Cambridge infants being approximately parallel to the 75th Tanner centile. Our findings in this regard are almost identical with those of Ounsted *et al.*, (1985) from Oxford. Indeed in the United Kingdom and elsewhere in the industrialized world it does seem as though there has been a gradual upward trend in head circumference throughout this century (Fig. 14). What this means in terms of physiological function we do not know but at least in the context of the present review it must mean that there is no anthropometric evidence to suggest impaired brain development in parallel with the

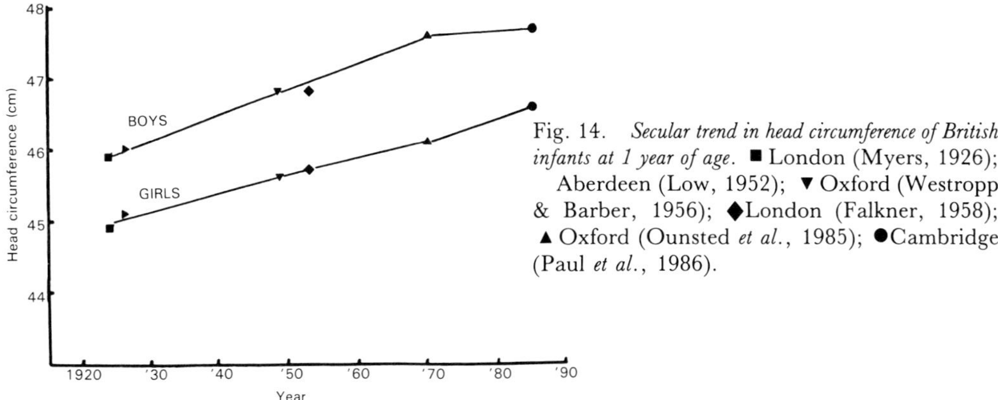

Fig. 14. *Secular trend in head circumference of British infants at 1 year of age.* ■ London (Myers, 1926); Aberdeen (Low, 1952); ▼ Oxford (Westropp & Barber, 1956); ◆London (Falkner, 1958); ▲ Oxford (Ounsted *et al.*, 1985); ●Cambridge (Paul *et al.*, 1986).

weight growth retardation. In this context it is interesting to note that an increase in mean IQ of British children over the past 50 years has recently been reported (Lynn *et al.*, 1987). The rise of about 1 standard deviation corresponds with the increase in head circumference shown in Fig. 14 which is also about 1 standard deviation, but it would be wrong to conclude that this implies a cause and effect relationship. Nevertheless this does provide scope for further research.

As far as the subcutaneous fat stores are concerned, a general conclusion in the Western World would probably be that smaller accumulations of fat are a good thing in that a tendency towards obesity is undesirable at any age. Whether there really is any link between infantile and adult obesity in man is however still very much an open question.

Many animal studies (Wallace, 1948; Clutton-Brock *et al.*, 1982; Lightfoot, 1984), but not all (for critical review see Allden, 1970), have led to the conclusion that early growth is crucial to maximum attained size. If this proves to be true of man also, is the growth 'retardation' we have been reporting likely to matter? Paediatric investigators in the UK and many other countries would again be inclined to say 'no' and that within reasonable limits, maximizing adult size is of little real practical significance. Not everyone would accept this view, however. For example, in China when we were discussing weaning, it was quite clear that our counterparts would not be interested in any practice which might reduce infant growth below the maximum, by however small a margin. Their primary consideration was the ultimate competitiveness of the nation in terms of sport! It was considered that the generally small size of the average Chinese person would have to change if they were ever to compete on even terms with the sprinters and other sportsmen and women from Africa, America and Europe. One could not help but be reminded of the fighting ability of the Scottish Red Deer, which is reputedly dependent on how fast the animals were able to grow in early life (Clutton-Brock *et al.*, 1982).

The reverse side of the coin has, however, been suggested by other animal studies. A less liberal food intake by rats in early life resulting in a slower rate of growth has been reported to enhance longevity (McCay *et al.*, 1935; see also this volume, Merry, p. 227). Sinclair (1955), 30 years ago, also speculated on the possibility that too rapid a maturation in children might be a cause of accelerated ageing. He stressed that insufficient thought had been given to the most desirable rate of growth.

He pointed out that this was not necessarily the maximum rate. He criticized the view that the infant of perfect nutriture was 'placid, rotund, red-faced and seated in contented contemplation of its folds of flesh', a depiction which presumably reflected contemporary ideals. This review by Sinclair is an excellent reference source to the earlier literature on diet in young animals and longevity.

Conclusion

Thus we return to the issues with which we started this discussion. It would be difficult, and indeed it would probably be unwise, to attempt to tailor a child's rate of growth in the same way that we do that of farm animals. We do not have sufficiently precise knowledge to do it properly, nor do we really know what to aim for. Is it possible that there is a trade-off in terms of longevity and quality of life in old age for athletic prowess in young adulthood? Only time and carefully conducted prospective longitudinal research is likely to provide the answer.

References

Allden, W. G. (1970): The effects of nutritional deprivation on the subsequent productivity of sheep and cattle. *Nutr. Abstr. Rev.* **40**, 1167–1184.

Bell, J. & Lay, P. M. (1968): The growth of Australian infants during the first year of life: a comparison 1933 and 1964. *Med. J. Aust.* **1**, 541–544.

Blaxter, K. L. (1961): Lactation and the growth of the young. In *Milk: the mammary gland and its secretion*, Vol II, eds S. K. Kon and A. T. Cowie, pp. 305–361. London: Academic Press.

Boggio, V., Lestradet, H., Astier-Dumas, M., Machinot, S., Suquet, M. & Klepping, J. (1984): Caracteristiques de la ration alimentaire des enfants français de 3 a 24 mois. *Arch. Fr. Pediatr.* **41**, 499–505.

Boulton, J. (1981): Nutrition in childhood and its relationships to early somatic growth, body fat, blood pressure and physical fitness. *Acta Paediatr. Scand.* Suppl. **284**.

Braude, R. (1954): Pig nutrition. In *Progress in the physiology of farm animals*, Vol 1, ed J. Hammond, pp. 40–53. London: Butterworths Scientific Publications.

Clutton-Brock, T. H., Guinness, F. E. & Albon, S. D. (1982): *Red deer: behaviour and ecology of two sexes*. Edinburgh: Edinburgh University Press.

Davies, D. P. (1973): Plasma osmolality and feeding practices of healthy infants in the first three months of life. *Brit. Med. J.* **2**, 340–342.

Department of Health and Social Security (1974): *Present-day practice in infant feeding*. Report on Health and Social Subjects, No. 9. London: HMSO.

Department of Health and Social Security (1980): *Present-day practice in infant feeding: 1980*. Report on Health and Social Subjects No. 20. London: HMSO.

Dewey, K. G. & Lonnerdal, B. (1983): Milk and nutrient intake of breast-fed infants from 1 to 6 months: relation to growth and fatness. *J. Pediatr. Gastroenterol. Nutr.* **2**, 497–506.

Doreau, M., Boult, S., Martin-Rosset, W. & Robelin, J. (1986): Relationship between nutrient intake, growth and body composition of the nursing foal. *Reprod. Nutr. Develop.* **26**, (2B), 683–690.

Falkner, F. (1958): Some physical measurements in the first three years of life. *Archs Dis. Child.* **33**, 1–9.

Fowler, V. R. (1981): The nutrition of the piglet. In *Recent advances in animal nutrition 1980*, ed W. Haresign, pp. 133–140. London: Butterworths.

Gracey, M. (1987): Normal growth and nutrition. *Wld. Rev. Nutr. Diet.* **49**, 160–210.

Hamill, P. V. V. (1977): *NCHS growth curves for children, birth to 18 years*. US Department of Health, Education and Welfare publication No. PHS 78–1650. Hyattsville, MD: National Centre for Health Statistics.

Health Education Council (1983): *Proposals for nutritional guidelines for health education in Britain.* Prepared for the National Advisory Committee on Nutrition Education. London: Health Education Council.

Hitchcock, N. E., Owles, E. N. & Gracey, M. (1982): Dietary energy and nutrient intakes and growth of healthy Australian infants in the first year of life. *Nutr. Res.* **2**, 13–19.

Hutchinson-Smith, A. N. (1973): Skinfold thickness in infancy in relation to birthweight. *Devel. Med. Child Neurol.* **15**, 628–634.

Kerr, G. A. (1972): Nutritional requirements of subhuman primates. *Physiol. Rev.* **52**, 415–467.

Knight, C. H., Maltz, E. & Docherty, A. H. (1986): Milk yield and composition in mice: effects of litter size and lactation number. *Comp. Biochem. Physiol.* **84A**, 127–133.

Kohler, L., Meeuwisse, G. & Mortensson, W. (1984): Food intake and growth of infants between six and twenty-six weeks of age on breast milk, cow's milk formula, or soy formula. *Acta Paediatr. Scand.* **73**, 40–48.

Kylberg, E., Hofvander, Y. & Sjolin, S. (1986): Diets of healthy Swedish children 4–24 months old. II Energy intake. *Acta Paediatr. Scand.* **75**, 932–936.

Lightfoot, A. L. (1984): Diets for early weaned pigs. In *Recent advances in animal nutrition*, 1984, ed W. Haresign and D. J. A. Cole, pp. 45–48. London: Butterworths.

Low, A. (1952): *Growth of children.* Aberdeen: University of Aberdeen.

Lynn, R., Hampson, S. L. & Mullineux, J. C. (1987): A longterm increase in the fluid intelligence of English children. *Nature* **328**, 797.

Martin, J. (1978): *Infant feeding 1975: attitudes and practices in England and Wales.* Office of Population Censuses and Surveys. London: HMSO.

Martin, J. & Monk, J. (1982): *Infant feeding 1980.* Office of Population Censuses and Surveys. London: HMSO.

McCay, C. M., Crowell, M. E. & Maynard, L. A. (1935): The effect of retarded growth upon the length of life span and upon the ultimate body size. *J. Nutr.* **10**, 63–79.

Ministry of Health (1959): Standards of normal weight in infancy. *Rep. Publ. Hlth. Med Subj. No. 99.* London: HMSO.

Myers, B. (1926): Statistics concerning the height, weight and other measurements of 1,400 London children. *Br. J. Child. Dis.* **23**, 87–107.

Oftedahl, O. T. (1984): Milk composition, milk yield and energy output at peak lactation: a comparative review. In *Physiological strategies in lactation*, ed M. Peaker, R. G. Vernon and C. H. Knight. Symposium of the Zoological Society of London No. 51, pp. 33–85. London: Academic Press.

Ounsted, M., Moar, V. A. & Scott, A. (1985): Head circumference charts updated. *Archs Dis Child.* **60**, 936–939.

Owen, G. M., Garry, P. J. & Hooper, E. M. (1984): Feeding and growth of infants. *Nutr. Res.* **4**, 727–731.

Paul, A. A., Ahmed, E. A. & Whitehead, R. G. (1986): Head circumference charts updated. *Archs Dis. Child.* **61**, 927–928.

Payne, P. R. & Wheeler, E. F. (1968): Comparative nutrition in pregnancy and lactation. *Proc. Nutr. Soc.* **27**, 129–138.

Prentice, A. M., Paul, A. A., Prentice, A., Black, A. E., Cole, T. J. & Whitehead, R. G. (1986): Cross-cultural differences in lactational performance. In *Human lactation 2: Maternal and environmental factors*, ed M. and P. Hamosh, pp. 13–44. New York: Plenum Press.

Richardson, F. D., Oliver, J. & Clark, G. P. Y. (1978): The pre-weaning and post-weaning growth of beef calves in relation to the amounts of milk and solid food consumed during the suckling period. *Rhod. J. Agric. Res.* **16**, 97–108.

Roberts, S. B., Cole, T. J. & Coward, W. A. (1985): Lactational performance in relation to energy intake in the baboon. *Am. J. Clin. Nutr.* **41**, 1270–1276.

Roede, M. J. & van Wieringen, J. C. (1985): Growth diagrams 1980. Netherlands third nationwide survey. *Tijdschr. v Soc. Gezondh.* **63**, 1–34.

Schluter, K., Funfack, W., Pachaly, J. & Weber, B. (1976): Development of subcutaneous fat in infancy. Standards for tricipital, subscapular and suprailiacal skinfolds in German infants. *Europ. J. Paed.* **123**, 255–267.

Sinclair, H. M. (1955): Too rapid maturation in children as a cause of ageing. In *Ciba Foundation colloquium on ageing*, ed G. E. Wostenholme and M. P. Cameron, pp. 194–208. London: J. & A. Churchill.

Tanner, J. M. & Whitehouse, R. H. (1973): Height and weight chart from birth to 5 years allowing for length of gestation. *Archs Dis. Child.* **48**, 786–789.
Tanner, J. M. & Whitehouse, R. M. (1975): Revised standards for triceps and subscapular skinfolds in British children. *Archs Dis. Child.* **50**, 142–145.
Wallace, L. R. (1948): The growth of lambs before and after birth in relation to the level of nutrition. *J. Agric. Sci.* **38**, 93–153.
Westropp, C. K. & Barber, C. R. (1956): Growth of the skull in young children. I. Standards of head circumference. *J. Neurol. Neurosurg. Psychiatr.* **19**, 52–54.
Whitehead, R. G. & Paul, A. A. (1984): Growth charts and the assessment of infant feeding practices in the western world and in developing countries. *Early Hum. Dev.* **9**, 187–207.
Whitehead, R. G. & Paul, A. A. (1987): Changes in infant feeding during the last century. In *Infant nutrition and cardiovascular disease*, Scientific Report No. 8, Medical Research Council Environmental Epidemiology Unit, Southampton, pp. 1–10.
Whitehead, R. G., Paul, A. A. & Ahmed, E. A. (1986): Weaning practices in the United Kingdom and variations in anthropometric development. In *Food for the weanling*, ed B. A. Wharton. *Acta Paediat. Scand.* Suppl. **323**, 14–23.
Whitehead, R. G., Paul, A. A. & Ahmed, E. A. (1988): DHSS present day infant feeding practice and its influence on infant growth. In *The physiology of growth*, Proc. SSHB Sym. No. 28. Cambridge: Cambridge University Press (in press).
WHO/FAO (1973): *Energy and protein requirements.* FAO Nutr. Meetings Rep. Ser. No. 52, WHO Tech. Re. Ser. No. 522. Food and Agriculture Organization, Rome and World Health Organization, Geneva.
Widdowson, E. M. (1970): Harmony of growth. *Lancet* **1**, 901–905.
Widdowson, E. M. (1983): Age, sex and nutrition. *BNF Nutr. Bull.* **8** (2), 117–132.
Widdowson, E. M. & McCance, R. A. (1960): Some effects of accelerating growth. I. General somatic development. *Proc. Roy. Soc. B.* **152**, 188–206.
Yates, N. G., Macfarlane W. V. & Ellis, R. (1971): The estimation of milk intake and growth of beef calves in the field by using tritiated water. *Aust. J. Agric. Res.* **22**, 291–306.
Yeung, D. L. (1983): *Infant nutrition: a study of feeding practices and growth from birth to 18 months.* Ontario: Canadian Public Health Association.

* * * * *

Discussion

Professor Care asked whether there had been a secular trend in the birth weights of infants which paralleled the interesting changes which Dr Whitehead had described relating to growth during infancy. He also commented on the weight change in calves. These of course are complicated by ruminal development. *Dr Whitehead* replied that there was some indication of a slight downward trend in birth weight especially in those sectors of the community in which the mothers' own weights seemed to be falling, but this was not statistically significant. In contrast there is an upward trend in skull size. As far as the rumen question is concerned much does depend on when the solids were given to the calves studied by Richardson but it was unlikely that the issue was a serious complication to the overall hypothesis being discussed.

Professor Care pointed out that the true stomach in the newborn calf is initially larger than the reticulo-rumen and the time which it takes for this situation to reverse and for the rumen to exceed the true stomach in size largely depends on the age at which solid food is introduced. *Dr Whitehead* then commented that perhaps the calf was not the best animal example that he could have taken to compare with the human situation but certainly the same phenomenon relating to the introduction of early food has been reported in a number of species including, the rat (Widdowson & McCance, 1960).

Professor Garrow questioned whether the cross-sectional data which Dr Whitehead had shown were applicable to the country as a whole in so far that Professor Holland's recent longitudinal studies do not show the secular change which one would expect. *Dr Whitehead* replied that Professor Holland's studies were carried out on older children and there was not time for the new phenomenon to have percolated through to them. Furthermore Professor Holland had no information on how his children had been fed or had grown during infancy. *Professor Garrow* wondered whether the cross-sectional survey data might not be complicated by changes in the nature of the population due to immigration. *Dr Whitehead* said that he did not think that this was likely. There was no evidence for this in the published literature either from Holland or Australia and this could certainly not explain the comparative data from Cambridge.

Dr Eastwood asked whether the size of the fontanelle gave any information of interest. *Dr Whitehead* commented that this had not been specifically examined.

Dr Tomkins asked whether in view of the interest in distribution of fat in adults there were any changes in the distribution of body fat among children. *Dr Whitehead* commented that the skin-folds on the back (subscapular skin-folds) were reduced in line with the triceps values. It was difficult in young children to carry out reproducible measures in other areas of the body and certainly there are no early data against which these could be compared.

Dr Bassett asked about compensatory growth and commented on experiments that he had undertaken in which he had held lambs at constant weight and subsequently fed them until the normal age of slaughter. He had found no differences in composition of the body at equal body weight at that time. *Dr Whitehead* said the view that early growth could compromise ultimate body size was not universally held but it was the majority view as described in the body of the text. One interesting possibility is that men whose growth was impaired in early life might carry on growing for a longer total period of time. Indeed there are some data for man indicating that growth could still take place at ages from 20–30 years.

15

Fibre in the diet

P. J. VAN SOEST

Introduction

Fibre has entered the limelight of popular nutrition, largely as a result of hypotheses advanced by Burkitt (1973) and Trowell (1975) regarding negative relationships between dietary fibre and human diseases. Formerly, the traditional attitude among human and monogastric animal nutritionists had been to treat fibre as a negative index of quality otherwise to be ignored as having no nutritional value, although nutritionists and physicians often recognized its worth as a natural remedy for constipation. Reversal of this attitude has been largely due to the discovery and recognition of the positive effects of dietary fibre and to the understanding of its metabolism which has resulted from recent dietary fibre research. There is also growing interest in analytical methodology for fibre fractions, and in the redefinition of the role of fibre in the caloric value of diets.

The fibre hypothesis stands as an alternative to that of other dietary factors—animal fat, cholesterol and protein—but it is difficult to compare the influence of dietary fibre and animal fats since human diets that are high in fibre tend to be low in animal products and *vice versa*. There is even some evidence that fibre protects against harmful effects of intake of animal products (Morris *et al.*, 1977). The negative association between intake of fibre and animal products leaves a chicken-and-egg argument as to whether animal products are the cause of disease or whether there is a fibre deficiency. Because humans tend to eat food to satiety, the increased intake of one component signifies some other dietary component must have necessarily decreased.

Dietary fibre has been defined as the complex macromolecular substances in food plants that are resistant to mammalian digestive enzymes. The definition has

Comparative Nutrition, ed K. Blaxter & I. Macdonald.

Table 1. *Responses of the fibre sources used in the Cornell Study (dry basis).* (Wrick *et al.*, 1983).

Component:	*Cabbage powder*	*Coarse bran*	*Fine bran*	*Wood cellulose*
Bulk volume (ml/g)	12.3	8.2	5.9	13.9
Particle size (μ)	484	744	173	143
Digestibility				
cellulose (%)	81[a]	41[b]	53[b]	20[c]
hemicellulose (%)	93[a]	58[b]	56[b]	50[b]

[abcd]Numbers with different superscripts are significant ($P<0.05$).

tended to focus on the polysaccharide components that are the dominant portion of the complex. However, significant amounts of resistant mineral, lipid, protein and polyphenolic components occur and modify the matrix polysaccharides with which they are associated. A description of the major components is given in Table 1 and the types or parts of food in which they occur. Because of the adopted definition, soluble polysaccharides including pectin and gums have been included in the dietary fibre complex, because these substances are also resistant to digestion. The definition is a compromise since these soluble materials are not fibrous in a physical sense. However, they can elicit responses in the digestive tract similar to the true insoluble matrix fibres. Bulk laxatives that contain large amounts of polysaccharide gums also fall into this class.

There has been criticism of this definition of dietary fibre on account of its emphasis upon carbohydrates and the overlooking of non-carbohydrate components that may have major effects. These include lignin, cutin, Maillard polymers (Van Soest, 1982), tannins and tannin-protein complexes (Wursch, 1979) that are also resistant to digestion. On the other hand the rigid definition of unavailable carbohydrate overlooks resistant and heat-damaged starches, some of which undoubtedly reach the large bowel (Stephen *et al.*, 1983) and can have a fibre-like effect; and also that all of these 'unavailable' carbohydrates may support substantial fermentation and contribute dietary metabolizable energy through absorbed volatile fatty acids (VFA).

Another related alteration occurs by way of the browning reactions elicited by baking, toasting and frying and also in the food industry in flaking and extrusion processing that can produce crisp browned products, eg chips, fritos, and various breakfast cereals (Van Soest & Robertson, 1977). The browning (Maillard) reaction involves the reaction of sugars with amino acids to form new lignin-like polymers that are indigestible and likely have fibre-like reactions. Mild toasting can greatly elevate the apparent lignin content of bread and also of breakfast cereals.

Fibre action and ruminant theory

The advancement of fibre as a preventive in human disease has led to suggestions for the mechanisms for such benefit. Fibre has been proposed to have benefit through effects on (1) passage of digesta, (2) colonic bacteria, (3) physical binding of indigestible fibre fractions, and (4) faecal composition. From these effects can be derived properties of dietary fibre that would be desirable and could provide a working basis for evaluation of fibre quality in human diets.

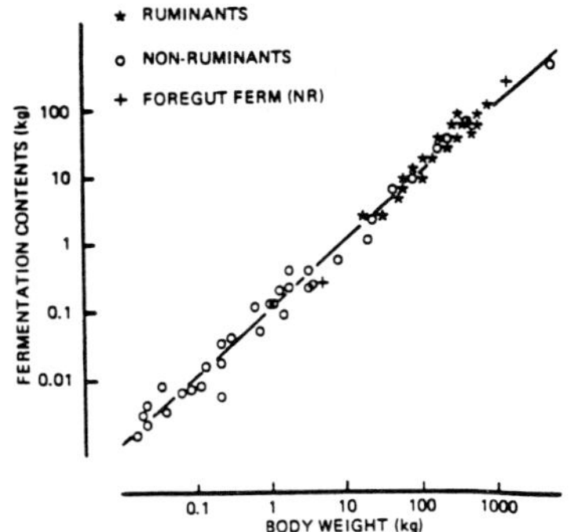

Fig. 1. *The log of wet fermentation contents regressed against log of body weight for African herbivores* (Demment & Van Soest, 1985). Foregut fermentors are defined as those who do not ruminate. Non-ruminants denoted in the figure are hindgut fermentors. The regression equation for all herbivores is log Y = 1.032 log X − 0.936, $r = 0.99$, $n = 59$. The regression slopes for ruminants and non-ruminants are not significantly different. The ruminant slope is 1.04. Regressions of this sort tend to overlook disparities characteristic of individual species (Demment & Van Soest, 1985).

Desirable effects of dietary fibre that have been postulated to have beneficial effects on human health include frequency of bowel movement and softness of the stool, the latter being associated with increased water content which reduces intracolonic pressure and therefore colonic stress and disease (Burkitt, 1973). These concepts have emphasized the water-holding capacity of fibre, and overlook the role that fibre has in supporting normal gut microorganisms.

The use of high-fibre diets in diabetes has allowed a reduction or elimination of insulin-dependency in many patients (Stevens *et al.*, 1985; Anderson & Bridges, 1982). This depends on the individual having a pancreas with some insulin secreting capability. Certain kinds of fibre are the most effective and appear to work in part by reducing the rate of absorption of sugar from a meal (Jenkins *et al.*, 1977). This places less immediate demand upon insulin. However, another factor is the fermentation of fibre in the colon. Propionic and isobutyric acids are among the major products from the fermentation. These acids are efficiently absorbed (McNeil *et al.*, 1978; Fleming *et al.*, 1983), enter the blood stream and are metabolized by liver into glycogenic products that do not require insulin for metabolic induction.

Ruminant-based theory integrates the previously mentioned concepts with the general theory of rumen function to which the fermentation in the large bowel has some resemblence (Van Soest, 1982). The hypothesis states that the action of fibre on the bowel is to a considerable extent mediated through the anaerobic microorganisms that grow on the fermenting fibre. Further there is a difference between brans (less fermentable) and vegetables, fruits and soluble types of dietary fibre (generally more fermentable) in regard to the microbial effect (Van Soest *et al.*, 1983). Stephen & Cummings (1980) have measured the microbial and residual dietary fibre components in faeces and shown different effects of cabbage and bran. Cabbage contributes less fibre to the faeces and more microbial matter, while the reverse is true for bran, less microbes and more faecal fibre.

Body size

While the focus of this paper is on the human species, comparison with other mammals is relevant for sources of models. The most intriguing aspect of fibre utilization in mammalian herbivores is body and gut size. The available data relating gastrointestinal contents have been summarized by Demment & Van Soest (1985) and are shown

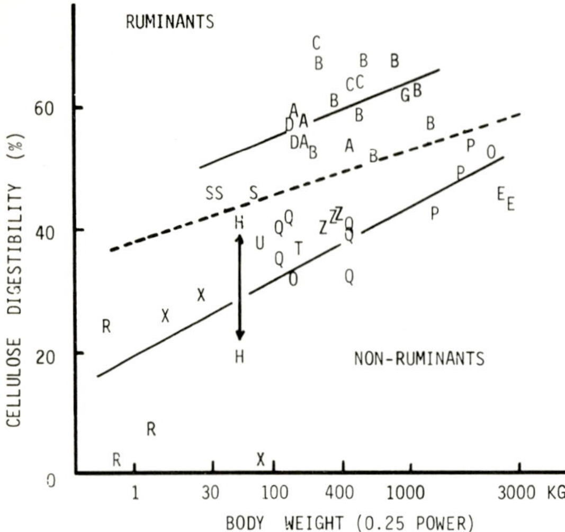

Fig. 2. *Relationship between body weight and cellulose digestibility in various animal species fed grass-based diets.* Identification of symbols: A, antelope; B, large bovids; C, camel; D, deer; E, elephant; G, giraffe, H, man; O, hippo; P, rhino; Q, horse; R, rodent; S, sheep and goats; T, tapir; U, pig; V, vole; X, panda; Z, zebra. Range of values on high-fibre cereal diets observed in man (H) is designated by arrows. Note that man is well within the scale of non-ruminant utilizers of cellulose. Weight scale is on the basis of one-quarter power. Data for man are restricted to those obtained from graminaceous cereal diets. Regression equation for ruminants denoted by upper solid line $y = 42.0 + 4.0x$; $r = 0.56$; 21 degrees of freedom. Dashed line separates ruminants from non-ruminants. Regression line for non-ruminants (lower solid line) is $y = 14.5 + 5.4x$; $r = 0.74$; 24 degrees of freedom (Van Soest, 1982).

in Fig. 1. Values for both ruminants and non-ruminants are shown to fall on the same regression line of similar power slope. Non-ruminants are classified into hindgut fermentors and foregut fermentors that do not ruminate. While there is a close relationship it must be remembered that logarithmic plots reduce apparent variation. There are significant interspecific differences in gut capacities. For example selector ruminants (deer, antelope) have smaller rumens than do grazers (sheep, cattle, bison, buffalo). Similar variation occurs within non-ruminants where the fermentation capacity varies from about 5 to 20% of body weight. These values are included in the figure.

The argument for association between retention digestibility and size is derived from the unitary slope of the logarithm of gastrointestinal capacity upon the logarithm of body weight, in contrast to the three-quarter power slope of the logarithm of heat production and energy requirements upon the logarithm of body weight. Theoretically gut turnover would be related to body weight raised to the difference between these powers, that is, equal to body weight to the one-quarter power for animals eating the same diet at equivalent requirement levels.

The capacity of mammalian herbivores to digest cellulose is related to their body size (Fig. 2). This effect is more evident in the case of non-ruminants than ruminants, which generally have greater capacity relative to size. From the position of man it is obvious that he is in the middle of the range. Small rodents have the poorest capacity and large rhinos, hippos and elephants the greatest.

Ruminants appear to be able to retain food residues longer than other animals of an equivalent size. Ruminant fermentation involves selective retention and comparatively fast passage of liquid relative to fibre. The difference between liquid and particulate passage is less in most other species. In man they are about equal, while in rabbits liquid is retained and fibre selectively ejected from the caecum leading to a low capacity for fibre digestion. The principal difference between ruminants and non-ruminants is that the ruminant is specialized in the utilization of cellulosic carbohydrates and has sacrificed maximal intake for optimal extraction of energy in cellulose. Other grazing non-ruminant herbivores (often larger animals) sacrifice digestive capacity for the sake of intake which, if sufficient, will override a low extraction rate. Small animals probably owe their poorer capacity to digest fibre to the fact that their energy requirements per unit of body weight are higher, necessitating faster passage and therefore lower fibre utilization. It is interesting that rodents are the main coprophagous group, suggesting that coprophagy may be an evolutionary response to the necessity of high passage rates, thus overcoming some of the limitations of short retention upon nutrient utilization. This characteristic renders the rat a most unsuitable model for human studies.

Microbial metabolism

In all animals the faeces are primarily composed of undigested fibre, microbes and microbial products. True endogenous matter is usually a minor fraction. In the case of highly digestible and fermentable diets, microbes become the dominant faecal component in all animals (Mason, 1984). Products of fermentation include volatile fatty acids (VFA), particularly acetic, propionic, butyric, isobutyric and isovaleric. These are produced along with some gas (CO_2, methane, hydrogen), and the growth and proliferation of the normal gut bacteria (Van Soest, 1982; 1984). The process can be expressed in an equation (McBurney *et al.*, 1987):

$$\begin{matrix}\text{hemicellulose, cellulose,} \\ \text{pectin or lactose}\end{matrix} + \begin{matrix}NH_3 \\ \text{or urea}\end{matrix} \rightarrow \begin{matrix}\text{microbes,} \\ \text{protein + lipid}\end{matrix} + \begin{matrix}\text{VFA or} \\ \text{lactate}\end{matrix} + \text{Gas}$$

The equation must balance according to rules of chemical stoichiometry (Wolin, 1981).

The VFA are normally absorbed directly across the colon wall in the form of free acid, thus relieving the acidity and maintaining the pH of the colon near 6, which is required by the normal fibre-digesting bacteria. The VFA are absorbed across the gut wall via the same mechanisms as in the rumen (McNeil *et al.*, 1978). This process has also been shown to occur in pigs, horses and dogs.

The VFA are probably not a major factor in increasing faecal water because they are largely absorbed (McNeil *et al.*, 1978). Volatile acid concentrations vary in human faeces (Ehle *et al.*, 1982) and probably reflect the balance between rate of production and absorption.

Urea and bicarbonate tend to flow into the colon, and the urea is hydrolyzed to ammonia and CO_2, the NH_3 supplying the nitrogen requirement for the growth of the fibre-digesting bacteria. Imbalances in equation 1 can lead to problems. For example, too rapid a fermentation (which could be from lactose or galactans from beans etc) leads to rapid gas and acid production; and too much acid, particularly lactic acid which can come from lactose or starch, can overpower the buffering mechanism and reduce pH of the colon with harmful effects on the normal cellulolytic bacteria. If the fibre intake is very low, the balance of equation 1 becomes altered. Because carbohydrate is deficient, the facultative bacteria switch to mucins and proteins which may derive from the gut lining and the mucins secreted by it. They no longer need urea since the nitrogen supply is now in excess of their needs. Putrefaction with the production of deaminated products and excess NH_3 results. This process is also

Table 2. *Stool characteristics and mean retention time in the Cornell Study* (Heller *et al.*, 1981; Wrick *et al.*, 1983).

	Basal	*Cabbage*	*Coarse bran*	*Fine bran*	*Cellulose*
Stool wt (g/d)	79[a]	87[a]	144[c]	111[b]	127[b]
Stool water (g/d)	59	68	112	82	95
% water	75.2[b]	78.1[c]	77.6[c]	73.5[a]	75.1[b]
Residual fibre (g/d)[1]	1.1[a]	3.1[b]	8.9[c]	8.3[c]	14.2[d]
Faecal nitrogen (g/d)	1.0[a]	1.1[a]	1.9[b]	1.1[a]	1.0[a]
Transit time (hr)	62[a]	64[a]	41[c]	57[a]	48[b]

[1]Measured as neutral-detergent fibre.
[abcd]Numbers with differing superscripts are significantly different ($P<0.05$).

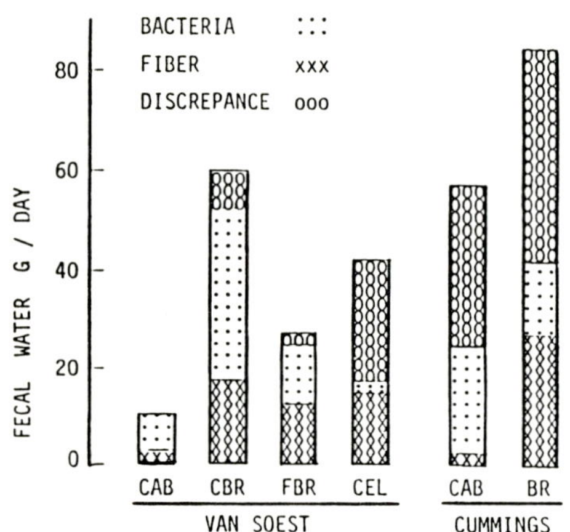

Fig. 3. *Histogram showing the calculated increments of water over controls in faeces based on the expected hydration capacities of residual dietary fibre and bacteria* (Table 3). Discrepance refers to the faecal water not accounted for after subtracting the amounts held by fibre and bacteria. Microbial mass was estimated in the Cornell Study by metabolic faecal nitrogen, in the Cummings experiment by a different procedure. (CAB = cabbage, CBR = course bran; FBR = fine bran; BR = bran).

associated with long retention and transit times. The excess amines and NH_3 are absorbed and must be detoxified by the liver and excreted via the kidneys (Visek, 1978). A similar problem may exist when vegetables with highly fermentable fibre are eaten. The substrate becomes exhausted; transit time is little affected and the colonic microbes may go for hours without dietary food resource. This constitutes the 'feast or famine' hypothesis (McBurney *et al.*, 1987).

Physical properties of fibre

Grinding and chemical refinement of fibre decreases its bulk volume and capacity to hold water and its ability to decrease transit time (Heller *et al.*, 1981; Van Dokkum *et al.*, 1983). In the Cornell Study (Heller *et al.*, 1980) fine bran actually decreased faecal water percentage and showed an insignificant effect upon transit time, in contrast to coarse bran (Tables 1 and 2).

The data support the opinion that unrefined foods in a coarse state are of real benefit. The different response between fine and coarse bran may account for some of the contradictory reports on the effects of fibre in studies where physical form may not have been adequately controlled (Van Dokkum *et al.*, 1983).

Table 3. *Physical properties and fermentability of some sources of dietary fibre.*

Source	*Cation exchange (meq/g)*	*Hydration (ml/g)*[a] *Dietary fibre*	*Faecal fibre*	*Unfermentable residue*[b] in vitro %
Cabbage	1920	2.8	2.3	9
Coarse bran	870	1.7	1.9	54
Fine bran	870	1.1	ND[c]	53
Wood cellulose	50	0.6	0.64	20–100[d]
Psyllium	30	0.9	3.1	72
Pectin	2270	11.0	—	0
Bacteria	—	4.0	—	—

[a]Hydration capacity of isolated fibres at 89 milliosmolar (McBurney *et al.*, 1985).
[b]Fermentation for 24 hr using human faecal inoculum (Horvath, 1983).
[c]Not determined. The value of 1.1 has been used in calculations for Fig. 2.
[d]The fermentibility of wood cellulose is highly variable depending upon donor of faecal inoculum. Digestion balances in the feeding study varied from 20 to 100% for wood cellulose recovered in faeces.

Stephen & Cummings (1980) calculated the incremental responses of microbial matter and water for cabbage and bran and postulated that the mechanisms for the two fibre sources in promoting faecal water differed, microbes dominating in the case of cabbage and undigested fibre in the case of bran. Their data are compared with those of the Cornell study in Fig. 3. The data are in agreement that cabbage is very fermentable, but the Cornell experiment showed a much smaller response. The finely ground wood cellulose and fine bran produced less water and bacteria but relatively equal fibre residues. The bacterial response was the least in the case of wood cellulose and like water response was poorest in the case of fine bran.

These results do not support the broad generalization that insoluble lignified sources of dietary fibre will uniformly promote faecal water through indigestible residue, and their microbial responses can also be highly variable. The generally poorer microbial responses of fine bran and wood cellulose may be the result of chemostatic effects where increased transit time reduces microbial efficiency. The microbial efficiency rises with faster transit because the voiding of a younger microbial population with less death and recycling of nutrients results in less VFA and more microbes in the case of shorter retention (Van Soest, 1981; 1984).

It has been suggested that water holding capacity promotes faecal response (McConnell *et al.*, 1974), though Stephen & Cummings disagreed with this (1980), pointing out that a high degree of fermentation may ruin this capacity. However, hydration capacity and cation exchange are positive factors in promoting fermentability (McBurney *et al.*, 1985) and if one considers the replacement of fermented fibre with produced microbes, the original hypothesis may still stand (McBurney *et al.*, 1985). A comparison of the physical properties of some sources of fibre is shown in Table 3.

Published results (McConnell *et al.*, 1974; Wrick *et al.*, 1983) show that dietary fibre sources are of unequal value as rated by hydration, stool volume and composition, and transit time, and have varying effects upon physiological responses (Table 4). Vegetables have the largest effects upon microbes, but less effect upon transit. Soluble gums have more effect in the upper tract upon gastric emptying.

Table 4. *Influence of type of fibre upon gastrointestinal responses.*

Fibre type	*Gastric emptying*	*Promote transit*	*Promotion of colonic fermentation*
Insoluble, lignified (coarse brans)	+	+ + + +	+ +
Vegetable or fruit fibre (pectinaceous)	+ +	+	+ + + +
Gums	+ + +	+	+ + +
Processed celluloses	+	+ +	Neg[a]

[a]Decreased fermentation relative to control.

Table 5. *Mineral balance (amounts per day) from the Cornell Study 1977* (12 male students) (Van Soest & Jones, unpubl).

	Diets				
	Coarse bran	*Fine bran*	*Solka floc*	*Cabbage*	*Low fibre control*
Ca (g)	0.36	0.33	0.45*	0.26*	0.40
Mg (g)	0.23**	0.24**	0.06*	0.21*	0.14
Fe (mg)	7.9**	8.2**	10.4	9.9*	11.3
Zn (mg)	1.9	3.1	– 1.0**	6.8*	4.4
Cu (mg)	– 0.05	– 0.09	– 0.35	+ 0.45[+]	0.06
Mn (mg)	– 2.2	– 1.4	– 4.4**	– 1.6	– 1.5

[+]$P<0.1$; *$P<0.05$; **$P<0.01$.

Mineral balances

Fibres are not equal in their effects upon metabolism (Table 5). Wood cellulose which has been added to bread is not a normal dietary constituent and has negative effects on mineral balance of copper, zinc, magnesium and manganese. However, none of the normal types of fibre such as that from bran and vegetable (cabbage) had this effect. Brans do not seem to have any consistent effect, positive or negative. Cabbage is positive except in the cases of iron and calcium.

Weight control and energy value

Weight control

Unsubstantiated claims have been made for fibre as a weight-reducing aid. While there are animal studies supporting such an effect, the relative level of fibre intakes that would cause lower energetic efficiency may be beyond that which is practical in human diets. There are even existing data which indicate that optimization of fibre intake in pigs, above a very low dietary fibre control, increased growth efficiency and weight gain (Kornegay, 1981). There is some evidence which suggests that an increased amount of fibre in the diet results in reduced intake over a period of days (Evans & Miller, 1975) and/or weight loss (Weinrich *et al.*, 1977), and that fibre helps people consciously restricting their intake to eat less (Mickelson *et al.*, 1979) and to lose weight (Yudkin, 1959; Mickelson *et al.*, 1979; Dodson *et al.*, 1981). A recent

Table 6. *Mean digestible energy intake before and after adjustment for carry-over effect and covariates* (Stevens, 1986).

Supplement	*Adjusted intake**[a] *(kcal/d)*	*Deficiency from control*
Control	2211	—
Psyllium	2054	157*
Bran	2154	57
Combination	2096	115*

[a]Mean daily energy intake over 14-day treatment periods.
*Different from control, $P<0.05$.

Cornell study with women (Stevens, 1986) indicates that consumption of Psyllium may reduce energy intake while wheat bran does not (Table 6). In the case of bran the reduction in dietary energy was offset by increased food intake.

The energy value of the fibre in a food is dependent upon its fermentability, so highly fermentable (digestible) fibres like those in fruits, vegetables (and pectin) probably yield more energy than the cereal brans that are more lignified and less fermentable. Wheat bran and psyllium yield about 1 kcal (4.18 kJ) per g by balance measurements in women (Stevens, 1986). By comparison the value of highly fermentable vegetable fibre and pectin would be about 3 kcal (12.5 kJ). Southgate & Durnin (1974) found that in bran-vegetable (mixed fibre) based diets dietary fibre contributed only 5% of the net dietary energy. However, in speaking of this, Southgate is careful to point out that energy is probably being traded—that is, the real absorption of energy in the form of VFA in the colon is really larger than observed, but that this effect is counterbalanced by large endogenous faecal losses which vary considerably with the type of dietary fibre.

References

Anderson, J. W. & Bridges, S. R. (1982): Short chain fatty acid metabolites of plant fiber after glucose metabolism of isolated rat hepatocytes. *Am. J. Clin. Nutr.* **34** (4), 840.

Burkitt, D. P. (1973): Some diseases characteristic of modern civilization. *Br. Med. J.* **1**, 274–279.

Cummings, J. H., Southgate, D. A. T., Branch, W. J., Wiggins, H. S., Houston, H. and Jenkins, D. J. A. (1979): Digestion of pectin in the human gut and its effect on calcium absorption and large bowel function. *Br. J. Nutr.* **41**(3), 477–485.

Demment, M. W. & Van Soest, P. J. (1985): A nutritional explanation for body-size patterns of ruminant and non-ruminant herbivores. *Am. Nat.* **125**, 641–672.

Dodson, P. M., Stocks, J., Holdsworth, G. & Galton, D. J. (1981): High-fibre and low-fat diets in diabetes mellitus. *Br. J. Nutr.* **46**, 289–294.

Ehle, F. R., Robertson, J. B. & Van Soest, P. J. (1982): Influence of dietary fibers on fermentation in the human large intestine. *J. Nutr.* **112**, 158–166.

Evans, E. & Miller, D. S. (1975): Bulking agents in the treatment of obesity. *Nutr. Metab.* **18**, 199–203.

Fleming, S. E., Marthinsen, D. & Kuhnlein, H. (1983): Colonic function and fermentation in men consuming high fiber diets. *J. Nutr.* **113**, 2535–2544.

Heller, S. N., Hackler, L. R., Rivers, J. M., Van Soest, P. J., Roe, D. A. & Lewis, B. A. (1980): Dietary fiber: the effect of particle size of wheat bran on colonic function in young adult men. *Am. J. Clin. Nutr.* **33**, 1734–1744.

Jenkins, D. J. A., Leeds, A. R., Gassull, M. A., Cochet, B. & Alberti, K. G. (1977): Decrease in postprandial insulin and glucose concentrations by guar and pectin. *Ann. Intern. Med.* **86**, 20.

Kornegay, E. T. (1981): Soybean hull digestibility by sows and feeding value for growing-finishing swine. *J. Anim. Sci.* **53**, 138–145.

Mason, V. C. (1984): Metabolism of nitrogenous compounds in the large gut. *Proc. Nutr. Soc.* **43**, 45–53.
McBurney, M. I., Horvath, P. J., Jeraci, J. L. & Van Soest, P. J. (1985): Effect of *in vitro* fermentation using human fecal inoculum on the water-holding capacity of dietary fibre. *Br. J. Nutr.* **53**, 17–24.
McBurney, M. I., Van Soest, P. J. & Chase, L. E. (1983): Cation-exchange capacity and buffering capacity of neutral-detergent fibres. *J. Sci. Fd. Agric.* **34**, 910–916.
McBurney, M. I., Van Soest, P. J. & Jeraci, J. L. (1987): Colonic carcinogenesis: the microbial feast or famine mechanism. *Nutr. Canc.* **10**, 23–28.
McConnell, A. A., Eastwood, M. A. & Mitchell, W. D. (1974): Physical characteristics of vegetable foodstuffs that could influence bowel function. *J. Sci. Fd. Agric.* **25**, 1457–1464.
McNeil, N. I., Cummings, J. H. & James, W. P. T. (1978): Short chain fatty acid absorption by the human large intestine. *Gut* **19**, 819–824.
Mickelson, O., Makdani, D. D., Cotton, R. H., Titcomb, S. T., Colmey, J. C. & Gatty, R. (1979): Effects of a high fiber bread diet on weight loss in college-age males. *Am. J. Clin. Nutr.* **32**, 1703–1709.
Morris, J. N., Marr, J. W. & Clayton, D. G. (1977): Diet and heart: a postscript. *Brit. Med. J.* **2**, 1307–1314.
Southgate, D. A. T. and Durnin, J. V. G. A. (1974): Calorie conversion factors. An experimental reassessment of the factors used in the calculation of the energy value of human diets. *Brit. Med. J.* **24**, 517–535.
Stephen, A. M. & Cummings, J. H. (1980): Mechanism of action of dietary fiber in the human colon. *Nature* **284**, 283–284.
Stephen, A. M., Haddad, A. C. & Phillips, S. F. (1983): Passage of carbohydrate into the colon. Direct measurements in humans. *Gastroenterology* **85**, 589–95.
Stevens, C. E. (1977): Comparative physiology of the digestive system. In *Duke's physiology of domestic animals*, ed M. J. Swenson, pp. 216–232. Ithaca State and London: Comstock.
Stevens, J. S. (1986): Dietary supplementation with wheat bran and psyllium gum: A clinical trial. PhD Thesis, Cornell University, Ithaca, NY.
Stevens, J., Burgess, M. B., Daiser, D. L. & Sheppa, C. M. (1985): Outpatient management of diabetes mellitus with patient education to increase dietary carbohydrate and fiber. *Diabetes Care* **8**, 359–366.
Trowell, H. (1975): Dietary changes in modern times. In *Refined carbohydrate foods and disease*, eds D. P. Burkitt and H. Trowell. London: Academic Press.
Van Dokkum, W., Pikaar, N. A. & Thissen, J. T. N. M. (1983): Physiological effects of fibre-rich types of bread 2. Dietary fibre from bread: digestibility by the intestinal microflora and water-holding capacity in the colon of human subjects. *Brit. J. Nutr.* **50**, 61–74.
Van Soest, P. J. (1981): Some factors influencing the ecology of gut fermentation in man. In *Gastrointestinal cancer: Endogenous factors*, Banbury Report 7, pp. 61–69. Cold Spring Harbor, New York: Cold Spring Harbor Laboratories.
Van Soest, P. J. (1982): *Nutritional ecology of the ruminant*, 374. Corvallis, Oregon: O & B Books, Inc.
Van Soest, P. J. (1984): Some physical characteristics of dietary fibers and their influence on the microbial ecology of the human colon. *Proc. Nutr. Soc.* **43**, 25–33.
Van Soest, P. J., Jeraci, J. L., Foose, T., Wrick, K. & Ehle, F. (1982): Comparative fermentation of fibre in man and other animals. In *Fibre in human and animal nutrition*, ed G. Wallace and L. Bell. Wellington, New Zealand: Royal Society of New Zealand.
Van Soest, P. J., Horvath, P. J., McBurnery, M. I., Jeraci, J. L. & Allen, M. S. (1983): Some in vitro and in vivo properties of dietary fibers from noncereal sources. In *Unconventional sources of dietary fiber*, ed I. Furda, pp. 135–141. I. Amer. Chem. Soc., Washington, DC.
Van Soest, P. J. & Robertson, J. B. (1977): What is fibre and fibre in food? *Nutr. Rev.* **35** (3): 12–22.
Visek, W. J. (1978): Diet and cell growth modulation by ammonia. *Am. J. Clin. Nutr.* **31**, 5216–5220.
Weinreich, J., Pedersen, O. & Dinesen, K. (1977): Role of bran in normals. Serum levels of cholesterol, triglyceride, calcium and total 3 alpha-hydroxycholanic acid, and intestinal transit time. *Br. J. Nutr.* **47**, 367–379.
Wolin, M. J. (1981): Fermentation in the rumen and human large intestine. *J. Dairy Sci.* **213**, 1463–1468.
Wrick, K. L., Robertson, J. B., Van Soest, P. J., Lewis, B. A., Rivers, J. M., Roe, D. A. & Hackler, L. R. (1983): The influence of dietary fiber source on human intestinal transit and stool output. *J. Nutr.* **113**, 1464–1469.
Wursch, P. (1979): Influence of tannin-rich carob pod fiber on cholesterol metabolism in the rat. *J. Nutr.* **109** (4), 685–692.
Yudkin, J. (1959): The causes and cure of obesity. *Lancet* **2**, 1135–1138.

Discussion

Dr Eastwood asked what factors determined the type of fermentation which took place in the subjects shown on Professor Van Soest's slides. *Professor Van Soest* stated that adaptation to the diets took place over several days and that it appeared that the determinant was the nature of the substrate more than the presence of particular organisms. The speciation of colonic microflora is difficult to alter by dietary means although numbers of organisms are affected.

Sir Kenneth Blaxter asked about the relationship between the volume of fermentation organs and body weight and was surprised that this was in fact a straight line with a factor of one. In the ruminant, gut contents amount to about 25% of body weight in the roughage-fed ruminant and considerably less, 5–6%, in an animal given a highly concentrated diet. It seemed remarkable that over such a wide range there was this proportionality. To this *Professor Van Soest* replied that the graph referred solely to fermentation contents in the gut and not to the whole digestive tract. The range of observed data is as wide as indicated by Sir Kenneth. However, such data will fit very well in a linear logarithmic plot as indicated by Professor Peters in his paper.

Professor Jackson asked for the evidence that digestion of mucin was solely a function of the colon, and how much was indeed digested there. *Professor Van Soest* stated that little was known about the quantity secreted. However, mucins appear to play an important role in the maintenance of gut microflora in the absence of requisite dietary substrates (work of Abigail Salyers, University of Illinois).

Dr Neale wondered about how far short-term experiments were relevant to the longer term problems relating to dietary fibre. Increasing the fibre consumption also increased the production of gas and it had been noted by survey methods that the intake of brown bread by the United Kingdom population has levelled off. He wondered whether this was related to gas production and a limitation by people of their intake for this reason. To the first question *Professor Van Soest* said that microbial adaptation to substrate appears to occur within a few days. In answer to the second question he described the fermentation process as leading to the production of carbon dioxide, hydrogen and methane and the probable absorption of some of these gases from the lumen of the gut and exhalation from the lungs. Flatus will depend on the rate of production and the nature of the dietary fibre.

Dr Thurnham asked Professor Van Soest, in reference to the paper by Professor Fraser on the previous day, to comment on the mechanism for the lowering of positive calcium balance by fibrous diets. *Professor Van Soest* indicated that binding of vitamin D, like cholesterol, by certain kinds of dietary fibre could be responsible. *Professor Kritchevsky* stated that there was binding of calcium which related to the presence of other compounds in the diet, and gave as an example oxalic acid. There were certainly complex interactions both in the short and the long term.

Dr Widdowson commented that with regard to binding of calcium, phytate could be important. *Professor Van Soest* commented that phytate is readily fermented and the resulting phosphates are less likely to bind calcium.

16

The retardation of ageing by diet: an animal model

B. J. MERRY

Introduction

The understanding of the biochemical mechanisms underlying ageing in man has proved a particularly intractable scientific problem. The ageing process, which is characterized by a progressive loss of homoeostatic control with time, is extremely complex, resulting from the interplay of subtle changes occurring simultaneously at the molecular, cellular, tissue and organ level. Further complexity arises at each of these levels as metabolic and homoeostatic compensations are made to accommodate age-induced disturbance of normal function. To distinguish the initiating biochemical event in any age change is therefore extremely difficult and this problem is often further exacerbated by the existence of underlying chronic pathology. While a species is characterized by an average lifespan, it is recognized that marked variation exists between individuals within a given species. Little is known of the factors which determine the rate of ageing between individuals or length of life between species. Attempts have therefore been made to develop experimental models in which the rate of ageing in laboratory animals can be manipulated in a predictable manner. Of a number of experimental strategies devised the most successful and reproducible have incorporated some form of dietary manipulation.

The beneficial effect of restricted feeding on survival in a laboratory rodent population has been known for many years (Osborne & Mendel, 1915; Osborne *et al.*, 1917). The effect is reproducible despite varying experimental designs and can be demonstrated not only in rodents but in fish and invertebrate species (Comfort, 1979; McCay *et al.*, 1939; Ross, 1969, 1972).

Comparative Nutrition, ed K. Blaxter & I. Macdonald. ©John Libbey 1988.

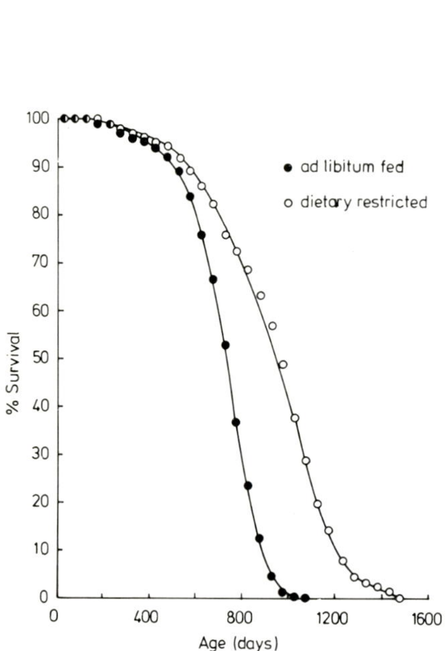

Fig. 1. *Survival profiles for CFY Sprague Dawley rats fed* ad libitum, *or on a restricted diet such that body weight was maintained at approximately 50% that of age-matched fully fed animals.* Group numbers, *ad libitum* = 623, diet-restricted = 948. Survival data are expressed in 50-day cohorts. Maximum lifespan achieved for *ad libitum*-fed animals was 1056 days, diet-restricted animals 1496 days.

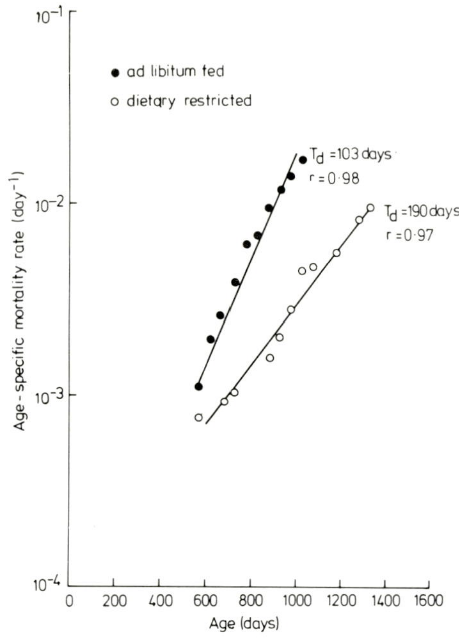

Fig. 2. *Transformation of the survival data of Fig. 1 by the Gompertz equation* $q_x = q_0 e^{\alpha x}$ *where*:

$q_x = d_x/hL_x$ is the death rate at age x,

d_x is the number of deaths between age x and age x + h,

L_x is the number alive at age x.

A plot of the logarithm of the death rate versus age is approximately linear. The rate of mortality is represented by the doubling time, $T_d = 0.693/\alpha$. The least squares method was used to fit the best straight line to the transformed data.

The dietary restricted model

Different experimental approaches have been adopted by a number of laboratories to induce chronic underfeeding in rodents and an extension in mean and maximum lifespan. These have involved varying the composition of the diet (ie reduced to 4% protein), which is then fed *ad libitum*, or more usually, the feeding of a normal balanced diet but on a limited basis, ie alternate day fasting and feeding. One of the simplest but most effective methods, which avoids repeated cycles of fasting and over-eating, is to limit access to the normal diet in rats so that the body weight is maintained at about 50% that of age-matched *ad libitum*-fed controls. Such a procedure, begun at weaning (21 days), will allow a continuous slow rate of growth to occur throughout life and results in a 36–42% extension in mean and maximum lifespan (Merry & Holehan, 1979, 1981) (Fig. 1). Transformation of the survival data from a number of laboratories by the Gompertz equation gives a time to double the rate of mortality in *ad libitum*-fed male rats of approximately 100 days, while in animals on restricted diet throughout postweaning life the figure is approximately 200 days (Holehan & Merry, 1986) (Fig. 2).

The greatest effect of underfeeding on subsequent survival is recorded when the regime is initiated either at weaning or in early adulthood and maintained throughout the postweaning lifespan (Yu *et al.*, 1982). Adult rodents can be successfully adapted to 56% of their normal food intake at one year of age if this is achieved gradually over about one month. Adult mice from two long-lived strains which were put on a restricted diet at one year showed an extension in mean and maximum lifespan of 10–20% (Weindruch & Walford, 1982).

The effect on lifespan of limited periods of restricted feeding followed by a return to full feeding has been more controversial. Dietary restriction for one year followed by *ad libitum* feeding was found not to extend lifespan in rats (Nolen, 1972). In a later study, however, using rats, mice and hamsters, it was reported that dietary restriction followed by a return to full feeding at one year was the most effective nutritional regimen for prolonging the lifespan in these species (Stuchlikova *et al.*, 1975). This conclusion was based not on maximum lifespan but on mean lifespan. Changes in the shape of the survival curve under different feeding regimes will markedly change the average survival without altering maximum lifespan significantly. The issue of whether the effects of a limited period of restricted feeding can accrue benefits for subsequent survival has been reinvestigated (Holehan & Merry, 1986). Survival of male rats returned to *ad libitum* feeding after periods of underfeeding ranging from seven days to one year was observed. It was concluded that during the first year of life, any beneficial effects of a limited period of underfeeding initiated at weaning were lost on return to full feeding. After approximately one year of restricted feeding a significant extension in maximum lifespan was observed although the effect was significantly less (10%) than recorded for rats on restricted diet throughout the whole of their postweaning lives. The effect of limited early periods of restricted feeding on subsequent survival is still a matter of controversy. Studies with the Fischer 344 rat, in contrast to the observations with the CFY Sprague Dawley, obtain significant increases in longevity after six months of restricted feeding before a return to full feeding (Yu *et al.*, 1985). It is now the consensus that the longer the postweaning period of dietary restriction, the greater the effect on subsequent longevity.

Composition of the diet

A survey of the numerous reports utilizing one of the many forms of dietary restriction to extend lifespan has failed to determine whether the beneficial effects obtained were due to the restriction of a particular dietary component. Conflicting conclusions have been drawn from studies designed to resolve this issue. Decreasing the intake of protein has been reported to increase longevity in rats, while other studies have yielded data which do not support this view (Miller & Payne, 1968; Ross & Bras, 1973, 1975; Nakagawa *et al.*, 1974; Barrows & Kokkonen, 1975; Leto *et al.*, 1976a,b; Payne, 1979). In a complex study using over 1600 COBS rats, Ross (1959) investigated the effects on subsequent survival of diets with varying protein and carbohydrate ratios. The results from this study were equivocal in their interpretation. Irrespective of the ratio of protein to carbohydrate, four energy-restricted diets significantly increased lifespan in rats compared to a commercial diet fed *ad libitum*. The high protein intake groups had markedly superior survival in the first half of life but the group fed low protein/low carbohydrate had the best late life survival. When this problem was reinvestigated by keeping energy intake the same, irrespective of protein content of the diet, it was found that reducing dietary protein decreased longevity (Davis *et al.*, 1983). Energy intake appeared to have a greater effect on survival than protein intake in this study. Moderate protein restriction in *ad libitum*-fed rats, in the absence of energy restriction, results in a significant increase in longevity, but the extent of this increase is much less than observed when a similar level of protein restriction is accompanied by energy restriction (Yu *et al.*, 1984).

A general criticism of attempts to separate the effects of energy and protein restriction on longevity in rodents has been made by Payne (1979). Energy intake modifies the amount of protein available for protein synthesis and as the severity of energy restriction is increased, more protein is utilized for energy purposes (Payne, 1979).

It is clearly established that high-fat diets decrease life expectancy but not life-span in rats, but increasing the fat content of the diet or altering the type has only marginal effects on survival characteristics (Harman *et al.*, 1976). The excess of minerals, vitamins and trace elements in laboratory diets and the design of experiments where vitamins and trace elements are added to diets fed on a restricted basis, indicates that restriction of vitamins and minerals are not involved in the effect of diet on longevity. Supplementation of the diet with vitamin E has a marginal effect on subsequent survival. The interpretation of studies using antioxidants such as vitamin E to extend maximum lifespan in rats is open to question for, to be effective, they have to be fed in doses which depress food intake (Comfort, 1979; Porta *et al.*, 1980).

Age-related pathology

It has been recognized from over 20 separate studies that the timing and incidence of age-related pathologies in the rat are exquisitively sensitive to the dietary history (Merry, 1987). It has been established that controlled underfeeding for prolonged periods in the postweaning life of rodent species results in an increased resistance to disease and a delay in the appearance of a wide spectrum of age-related pathologies (Cheney *et al.*, 1980). It is the consensus, however, that this effect on the timing of age-related pathology does not fully explain the extension of lifespan observed (Moment, 1982).

The effect of dietary restriction is most noticeable on the incidence of chronic glomerulonephritis, myocardial fibrosis, peribranchial lymphocytosis, periarteritis, prostatitis and endocrine hyperplasias in rats (Ross, 1959, 1964; Berg, 1960; Maeda *et al.*, 1985). The reduction in incidence of these pathologies can be as much as 50–90% and the cases which do develop are usually mild and seen at very late ages. Many of the reports related to chronic underfeeding and pathology have concentrated on the incidence of neoplastic lesions, on which the protein content of the diet has a complex action. Some types of tumour are commonest at high protein intakes while others increase in frequency when the protein intake is low (Payne, 1979). In rats on restricted diets there is a reduction in frequency of tumours of the pituitary gland, lung and pancreatic islet cells but not in the incidence of tumours of the thyroid gland, urinary bladder and tumours of soft tissue origin, although their appearance was delayed. Malignant epithelial tumours were also more common in rats on restricted diets (Ross & Bras, 1971). If the onset of restricted feeding is delayed to six months of age it is as effective as food restriction initiated at six weeks in slowing the progression of age-related pathology, although significant differences between survival curves are seen (Yu *et al.*, 1985).

In $B10C_3F_1$ and B6 mice in which underfeeding was delayed until 12–13 months of age, the formation of spontaneous lymphoma was decreased and the proportion of mice bearing multiple tumours significantly reduced (Weindruch & Walford, 1982).

Molecular studies in B6/1pr, C3H/1pr and MRL/1pr mice and in Fischer-344 rats, maintained on restricted feeding (up to 50%), revealed greatly diminished levels of mRNAs for several oncogenes (c-myc, v-myc, v-fos, v-abl, and v-raf). Conversely spleen and lymph node cells from mice fed low-fat, high energy or high-fat, high energy diets showed significantly higher levels of oncogenes expression (Khare, *et al.*, 1986; 1987).

It is a characteristic of the MRL/1 autoimmune-prone mouse strain that both males and females develop lymphoproliferative disease, autoimmunity and a rapidly progressive fatal renal disease. When fed *ad libitum* they live approximately six months, but lifespan is doubled when diet is restricted, even when the restricted feeding regimen is not implemented until after the onset of the disease. While such delayed dietary restriction dramatically affects the expression of the renal pathology and autoimmune disease, the mechanism of the protective action is not understood, for neither the formation of anti-DNA nor antigen-antibody complexes is reduced by dietary restriction (Kubo *et al.*, 1984). Restricted feeding enhances the synthesis of interleukin 2 in lymph node cells from normal rats (Richardson & Cheung, 1982) and MRL/1 mice. Autoimmune-prone mice strains characteristically have very deficient production of interleukin 2 (Altman *et al.*, 1981).

The delayed appearance and enhanced resistance to many age-related pathologies observed in rodents on chronically restricted diets has led to the detailed assessment of immunological ageing in these animals. The general response observed is a prolonged maintenance of T-cell-mediated function, with higher T- and B-cell proliferative response to mitogens. An inhibition of spontaneously active suppressor cells and maintenance of inducible suppressor cells with age is recorded, associated with a higher proportion of T-helper and T-suppressor cell populations. Restricted feeding prevented the rise in Ly-1 B-cells (normally increased four- or five-fold) in autoimmune-prone mice, and is also known to increase levels of IgM autoantibodies in both normal and autoimmune-prone mice (Hayakawa *et al.*, 1984). In food-restricted mice the Ly-1 B-cells remain at the 2–5% level whereas in *ad libitum*-fed or high-fat-fed mice these cells represented 15–25% of B-cells in B/W mice 8–10 months old (Fernandes, G., unpublished). In addition, the effect of dietary restriction in suppressing the development of autoimmunity appears to be due to the maintenance of a higher proportion of Lyt-2^+ (T-suppressor) cells. Enhanced 'natural killer' cell activity, which is generally correlated with the prevention of tumours, is also observed in rodents on dietary restriction.

While the overall incidence of spontaneous tumours is significantly depressed in rats on chronically restricted diets, protection against the initiation of tumours by exogenous carcinogens is also apparent. Pashko & Schwartz (1983) using

Table 1. *Effects of dietary restrictions on MAM-induced intestinal tumours.** From Pollard *et al.* (1984). Reprinted with permission.

Group	No. of rats	L-485 diet	Interval (days) to Restriction	Interval (days) to Autopsy	Average body wt (g)	No. of rats with tumours/ no. of rats at risk	Total no. of tumours	Average no. of tumours/ rat	P value
A	11	*Ad libitum*		140	460	10/11	30	2.72	<0.0001
	10	12 g/day	10	140	320	3/10	4	0.4	
B	8	*Ad libitum*		140	382	6/7	11	1.57	NS
	7	12 g/day	63	140	308	7/7	16	2.2	
C	10	*Ad libitum*		140	431	6/10	14	1.4	NS
	10	*Ad libitum/* alternate days	8	140	341	6/10	11	1.1	
D	10	*Ad libitum*		140	418	9/10	20	2.0	NS
	10	*Ad libitum/* alternate days	31	140	385	6/9	18	2.0	

*Weanling male S-D rats were inoculated sc once with MAM (30 mg/kg of body weight). Thereafter, groups were fed either *ad libitum* or restricted diet until d 140, when they were killed and examined.

male A/J mice recorded the binding of [^{3}H]-dimethylbenz(a)anthracene (DMBA) to the DNA from skin at five, seven and ten weeks after the start of restricted feeding (60% of *ad libitum* intake). The mutagenic action of this carcinogen is mediated through the conversion to reactive epoxides that bind covalently with DNA, and significantly reduced binding of [^{3}H]DMBA to skin DNA was observed in animals on a restricted diet. Similar protection against the formation of intestinal tumours by the carcinogen, methylazoxymethanol (MAM) in the Lobund Sprague-Dawley rat on a restricted diet has been demonstrated (Pollard *et al.*, 1984). Fully-fed male Lobund rats show a high percentage of grossly visible tumours in the colon and small intestine 20 weeks after a single subcutaneous injection of MAM. Significantly fewer tumours are seen when rats are fed 75% of the *ad libitum* food intake ten days after exposure to MAM (Table 1). Delayed onset of underfeeding until 63 days after exposure to MAM was ineffective in preventing tumour development. Paradoxically, alternate day fasting and feeding, a strategy frequently employed to induce restricted feeding and extended longevity, was ineffective in preventing MAM-induced tumours. It was the conclusion of the authors that the moderate degree of dietary restriction used did not depress the metabolic state and the restricted feeding was acting in a suppressive rather than a chemopreventive manner.

The major causes of death associated with ageing in the human population are pathologies associated with the cardiovascular system in which the development of hypertension is a major predisposing factor. Systolic blood pressure rises with age in laboratory rat populations from 100 mmHg at six months to over 140 mmHg at two years and older. Chronic dietary restriction did not modify this age-related increase in systolic blood pressure (Yu *et al.*, 1985) (Fig. 3). Several rodent models of essential hypertension have been developed through selective breeding. The spontaneously hypertensive (SH) rat which has been selectively bred from the Kyoto Wistar (WKY)

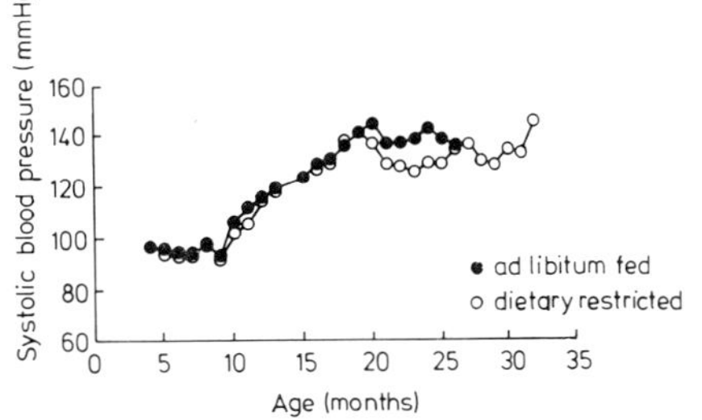

Fig. 3. *Systolic blood pressures with age in rats fed* ad libitum *or diet-restricted (60% of the mean caloric intake of* ad libitum *group) from 6 weeks.* Group numbers, *ad libitum* = 130, dietary restricted = 110. (Redrawn with permission from Yu *et al.* [1985]).

normotensive strain provides a good model since the hypertension is spontaneous in 100% of animals, increases in severity with age, is more severe in males and is associated with pathologies involving the heart, brain and kidneys similar to those found in the human condition. The hypertension develops before maturity, undergoes a secondary slower increase throughout life, with death resulting at about 18 months compared to 24 months in the WKY normotensive control. The early death is attributed to six specific lesions: renal interstitial fibrosis, myocardial oedema, fatty infiltration of the myocardium, atrial thrombosis, adrenal congestion and adrenal vacuolization (Lloyd & Boyd, 1981). Restriction of food intake (40% of the normal diet) from time of weaning in both the WKY and SH rats significantly increased both mean and maximum lifespan. Mean lifespan in normotensive animals was increased by eight months (from 24 to 32 months) while mean lifespan of the SH rats was increased by over 12 months (from 18 to over 30 months). Maximum lifespan in the WKY rat was increased from approximately 30 months to 38 months while that of the SH rat was increased from 22–23 months to 36–37 months. The extension of lifespan in the SH rat was accompanied by a decrease in the specific lesions normally associated with the hypertensive state to a level not significantly different to that observed in the WKY normotensive control on dietary restriction. Dietary restriction did not, however, modify the development of the hypertensive condition, an observation in agreement with the failure of restricted feeding to modify the age-related increase in blood pressure in normotensive Fischer 344 rats (Lloyd, 1984; Yu *et al.*, 1985). The mechanism by which restricted feeding protects against the development of hypertension-induced tissue damage in the SH rat remains to be explained.

In a somewhat similar manner chronic dietary restriction has been shown to protect KdKd mice from the development of genetically-determined renal disease. The renal disease of KdKd mice is similar to nephronophthisis in man and is inherited as an autosomal recessive located in linkage group X (Lyon & Hulse, 1971). The kidneys appear normal at birth but early in life progressive kidney disease develops, with proteinuria present by ten weeks followed by polydipsia. Autoimmunity toward erythrocytes develops and the KdKd mice die between seven and nine months of age. Restricting energy intake from 60 days decreased the appearance of the renal disease and inhibited the development of autoimmunity. Over 50% of animals lived to 500 days but when restricted mice were returned to a higher energy intake at 240 days there was rapid development of renal disease and death within eight weeks (Table 2). Restricted protein intake alone did not affect survival nor did it inhibit the development of kidney disease (Fernandes *et al.*, 1978).

Table 2. *Influence of dietary restriction on longevity of KdKd mice.* Reprinted with permission from Fernandes *et al.*, (1978).

kcal/d	*Protein (%)*	*No. of mice**	*240 d*	*Survivors/total 300 d*	*500 d*
I. *Ad libitum*	17	15	4/15	0/15	0
II. 16	22	20	1/20	0	0
III. 16	6	20	2/20	0	0
			→	0/9 (16 kcal)	0
IV. 8	22	20	20/20		
			→	9/9 (8 kcal)	5/9

*Entering study at 60 days.

It is not understood how restricted feeding acts to suppress genetically-determined pathology or inhibit the development of spontaneous or carcinogen-induced tumours. Restricting the caloric intake appears much more important in modifying the development of disease than restricting the level of protein intake in the diet.

Mechanisms by which dietary restriction modifies ageing in rats

The effect of dietary restriction in displacing the survival curve to the right, so increasing both life expectancy (mean lifespan) and maximum lifespan, has led to the conclusion that diet influences longevity in rodents by slowing the rate of ageing. Restricted feeding not only delays and suppresses the appearance of age-related pathology, it also retards physiological ageing (Holehan & Merry, 1986). Studies of varied physiological and biochemical systems which demonstrate age-related changes suggest that animals maintained on a restricted diet are retained in a physiologically younger condition than age-matched, fully-fed controls. The basic molecular mechanism by which dietary restriction can have such a wide-ranging effect on physiological ageing and its associated pathology has proved extremely elusive to determine.

Based on the original idea of Rubner (1908) it became clear that an inverse correlation could be constructed between lifespan and metabolic rate in mammals, giving rise to the idea that there is a total lifetime energy expenditure of about 0.86 MJ (200 kcal) per gram body weight. Although most mammalian species have about the same lifespan energy expenditure, primates are higher with an average of 2.10 MJ (488 kcal) per gram. Detailed analysis of 77 mammalian species has since revealed three major groupings of lifespan energy expenditure (Cutler, 1983). This concept has been adapted in a hypothesis to explain the action of diet on mammalian ageing. Sacher (1977) proposed that dietary restriction reduced the metabolic rate, thereby allowing an animal a longer chronological period before reaching this theoretical maximum of total energy expenditure per unit mass of tissue. Support for this idea was based on an analysis of the survival data from a study utilizing five different diets of varying calorific value (Ross, 1969). Sacher calculated that lifetime energy expenditure between groups varied by only 5% from 0.43 MJ (102 kcal) per gram body weight. This concept was further developed to suggest that decreased metabolic rate would result in a decreased rate of free radical generation thereby providing for a slower rate of tissue damage and reduced rate of ageing (Harman, 1981). Analysis of dietary and survival data from other studies have yielded contradictory conclusions, with rats on dietary restriction utilizing more energy per gram body mass in a lifetime than *ad libitum*-fed controls (Masoro *et al.*, 1982; Holehan, 1984). Direct evaluation of the metabolic rate in six-month-old fully-fed and diet-restricted rats over 24-hour periods under normal housing conditions gave values of 0.57 MJ (136 kcal) and 0.60 MJ (143 kcal) per kg lean body mass per day respectively. Observations on mitochondrial recovery in mice on restricted diet from weaning suggested a more efficient uncoupling and recovery in such animals, which was interpreted to mean a reduction of free radical generation in the intact animal and reduced mitochondrial damage with time. Dietary restriction appeared to postpone the onset of age-related losses of mitochondria by slowing mitochondrial damage and turnover throughout life (Weindruch *et al.*, 1980). The activity of the free radical scavenger superoxide dismutase is inversely related to the protein level of the diet, while lipid peroxidation activity in liver homogenates is positively correlated with the protein intake. Thus in animals with extended lifespans resulting from feeding a diet low in protein (4%), enhanced superoxide dismutase activity in hepatocytes and alveolar macrophages is associated with a reduced capacity for lipid peroxidation (Watson *et al.*, 1976). The cellular biomarker of ageing, lipofuschin, a product of lipid peroxidation, is reduced in heart and brain tissue of mice maintained on a diet containing 4% protein (Enesco & Kruk, 1981).

These studies show that chronic dietary restriction does not increase longevity by reducing the metabolic rate, although decreased generation of, and increased protection against free radicals may play some part in slowing down the rate of ageing. This conclusion has been confirmed by observations of core body temperature recorded by rectal probes. In the first year of life, during periods prior to meal feeding, core temperature of rats on restricted diets does fall by up to 2°C, but post-prandially and during the later stages of life, higher core temperatures are recorded in experimental compared to control fully-fed animals (Holehan & Merry, 1986).

The activity levels of individual enzymes in a variety of tissues show no clear trend with ageing or under restricted feeding conditions. This failure to find a consistent trend in enzyme activity is a common observation and reflects the complexity of metabolic adaptations invoked to maintain homoeostasis in ageing animals. The activity levels of individual enzymes represent a balance between synthesis and degradation rates. Many of the conflicting conclusions derived from studies on specific activity levels may be resolved by observations on protein turnover. This idea has been extended to suggest that dietary restriction may influence the ageing process by retarding the progressive age-related decrease in the rate of protein turnover (Richardson & Cheung, 1982). The consequences of reduced protein turnover with age would be first, a reduced ability to adapt metabolically to environmental challenge, and second, an increased cellular load of damaged protein as the 'dwell' time increased (Adelman & Dekker, 1985).

Comparison of the labile component of glucose-6-phosphate dehydrogenase in young and old, fully-fed and food-deprived mice (40 hr), revealed a 50% decrease in the proportion of labile enzyme in brain, spleen and liver of food-deprived animals (Wulf & Cutler, 1975). Mice fed a restricted diet (80% for 15 days, then 60% of the *ad libitum* intake for a further 55 days) from 23.5 months of age showed significant

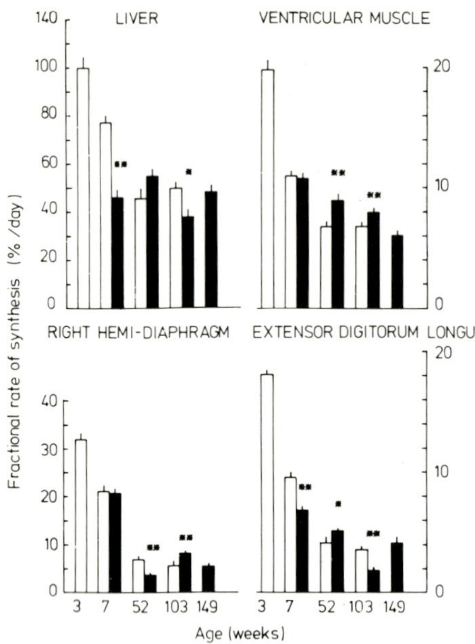

Fig. 4. *Fractional rates of protein synthesis with age determined* in vivo *for liver, ventricular muscle, right hemi-diaphragm and extensor digitorum longus muscle for rats maintained either on* ad libitum *feeding (□), or restricted feeding (■) as specified in Fig. 1.* Means and s.e.m. are shown for 5 animals for each age and experimental group. Statistical differences between the means for control and diet-restricted animals at each age were evaluated using Student t-test ($^*P<0.025$, $^{**}P<0.01$). (Data from Merry *et al.*, 1987; Goldspink *et al.*, 1986; 1987).

alterations in the proportion of heat-labile aminoacyl-tRNA synthetases in liver and brain. Prior to restricted feeding approximately 35 and 25% of leucyl- and tyrosyl-tRNA synthetases in the brain and liver, respectively, were heat-labile. After 40 and 70 days of restricted feeding the percentage of heat-labile enzyme had decreased to about 20 and 10% in the brain and to undetectable or very low levels in the liver (Takahashi & Goto, 1987).

Protein synthesis and turnover have been studied both *in vitro* and *in vivo* in a number of tissues from diet-restricted rats. A significantly higher rate of protein synthesis has been recorded in suspensions of freshly isolated kidney cells and cell-free homogenates of testis and spleen lymphocytes from diet-restricted rats (60% of *ad libitum* intake) (Richardson & Cheung, 1982; Richardson, 1985). The age-related decline in testicular protein synthesis observed between 12 and 19 months is inhibited by restricted feeding, and mitogen-induced protein synthesis and interleukin-2 production are similarly increased. The absolute rate of protein synthesis for hepatocytes isolated from rats fed *ad libitum* decreased 55% between 2.5 and 19 months but in cells from rats maintained on 60% of the normal diet, protein synthesis rates decreased only slightly with age and were significantly higher than recorded in cells from age-matched fully-fed animals. Thus the general conclusion from studies *in vitro* was that dietary restriction retarded the normal age-related decline of protein synthesis and degradation and therefore of protein turnover.

This finding has been confirmed at the level of the whole animal by studies conducted *in vivo* in rats (Lewis *et al.*, 1985). *In vivo* protein synthesis within discrete tissues from diet-restricted animals has revealed a more complex and varied response (Fig. 4). Protein turnover in the ventricular muscle of the heart and the small intestine closely followed the response observed for the whole animal but the general effect on skeletal muscle, lung and large intestine was a lowering of the rate of protein turnover

(Goldspink *et al.*, 1986; El Haj *et al.*, 1986; Goldspink *et al.*, 1987). In contrast to the *in vitro* observations, protein synthesis in the liver when measured by two distinct techniques *in vivo* was depressed at all ages when compared with control tissue (Merry & Holehan, 1986; Merry *et al.*, 1987). Turnover rates for hepatic proteins could not be calculated in this study because it is not known what proportion of the total protein synthesized is exported from the liver of rats, as a factor of age and dietary restriction.

Experimental support for enhanced rates of protein turnover in rodents on chronic dietary restriction has been reported from both *in vivo* and *in vitro* studies, although the data from the *in vivo* work are less conclusive in supporting the idea that a general increase in the rate of protein turnover is induced by restricted feeding.

Protein synthesis and degradation rates are subject to hormonal control and it has been proposed that at least part of the reduction in the rate of protein synthesis with age results from a decline in growth hormone (GH) secretion. In the skeletal muscle of old *ad libitum*-fed rats, protein synthesis can be restored by GH administration (Sonntag *et al.*, 1985). Growth hormone pulse amplitude and mean plasma concentrations can also be restored in old rodents by L-dopa, a precursor of brain catecholamines. Growth hormone in young rats is secreted in pulses every three to four hours and this periodicity of GH release is maintained in young diet-restricted rats (Merry & Holehan, 1985).

Although the frequency of release of GH is unaffected in rats on restricted diet, peak duration is reduced. It is not possible, however, to enhance the growth rate in these animals by exogenous GH administration (Merry & Holehan, 1985). No detailed studies of GH secretion in old diet-restricted rats have been published, but since GH release is dependent upon the turnover of the hypothalamic catecholamines, which is preserved in old diet-restricted animals, GH secretion may also be enhanced with age in these animals (Merry & Holehan, 1985; Sonntag *et al.*, 1985).

Many theories which attempt to explain the action of diet on ageing in rodents have postulated a central role for the neuroendocrine system, since it is known to regulate cellular metabolism in all tissues and exerts a critical control of the timing of gene expression. Dietary levels of specific amino acids have been shown to modify the synthesis and turnover rates of particular monoaminergic neurotransmitters in rodents (Fernstrom & Wurtman, 1971). It can be envisaged that dietary restriction operates through a complex neuroendocrine response mediated by monoamine neurotransmitters in the hypothalamus, the synthesis and turnover of which respond directly to serum concentrations of essential amino acids. The effect is amplified through a change in the profile of pituitary hormone secretion with ageing. This idea is supported by detailed studies of the endocrine response to chronic dietary restriction and retarded reproductive ageing observed in underfed rodents (Merry & Holehan, 1985; Holehan & Merry, 1986). Experimental data to support retarded brain ageing and the role of the neuroendocrine system in the diet-restricted model have been reviewed elsewhere (Merry & Holehan, 1988). Further support for this idea is provided by the extensive studies of Everitt who has developed a rodent model of retarded ageing based on early surgical hypophysectomy linked to specific endocrine support (Everitt *et al.*, 1980). The relationship between the anti-ageing actions of hypophysectomy and food restriction is still unclear although the possibility exists that it is an alternate stratagem to induce restricted feeding.

Conclusions

It is feasible to retard the rate of ageing and the appearance of age-related pathology in rodents by means of simple routine dietary manipulations. Such a procedure retards the decline in immunological surveillance with age while at the same time affording the animal protection against the development of autoimmune disease and the expression of inherited pathology. A slower rate of physiological and biochemical ageing is observed in rodents on restricted diet throughout their postweaning life, although beneficial effects on survival are seen if restricted feeding is delayed until mid-life. The manipulation of ageing by diet within the Mammalia has only been reported for short-lived rodent species. It is, however, the most successful animal model of retarded ageing and provides a unique opportunity to investigate the biochemical controls of mammalian ageing. It is not understood how diet can modify both the rate of ageing and the onset of age-related pathology, but two hypotheses have been formulated which seek to explain the operative effect of restricted feeding. The retention of a higher rate of protein turnover to advanced age would protect against the accumulation of labile or damaged proteins while maintaining a fine degree of metabolic control. A complex neuroendocrine response would provide for the retention of a functional immune system to advanced age and would explain delayed physiological ageing.

It is possible that the neuroendocrine system plays a major role in the control of protein turnover with ageing in the diet-restricted rodent but more experimental data are required before these two hypothesis can be resolved.

References

Adelman, R. C. & Dekker, E. E., eds (1985): Modification of proteins during aging. In *Modern aging research*, vol. 7. New York: Alan R. Liss.

Altman, A., Theofilopoulos, A. N., Weiner, R., Katz, D. H. & Dixon, F. J. (1981): Analysis of T cell function in autoimmune murine strains. *J. Exp. Med.* **154**, 791–808.

Barrows, C. H., Jr. & Kokkonen, G. (1975): Protein synthesis, development, growth and life span. *Growth* **39**, 525–533.

Berg, B. N. (1960): Nutrition and longevity in the rat. I. Longevity and onset of disease with different levels of food intake. *J. Nutr.* **71**, 255–263.

Cheney, K. E., Liu, R. K., Smith, G. S., Leung, R. E., Mickey, M. R. & Walford, R. L. (1980): Survival and disease patterns in C57BL/6J mice, subjected to undernutrition. *Exp. Gerontol.* **15**, 237–258.

Comfort, A. (1979): *The biology of senescence*, 3rd edn. Edinburgh and London: Churchill Livingstone.

Cutler, R. G. (1983): Superoxide dismutase, longevity and specific metabolic rate. *Gerontology* **29**, 113–120.

Davies, T. A., Bales, C. W. & Beauchene, R. E. (1983): Differential effects of dietary caloric and protein restriction in the ageing rat. *Exp. Gerontol.* **18**, 427–435.

El Haj, A. J., Lewis, S. E. M., Goldspink, D. F., Merry, B. J. & Holehan, A. M. (1986): The effect of chronic and acute dietary restriction on the growth and protein turnover of fast and slow types of rat skeletal muscle. *Comp. Biochem. Physiol.* **85A**, 281–287.

Enesco, H. E. & Kruk, P. (1981): Dietary restriction reduces fluorescent age pigment accumulation in mice. *Exp. Gerontol.* **16**, 357–361.

Everitt, A. V., Seedsman, N. J. & Jones, F. (1980): The effects of hypophysectomy and continuous food restriction, begun at ages 70 and 400 days, on collagen ageing, proteinuria, incidence of pathology and longevity in the male rat. *Mech. Ageing Dev.* **12**, 161–172.

Fernandes, G., Yunis, E. J., Miranda, M., Smith, J. & Good, R. A. (1978): Nutritional inhibition of genetically determined renal disease and autoimmunity with prolongation of life in kd/kd mice. *Proc. Natl. Acad. Sci. USA* **75**, 2888–2892.

Fernstrom, J. D. & Wurtman, R. J. (1971): Effect of chronic corn consumption on serotonin content of rat brain. *Nature* **234**, 62–64.

Goldspink, D. F., El Haj, A. J., Lewis, S. E. M., Merry, B. J. & Holehan, A. M. (1987): The influence of chronic dietary intervention on protein turnover and growth of the diaphragm and extensor digitorum longus muscles of the rat. *Exp. Gerontol.* **22**, 67–78.

Goldspink, D. F., Lewis, S. E. M. & Merry, B. J. (1986): The effects of ageing and chronic dietary intervention on protein turnover and the growth of ventricular muscle in the rat heart. *Cardiovasc. Res.* **XX**, 672–678.

Harman, D. (1981): The aging process. *Proc. Natl. Acad. Sci. USA* **78**, 7124–7128.

Harman, D., Hendricks, S., Eddy, D. E. & Siebold, J. (1976): Free radical theory of aging: Effect of dietary fat on central nervous system function. *J. Am. Geriat. Soc.* **24**, 301–307.

Hayakawa, K., Hardy, R. R., Honda, M., Hertzenberg, L. A. & Steinberg, A. D. (1984): Ly-1 B cells: Functionally distinct lymphocytes that secrete IgM autoantibodies. *Proc. Natl. Acad. Sci. USA* **81**, 2494–2498.

Holehan, A. M. (1984): *The effect of ageing and dietary restriction upon reproduction in the female CFY Sprague-Dawley rat.* PhD Thesis, University of Hull, UK.

Holehan, A. M. & Merry, B. J. (1986): The experimental manipulation of ageing by diet. *Biol. Rev.* **61**, 329–368.

Khare, A., Freidrichs, W., & Fernandes, G. (1986): Paper presented at the International Symposium on Nutritional Regulation of Immunity and Infection. Toronto, Canada (abstr).

Khare, A., Laganier, S., Yu, B. P., Sandberg, L., Friedric, B. (1987): Effect of food restriction and aging on immune cell fatty-acids, functions and oncogene expression in SPF Fischer-344 rats. *Fed. Proc.* **46**, 567.

Kubo, C., Day, N. K. & Good, R. A. (1984): Influence of early or late dietary restriction on life span and immunological parameters in MRL/Mp-Ipr/Ipr mice. *Proc. Natl. Acad. Sci. USA*. **81**, 5831–5835.

Leto, S., Kokkonen, G. C. & Barrows, C. H. (1976a): Dietary protein, life-span and biochemical variables in female mice. *J. Gerontol.* **31**, 144–148.

Leto, S., Kokkonen, G. C. & Barrows, C. H. (1976b): Dietary protein, life-span and physiological variables in female mice. *J. Gerontol.* **32**, 149–154.

Lewis, S. E. M., Goldspink, D. F., Phillips, J. G., Merry, B. J. & Holehan, A. M. (1985): The effects of aging and chronic dietary restriction on whole body growth and protein turnover in the rat. *Exp. Gerontol.* **20**, 253–263.

Lloyd, T. (1984): Food restriction increases lifespan of hypertensive animals. *Life Sci.* **34**, 401–407.

Lloyd, T. & Boyd, B. (1981): Development and regulation of hypertension in the spontaneously hypertensive rat: enzymatic and nutritional studies. In *Function and regulation of monoamine enzymes: Basic and clinical aspects*, ed E. Usolin, N. Weiner and M. B. H. Youdin, pp. 843–854. London: Macmillan Press.

Lyon, M. F. & Hulse, E. V. (1971): An inherited kidney disease of mice resembling human nephronophthisis. *J. Med. Genet.* **8**, 41–48.

McCay, C. M., Maynard, L. A., Sperling, G. & Barnes, L. L. (1939): Retarded growth, lifespan, ultimate body size and age changes in the albino rat after feeding diets restricted in calories. *J. Nutr.* **18**, 1–13.

Maeda, H., Gleiser, C. A., Masoro, E. J., Murata, I., McMahan, C. A. & Yu, B. P. (1985): Nutritional influences on ageing of Fischer 344 rats: Pathology. *J. Gerontol.* **40**, 671–688.

Masoro, E. J., Yu, B. P. & Bertrand, H. A. (1982): Action of food restriction in delaying the aging process. *Proc. Natl. Acad. Sci. USA* **79**, 4239–4241.

Merry, B. J. (1987): Food restriction and the aging process. In *Biological age and aging risk factors*, ed A. Ruiz-Torres, pp. 259–272. Madrid: Technipublicaciones, SA.

Merry, B. J. & Holehan, A. M. (1979): Onset of puberty and duration of fertility in rats fed a restricted diet. *J. Reprod. Fert.* **57**, 253–259.

Merry, B. J. & Holehan, A. M. (1981): Serum profiles of LH, FSH, testosterone and 5 α-DHT from 21 to 1000 days of age in *ad libitum* fed and dietary restricted rats. *Exp. Geront.* **16**, 431–444.

Merry, B. J. & Holehan, A. M. (1985): The endocrine response to dietary restriction in the rat. In *The molecular biology of aging, vol. 35, Basic Life Sciences*, ed A. D. Woodhead, A. D. Blackett and A. Hollaender, pp. 117–141. New York: Plenum Press.

Merry, B. J. & Holehan, A. M. (1988): Dietary restriction and the neuroendocrinology of ageing. In *Monograph series: Interdisciplinary topics in gerontology*, ed A. V. Everitt and J. R. Walton. Basel: S. Karger. (in press).

Merry, B. J., Holehan, A. M., Lewis, S. E. M. & Goldspink, D. F. (1987): The effects of ageing and chronic dietary restriction on *in vivo* hepatic protein synthesis in the rat. *Mech. Ageing. Dev.* **39**, 189–199.

Miller, D. S. & Payne, P. R. (1968): Longevity and protein intake. *Exp. Gerontol.* **3**, 231–234.

Moment, G. B. (1982): Theories of aging: an overview. In *Testing the theories of aging*, ed R. C. Adelman and G. S. Roth, pp. 1–23. Boca Raton, Florida: CRC Press.

Nakagawa, I., Sasaki, A., Kajimoto, T., Fukuyama, T., Suzuki, T. & Yamada, E. (1974): Effect of protein nutrition on growth, longevity and incidence of lesions in the rat. *J. Nutr.* **104**, 1576–1583.

Nolen, G. A. (1972): Effects of various restricted dietary regimes on the growth, health and longevity of albino rats. *J. Nutr.* **102**, 1477–1494.

Osborne, T. B. & Mendel, L. B. (1915): The resumption of growth after long continued failure to grow. *J. Biol. Chem.* **23**, 439–454.

Osborne, T. B., Mendel, L. B. & Ferry, E. L. (1917): The effect of retardation of growth upon the breeding period and duration of life in rats. *Science* **45**, 294–295.

Pashko, L. L. & Schwartz, A. G. (1983): Effects of food restriction, dehydroepiandrosterone, or obesity on the binding of ^{3}H-7, 12-dimethylbenz(a)anthracene to mouse skin DNA. *J. Gerontol.* **38**, 8–12.

Payne, P. (1979): Ageing and nutrition. In *Drugs and the elderly*, ed J. Crooks and I. H. Stevenson, pp. 39–47. London: Macmillan Press.

Pollard, M., Luckert, P. H. & Pan, G.-Y. (1984): Inhibition of intestinal tumorigenesis in methylazoxymethanol-treated rats by dietary restriction. *Cancer Treatment Rep.* **68**, 405–408.

Porta, E. A., Joun, N. S. & Nitta, R. T. (1980): Effects of the type of dietary fat at two levels of vitamin E in Wistar male rats during development and aging. I. Lifespan, serum biochemical parameters and pathological changes. *Mech. Ageing Dev.* **13**, 1–39.

Richardson, A. (1985): The effect of age and nutrition on protein synthesis by cells and tissues from mammals. In *Handbook of nutrition in the aged*, ed R. R. Watson, pp. 31–48. Boca Raton, Florida: CRC Press.

Richardson, A. & Cheung, H. T. (1982): The relationship between age-related changes in gene expression, protein turnover, and the responsiveness of an organism to stimuli. *Life Sci.* **31**, 605–613.

Ross, M. H. (1959): Protein, calories and life expectancy. *Fed. Proc.* **18**, 1190–1207.

Ross, M. H. (1964): Nutrition, disease and length of life. In *Diet and body constitution*, ed G. E. W. Wolstenholme and M. O'Connor, pp. 91–193. London: Ciba Foundation Study Group, number 17.

Ross, M. H. (1969): Aging, nutrition and hepatic enzyme activity patterns in the rat. *J. Nutr. Suppl.* **1**, **97**, 563–602.

Ross, M. H. (1972): Length of life and caloric intake. *Amer. J. Clin. Nutr.* **25**, 834–838.

Ross, M. H. & Bras, G. (1971): Lasting influence of early caloric restriction on prevalence of neoplasms. *J. Nat. Cancer Inst.* **47**, 1095–1113.

Ross, M. H. & Bras, G. (1973): Influence of protein under and over nutrition on spontaneous tumor prevalence in the rat. *J. Nutr.* **103**, 944–963.

Ross, M. H. & Bras, G. (1975): Food preference and length of life. *Science* **190**, 165–167.

Rubner, M. (1908): *Das Problem der Lebensdauer und seine Beziehungen zu Wachstrum und Ernahung*. Muchen: R. Oldenbourg.

Sacher, G. A. (1977): Life table modification and life prolongation. In *Handbook of the biology of aging*, ed C. E. Finch and L. Hayflick, pp. 582–638. New York: Van Nostrand Reinhold Company.

Sonntag, W. E., Hylka, V. W. & Meites, J. (1985): Growth hormone restores protein synthesis in skeletal muscle of old male rats. *J. Gerontol.* **40**, 689–694.

Stuchlikova, E., Juricova-Horakova, M. & Deyl, Z. (1975): New aspects of the dietary effect of life prolongation in rodents. What is the role of obesity in aging? *Exp. Gerontol.* **10**, 141–144.

Takahashi, R. & Goto, S. (1987): Influence of dietary restriction on accumulation of heat-labile enzyme molecules in the liver and brain of mice. *Arch. Biochem. Biophys.* **257**, 200–206.

Watson, R. R., Rister, M. & Baehner, R. L. (1976): Superoxide dismutase activity in polymorphonuclear leucocytes and alveolar macrophages of protein malnourished rats and guinea pigs. *J. Nutr.* **106**, 1801–1808.

Weindruch, R. L., Cheung, M. K., Verity, M. A. & Walford, R. L. (1980): Modification of mitochondrial respiration by aging and dietary restriction. *Mech. Ageing Dev.* **12**, 375–392.

Weindruch, R. H. & Walford, R. L. (1982): Dietary restriction in mice beginning at 1 year of age: effect on life-span and spontaneous cancer incidence. *Science* **215**, 1415–1418.

Wulf, J. H. & Cutler, R. G. (1975): Altered protein hypothesis of mammalian aging processes—I. Thermal stability of glucose-6-phosphate dehydrogenase in C57BL/6J mouse tissue. *Exp. Gerontol.* **10**, 101–117.

Yu, B. P., Masoro, E. J., Murata, I., Bertrand, H. A. & Lynd, F. T. (1982): Life span study of SPF Fischer 344 male rats fed *ad libitum* or restricted diets: Longevity, growth, lean body mass and disease. *J. Gerontol.* **37**, 130–141.

Yu, B. P., Wong, G., Lee, H.-C., Bertrand, H. & Masora, E. J. (1984): Age changes in hepatic metabolic characteristics and their modulation by dietary manipulation. *Mech. Ageing Dev.* **24**, 67–81.

Yu, B. P., Masoro, E. J. & McMahan, C. A. (1985): Nutritional influences on aging of Fischer 344 rats: I. Physical, metabolic and longevity characteristic. *J. Gerontol.* **40**, 657–670.

* * * * *

Discussion

Professor Stock returned to the over-feeding experiments which he had conducted using the cafeteria method of feeding. He argued that just as restricted feeding retarded ageing so over-feeding should accelerate ageing. Survival in cafeteria-fed animals was similar to the normal controls and he did not observe accelerated ageing in these animals, though a considerable increase in weight was observed. *Dr Merry* commented that to his knowledge no mammalian model of accelerated ageing had been developed. In both the cafeteria-feeding and diet-restricted feeding experiments it is extremely difficult to achieve a consensus as to what constitutes the appropriate control animal, since *ad libitum*-fed animals are recognized as being over-fed.

Dr Eastwood raised the matter of immigrant populations and comparisons of mortality. *Dr Merry* commented that it was difficult in studies of this type to be certain that it was the change in dietary habit which was responsible for the change in survival statistics although this factor appears to be the most likely explanation.

Dr Elia raised the problem about the treatment of the patient with cancer. In clinical practice it is usual to combat the decline in weight by improving nutritional status and wondered whether there was any effect here which was of concern. In particular would there be a change in tumour growth and what practice should in fact be adopted? *Dr Merry* replied that the situation of retarded tumour development in the animal model and the human patient were not comparable. In the human condition the tumour is not usually seen by the clinician until it has reached an advanced stage whereas in the diet-restricted animal model tumour growth and retarded immunological ageing have been initiated quite early in life. In experiments with tumour induction by exogenous carcinogens, tumour suppression is only feasible if restricted feeding is implemented early in the growth of the tumour and is not effective if delayed beyond a certain point. The data necessary to extrapolate from the animal model to the clinical situation were not available.

17

Is man unique?

ANTON C. BEYNEN

Introduction

From the outset of this communication I wish to qualify its title further into 'Is man unique, in terms of nutritional properties, when compared to experimental animals?'. The answer is yes or no, depending on the properties of man to be compared with those of experimental animals. It also depends on the degree of detail of the comparison. In an attempt to discuss the simultaneous uniqueness and universality of man, one approach would be to describe various examples of these opposite characteristics. However, I would like to focus on trends in the use of animals for human nutrition research. I shall put forward two suggestions. First, in experimental nutrition research man is becoming *more* unique in scientific terms. Secondly, man is becoming *less* unique in ethical terms.

Animal experimentation

The relationship between man and animal depends on the cultural and intellectual environment of the society concerned. Man uses animals for transportation, protection, companionship, and as a source of food. In the past few centuries animals have also become a tool in biomedical research. In many countries the use of animals for scientific purposes has been legalized. However, animal use is subject to various provisions so as to protect animals from cruelty and to provide humane treatment. The legislation governing animal experimentation continues to be refined (Hollands, 1986; Van Zutphen *et al.*, 1986).

Comparative Nutrition, ed K. Blaxter & I. Macdonald. ©John Libbey 1988.

The use of animals for research is an emotive subject. In the debate on animal experiments at least three views play an important role. Animal experimentation would violate the rights of animals (Regan, 1983), and imposes suffering on animals (Singer, 1977). Animal experimentation would be necessary for the acquisition of knowledge from which stems the welfare of both mankind and animals (Paton, 1984). The majority of the general public probably approves animal experimentation as controlled by law. In December 1985 there was a referendum in Switzerland on the use of animals in research. A demand for a complete ban of animal experimentation was rejected by a two-to-one majority (Dickson, 1985).

The total number of animals used in the United Kingdom in 1982 was 4.2 million (Home Office, 1982). For the United States in 1980 and the Netherlands in 1986 these figures were 20–70 and 1.2 million, respectively (Institute for Laboratory Animal Resources, 1980; Sectie Dierproeven van de Veterinaire Hoofdinspectie van de Volksgezondheid, 1986). As a rough guide, this is equivalent to one animal per ten residents per year in each of these countries. Put in another way, seven animals are used for each of us during our lifetime. Mice and rats represent about 80% of the total animals used. About half of the animals are used for the control of vaccines and sera, and for toxicological research. Thus governmental regulations dictate about 50% of total animal use.

There are no data available on the number of animals used in human nutrition research. In volumes 35–38 of the *American Journal of Clinical Nutrition*, which is a journal that particularly focuses on human nutrition research, 76 (17%) of the original research papers involved animal studies. About half of these papers dealt with aspects of lipid or mineral metabolism.

Why use animals in human nutrition research?

Thus animals are used for human nutrition research. The major disadvantage lies in the fact that animals are not humans, and therefore extrapolation of animal data to man has to be done with great caution. In a workshop on the suitability of animal models for research in human nutrition during the XIII International Congress of Nutrition in Brighton, 1985, one of the questions addressed was: 'Why use animal models in human nutrition research?'. All participants agreed on the following points: greater control over the variables (including diet) being studied; reduction of the variability between subjects; more ability to carry out demanding and invasive studies; ability to carry out lifespan (endpoint) and multigeneration studies; use of the specific sensitivity of animals at the species, strain or individual level, and reduction of cost (Beynen & West, 1986).

General considerations in the choice of animal model

The appropriate choice of the animal for the experiment strongly influences the relevance of the outcome for human nutrition (Erbersdohler, 1981; Widdowson, 1986). Criteria for the selection of animal models can be divided into those of a practical and those of a scientific nature. In the above-mentioned workshop in Brighton

Table 1. *Species of animals used in papers published in volumes 35–38 of* The American Journal of Clinical Nutrition. *17% (76) of the original research papers involved animal studies.*

Species	*Number of papers*
Rat	51
Mouse	6
Monkey	5
Dog	4

(Beynen & West, 1986) we addressed the question: 'What are the criteria for the choice of animal models in human nutrition research?'. All participants agreed on the following points. The animal must exhibit, as closely as possible, the biological phenomenon to be examined or it must be possible to induce such a phenomenon. The animal husbandry used must not impose unreasonable constraints on the animal, on the experimental design or on the investigator. The experience (in both meanings of the word) of research workers plays a role in the choice of animal model to be used. The availability and price of animals also plays a role.

Screening of journals concerned with human nutrition research shows that the rat is the most favourite model (Table 1). Advantages and limitations to the use of rats have been discussed by Yang & Mickelsen (1974). The discussion centred almost essentially upon practical aspects rather than scientific considerations. Giesecke (1986) compared various animal species, including man, with respect to features of digestion and intermediary metabolism, and concluded that the rat is among the species most dissimilar to man. It could be suggested that the selection of animal models for human nutrition research is often based on practical rather than scientific reasons. Clearly, this does not serve optimally the advancement of human nutrition science. Below I suggest that the process of selecting the most suitable animal becomes more important than it has been in the past.

Changes in human nutrition research and its impact on the use of animal models

The problems addressed in human nutrition research have changed over the years. Much of the experimental work in the first half of this century was aimed at identifying constituents in the diet essential for maintaining optimal body function. Many critical discoveries, particularly concerning vitamins, minerals and trace elements, have been made. The use of animals has certainly speeded up the process of discovery of these nutrients as well as the pathways of their metabolism. With animals the effects of a single deficiency and its development could be studied. At any time during the experiment the animal could be killed and tissues studied, or the effects of rehabilitation followed. Such experiments can never be done in humans. Thus the initial work was qualitative in nature, directed at 'simple' nutritional disorders and elucidation of metabolic pathways.

The great challenge of human nutrition research now lies in work of a quantitative nature. Objective of research is to determine the relative or absolute contribution of mechanisms which are generally known to exist. Important questions are: what are the optimal levels of nutrients in the diet so as to prevent multifactorial diseases

Table 2. *Approximate intakes of cholesterol generally used in cholesterol feeding trials.*

Species	*Dietary cholesterol load (g/100 g dry matter)*	*Cholesterol intake (mg/kg body wt/d)*
Man (66.7 kg)	0.2	15
Rabbit (2.5 kg)	0.5	200
Rat (0.25 kg)	2.0	1200

such as coronary heart disease, cancer, diabetes, mental retardation etc. The change in the nature of problems being studied has profound implications for the use of animals in general, and the choice of animal models in particular. There are few qualitative species differences in metabolism. In contrast, most species differences are quantitative, due to differences in size, rate of metabolism, growth, maturation, and reproduction, and hence, nutrient requirements.

For qualitative studies it may be an advantage when animal models have exaggerated or dissimilar metabolic or anatomic characteristics to those of man. Rapid growth and small size of various animals has been shown to be crucial for accelerated identification of essential nutrients. However, for quantitative studies, metabolic or anatomic features of animal models should be as similar as possible to those of man. Thus man becomes more unique in scientific terms. This implies that human beings would be the ideal subjects of study to shed more light on the present problems in human nutrition research. However, practical as well as ethical considerations make it impossible to use human beings in various types of work.

The change from qualitative to quantitative work in human nutrition research results in the extrapolation of animal data to man becoming more difficult, and the choice of animal model becoming more crucial. The problem of extrapolation is well known, and so is the principle that ultimately all hypotheses generated as a result of animal experiments will have to be tested in man. Depending on the nature of the problem under study testing in man can either be done directly or is impossible. I shall illustrate this by comparing research on coronary heart disease with that on cancer.

For heart disease, much of the research in animals is directed towards the measurement of risk indicators, such as the concentration of serum cholesterol and blood pressure. If one's sincere concern is with human nutrition, this work should be carried out with humans. Many investigators (including myself until recently) continue to use animals for studies that can be done in humans. Consequently, animals are sacrificed unnecessarily, and time and resources are wasted. Obviously, studies on the diet-induced endpoints of the disease, such as atherosclerosis, cannot easily be done in humans. Likewise, there may be reasons to perform fundamental research on cholesterol metabolism and control of blood pressure in animals.

So far, opportunities in cancer research are limited. Reversible risk indicators are unknown, and experimental nutrition research in this area must focus on the endpoint of the disease, that is tumour formation. Thus investigators have to rely on animals as subjects of study.

I wish to draw attention to the occasional use of 'extreme' diets in animal studies. This relates to the fact that most investigators find pronounced effects more easy and interesting to induce and study. The feeding to animals of diets which are unrealistic for man can interfere with extrapolation. In cholesterol feeding experiments with humans, realistic loads are up to 1000 mg of cholesterol per day, which is equivalent to the daily consumption of four egg yolks. Cholesterol intake is then about 15 mg/kg body weight per day. However, in studies with rabbits and rats intakes are often 10 and 80 times higher (Table 2). At such high intakes compensatory mechanisms fail (Beynen, 1988), and cholesterol will accumulate in the body, especially the liver. This may cause liver damage and diminished liver function (Beynen *et al.*, 1986), which in turn could lead to biased interpretation of experimental results. It will also interfere with the extrapolation of the experimental outcome to man.

Ethical considerations and animal experimentation

The attitude of scientists toward animals may be changing. Although animal studies are within the law, many scientists are discussing the moral implications of animal experimentation. The growing interest and concern of part of the general public has not only resulted in legislation controlling animal treatment but also in scrutinizing the admissibility of animal experiments on ethical grounds. In July 1979, local ethical committees for the review of animal experiments became mandatory in Sweden. Institutional animal care committees have also been in existence for several years in Canada. In the United States, the National Institutes of Health, the major grant-awarding body for biochemical research in this country, requires ethical review of research which is submitted for funding. It is anticipated that animal experiment review committees will also become compulsory in other countries (Britt, 1984). Clearly, such committees further trigger ethical reflections by scientists. In fact, the scientist who has designed the projected experiment has been the first to balance the importance of the research project (certainty of scientific or medical benefit), the methodology proposed and the anticipated discomfort of the animals. Subsequently, the ethical committee will also judge the admissibility of the experiments proposed. The committees generally consist of scientists, laboratory animal technicians and lay-persons (Britt, 1984).

Apart from the influence of the existence of ethical committees, there may also be a change in attitude of scientists imposed by training. In the Netherlands a course on laboratory animal science is now compulsory for scientists carrying out animal experiments (Van Zutphen *et al.*, 1986). In this course technical aspects of animal experimentation are taught, and the moral implications discussed. Thus students are actually trained to weigh the issues of animal experiments, and to take on public accountability. It is expected that similar courses may also become mandatory in other countries. Thus there will be a growing ethical concern among scientists about animal experimentation. As a result, man becomes less unique in ethical terms, when compared to animals.

I wish to give an example of how recognizing that animals have intrinsic worth can affect animal experimentation. In the course of our studies on diet-induced formation of gallstones in mice we decided to assess carefully the degree of discomfort in gallstone-bearing mice (Beynen *et al.*, 1987). Superficial examination of the animals did not show abnormality, but we found it difficult to see that animals with expanded gallbladders containing large numbers of gallstones (with diameters ranging from 0.1 to 0.8 mm) would not endure discomfort. Thus discomfort was assessed by clinical

Table 3. *Mean frequency distribution of scores from assessment of stance and response to palpation in gallstone-bearing mice.* After Beynen *et al.* (1987).

	Score on a 0–3 scale							
	Mice without gallstones (n = 47)				*Mice with gallstones (n = 73)*			
	0	1	2	3	0	1	2	3
Stance	91	9	1	0	82	16	2	0
Palpation	92	6	1	1	65	21	11	4

Score: 0 = normal; 3 = abnormal.

examination and assigning scores per individual animal to parameters such as activity, stance, hair coat, position of eyes, discharge from eyes and nose, cleanliness of anal orifice, condition of tail, condition of paws and ears, and response of palpation of the right hypochondrium. Scoring was performed in random order, independently and 'blind' by three veterinarians.

There was considerable between-assessor variation in the assignment of scores to the variables used to assess discomfort. Out of the nine variables, only stance and response to palpation tended to be abnormal in the gallstone-bearing mice. Table 3 presents the mean frequency distribution of the scores from the assessment of stance and palpation of the right hypochondrium. The difference between the frequency distributions of stance scores did not reach a level of statistical significance. The response to palpation, however, was significantly altered. Thus in the gallstone-bearing mice the incidence of abnormal responses to palpation, such as squeaking and exaggerated muscular responses, was significantly higher than in their gallstone-free counterparts.

We concluded that mice with gallstones experienced pain upon palpation. They might have experienced pain continuously as the stance of the animals tended to be abnormal. We are well aware of the limitations of this study, and realize that it does not prove unequivocally that induction of gallstones causes discomfort or pain. However, we tentatively conclude that discomfort is involved, which should be taken into account in any projected work in which gallstone induction in animals may occur. This prompts us to study in future work the effects of diet on risk indicators for gallstone formation, rather than the endpoint, that is the formation of stones. In practice, this means that we shall study the effects of diet on lithogenicity of bile fluid. Of course, the animals have to be killed to take bile samples, but they may not endure discomfort during the course of this experiment.

Conclusions

The major disadvantage of the use of animals for human nutrition research lies in the fact that animals are not humans. Species differences can be involved, and extrapolation of animal data to man has to be done with great caution. The gap between animals and humans is broader for quantitative than for qualitative studies. Since emphasis has switched from qualitative to quantitative studies, the selection of animal models is more crucial than it was in the past.

Of course, it cannot be proven (or disproven) that without the use of animals our knowledge of human nutrition would be less. I feel that it can be stated that animals do have a place in human nutrition research. The use of animals has generated a host of ideas and hypotheses. Undoubtedly, it has speeded up the discovery process. In addition, certain studies simply cannot be carried out in humans, such as controlled experiments on the effects of diet on endpoints of chronic disease. The outcome of these experiments is necessary to understand the aetiology of diseases, and to formulate ways of prevention. The use of animals is of importance in making an educated guess in this respect. This type of nutrition research is similar to certain aspects of toxicological research. We want to determine empirically the optimal level of individual constituents in the diet of man but the results of animal experiments do not predict fully the situation for man. However, information on animals do reduce the risk of coming to wrong decisions.

I feel that scientists have obligations to the advancement of knowledge, to man and to experimental animals. If we are concerned with human nutrition we should first consider whether humans can be used as subjects of study. The use of human beings gets round the extrapolation gap between animals and man. If humans cannot be used, the best animal model available should be chosen. I wish to reiterate the guidelines for animal experimentation which were agreed upon during the workshop in Brighton (Beynen & West, 1986): only those experiments to be carried out which have potential to contribute useful knowledge — as seen by outside observers possibly comprising a committee capable of providing peer review; use of the minimum number of animals consistent with statistical analysis of the results anticipated (journal editors should help here!), and reduction of discomfort to animals as far as possible. It should not be implied that experimental animals always suffer discomfort. Any intervention should be within acceptable limits established by investigators and society as a whole.

References

Beynen, A. C. (1988): Animal models for cholesterol metabolism studies. In *New developments in biosciences: their implications for laboratory animal science*, eds A. C. Beynen and H. A. Solleveld, pp. 279–288. Dordrecht, Boston and Lancaster: Martinus Nijhoff Publishers.

Beynen, A. C., Baumans, V., Bertens, A. P. M. G., Havenaar, R., Hesp, A. P. M. & Van Zutphen, L. F. M. (1987): Assessment of discomfort in gallstone-bearing mice: A practical example of the problems encountered in an attempt to recognize discomfort in laboratory animals. *Lab. Anim.* **21**, 35–42.

Beynen, A. C., Danse, L. H. J. C., Van Leeuwen, F. X. R. & Speijers, G. J. A. (1986): Cholesterol metabolism and liver pathology in inbred strains of rats fed a high-cholesterol, high-cholate diet. *Nutr. Rep. Int.* **34**, 1079–1087.

Beynen, A. C. & West, C. E. (1986): The suitability of animal models for research in human nutrition: a workshop report. In *Proceedings XIII International Congress of Nutrition*, eds T. G. Taylor and N. K. Jenkins, pp. 58–59. London: John Libbey & Company Ltd.

Britt, D. (1984): Ethics, ethical committees and animal experimentation. *Nature* **311**, 503–506.

Dickson, D. (1985): Swiss voters reject ban on vivisection. *Science* **230**, 1257.

Erbersdohler, H. (1981): Zur Übertragbarkeit ernährungsphysiologischer Daten aus Tierversuchen auf den Menschen. *Ernährungs-Umschau* **28**, 15–19.

Giesecke, D. (1986): Species differences relevant to nutrition and metabolism research. In *Clinical nutrition and metabolic research*, eds G. Dietze, A. Grünert, G. Kleinberger and G. Wolfram, pp. 311–328. Basel: Karger.

Hollands, C. (1986): The animals (scientific procedures) act 1986. *Lancet* **2**, 32–33.

Home Office (1982): *Statistics of experiments on living animals (Cmnd 8986)*. London: HMSO.
Institute for Laboratory Animal Resources (1980): *International survey on the supply quality and use of laboratory animals (NIH Public. No. 80-2091)*. Washington DC: US Department of Health and Human Services.
Paton, W. (1984): *Man and mouse*. Oxford: Oxford University Press.
Regan, T. (1983): *The case for animal rights*. Berkeley, CA: University of California Press.
Sectie Dierproeven van de Veterinaire Hoofdinspectie van de Volksgezondheid (1986): *Zo Doende 1986*. Rijswijk: Ministerie van Welzijn, Volksgezondheid en Cultuur.
Singer, P. (1977): *Animal liberation*. New York: Avon Books.
Van Zutphen, L. F. M., Beynen, A. C. & Rozemond, H. (1986): Dutch legislation. *Nature* **321**, 556.
Widdowson, E. M. (1986): Animals in the service of human nutrition. *Nutr. Rev.* **44**, 221–227.
Yang, M. G. & Mickelsen, O. (1974): Laboratory animals in nutritional research. In *Methods of animal experimentation, Volume V. Nutrition, aging, and artifical organs*, ed W. I. Gay, pp. 1–40. New York and London: Academic Press.

* * * * *

Discussion

Sir Kenneth Blaxter in opening the discussion said that there was a second dimension of moral dilemma if the general public, as evidenced by the survey in Switzerland, stated that it was ethical to use an animal model to deal with the problems which confront man and then as scientists we state that there is no adequate model that we can use. How can we justify the situation? It almost sounds like a confidence trick. *Professor Beynen* agreed that this problem was a real one.

Professor Conning took up the general issue, stating that toxicologists had grappled with the broad ethical problems in relation to the needs of preventive medicine for some time. Experimental toxicologists use animal studies to identify the specific cellular mechanisms which result in the toxicity under study. The animal is thus used to analyse the biochemical processes that together result in the toxic effect. Nutritional science could well benefit from the same approach because at the cellular level there are many similarities of response between species which could constitute valuable clues to the responses of man. *Professor Beynen* agreed but pointed out that when dealing with nutrients, much more emphasis was placed on the quantitative aspects. There is a need to specify the amounts that constitute an adequate diet. *Professor Conning* suggested that this might be easier if the function were more precisely defined.

Dr Campbell Brown said that the last speaker had omitted to include consideration of the importance of human studies between ethnic groups, which often provide situations which could be used as natural experiments, reflecting both the differences in gene pools and the adaptations made by each group to their varying environments. Controlled animal experiments may identify causal factors.

Sir Christopher Booth summarized the situation from an historical perspective. In studies in the early part of the present century infection had been the main cause of mortality and morbidity and here animal work had been essential and highly effective. In the 1930s the elucidation of the role of the vitamins and hormones could also use animal models with very considerable success. At the present time, with the current interest in genetic research, it appeared that the animal of choice was not an animal at all but *E. coli*. Contemporary problems relating to degenerative diseases of various sorts, such as osteoarthritis, cardiovascular disease and so on, do not comprise a single model which can be applied to all such conditions, nor can the laboratory animal be used in the same way as it was in the period of the discovery of the vitamins and hormones. *Professor Beynen* replied that this agrees with what he had described as a change from qualitative to quantitative problems in human nutrition research.

Professor Forbes pointed out that it is normal in experimental work to use greater numbers of smaller animals. Indeed it appeared that the scale of experimentation was such that a plethora of mice and rats were used when a smaller number would be adequate. He suggested somewhat frivolously that experimenters considered the worth of an animal to be proportional to the three-quarters power of their mass.

Dr McCracken made the point that many of the problems encountered in relation to nutrition and human health were of a multi-factorial nature and required a multi-disciplinary approach. However, the scientific literature abounded with studies which could not be adequately interpreted because of a failure to quantify precisely some important dependent variable. There was a strong case, both in terms of improvement of scientific knowledge and the efficient use of experimental animals and resources, for increased development of multi-disciplinary teams and/or increased inter-laboratory collaboration.

General discussion

Professor Waterlow commented that while mechanisms of energy transduction appear common to all species there is perhaps little information about the variability of animals within species with respect, for example, to basal metabolic rate.

Sir Kenneth Blaxter pointed out that work with domesticated species indicated that variability in fasting metabolism was of the same order as that in man.

Professor Waterlow continued by asking how far there was evidence in animals of adaptability of metabolism to different nutritional circumstances, a subject of considerable interest in the field of human nutrition at the present time.

Sir Kenneth Blaxter replied that Marston's early work in Australia had shown adaptation of the basal metabolic rate to undernutrition in sheep and there was considerable evidence of adaptation to different types of diet.

Dr McCracken commented that even in the highly selected laboratory rat there was evidence of considerable variability. In cafeteria feeding, for example, his results showed a two-fold range of intake of rats of the same age and weight.

Dr Eastwood commented that 80% of individuals marry spouses who were born within 30 miles of themselves, suggesting that the human population was a locally breeding one. The real problem now was not so much whether an animal was a good model of human deficiency syndromes but whether there were similarities of response to over-nutrition. Studies of tissue responses might be more rewarding in a search for similarities.

Sir Christopher Booth asked what evidence there was for adaptation and how far appetite control was involved.

To this Professor Garrow replied that most trials to unravel such effects had been of short duration. Studies in New York of six weeks' duration had shown an initial similarity in N metabolism in subjects but that subsequently a considerable divergence emerged. The short duration of many human experiments is a real problem.

Sir Christopher Booth asked how far overindulgence was specifically a human problem, either innate or a product of our industrialized society.

Sir Kenneth Blaxter contended that all species, given confinement, freedom from stress and an abundance of food would become obese, and wondered whether this generalization could be supported.

Dr Peters pointed out that African bushmen work procuring food for only a few hours a day and then laze about. They remain thin. They could spend 4–8 hours collecting food and probably become fat but do not chose to do so.

Dr Prentice pointed out that there are times of the year for native populations when food is scarce and undernutrition a commonplace occurrence. Reproduction continues in these circumstances.

Dr Campbell Brown mentioned the situation in Quatar which has seen enormous changes in disposable income during the last 20 years. Mature onset diabetes is six times more prevalent in Asians living there than among Europeans. Diabetes in the population in Quatar and Kuwait presents a new pathology and clinical syndrome compared with Europe and suggests that this represents an adaptation.

Dr McCracken thought that the answer to Peters' comment about the bushmen related to motivation of the population and availability of food. In western societies food is easily obtained at little cost in terms of energy expenditure. Even the pig, which is generally regarded as being a glutton, reduces its intake of food *ad libitum*, if constraints are placed on the ease of accessibility. This illustrates the importance of psychological factors.

Dr Eltringham replied to Sir Kenneth Blaxter's contention that all animals can become fat. The wild animals of Africa are usually living close to their carrying capacity and consequently are often in negative energy balance particularly in the dry season. They rarely have the opportunity in the wild of overfeeding. However, the work that he and his colleagues have done shows that captive wildlife will certainly become very fat when given access to good food over long periods.

Dr Prentice pointed out that the allometry of body fat showed very poor interspecies correlations but, even so, man appeared to be a very fat animal. He suggested that the high fat content of man might have evolutionary significance and that, subjected to dietary deprivation, fat has a survival value.

On the ability of man to deposit fat, Professor Waterlow drew attention to the situation in the Cameroons. At certain seasons young men are set aside, not allowed to work, given free access to the women of the tribe and enormous amounts of food. They gain about 50 kg body weight and this is lost during the hungry season. Fat thus has a buffering effect and presumably a survival value (information from Dr. I. de Garine, Paris).

Professor Garrow continued by referring to the Pima Indians of Arizona who are fat and diabetic. The obesity is not genetic but the high incidence (50% in females and 40% in males) of diabetes could well be. Such a gene would be of little significance in a situation of limited food supply. 'Civilisation' resulted in more food being available and an increased incidence of diabetes. The human species has for most of evolution been limited by its food supply.

Professor Stock said that he doubted whether large deposits of fat had any survival value. During the reproductive phase of life people and wild animals are lean, and fat is largely laid down later in life. There are no discernible selection pressures on fatness.

Dr Peters pointed out that it was all too easy to postulate selectionist arguments to justify evolutionary hypotheses and few of these could be substantiated. To illustrate the point he said it could be postulated that fat had survival value as a storage organ for fat soluble toxins, so that potentially dangerous metabolites and contaminants could be sequestered, like DDT, thus allowing man to reach a great age and be fat at the same time!

Sir Christopher Booth then called for comments on ageing. Sir Kenneth Blaxter asked whether the old theory, due to Rubner, that since between species, metabolic rate increased with body weight to the power of 0.75 and longevity with the power of 0.25, every gram of cells, irrespective of species, is destined to burn the same amount of fuel—or to generate the same amount of ATP, applied to dietary restriction.

Dr Merry replied that total life span energy expenditure per g of lean tissue by restricted animals was greater than that of controls.

Dr Eastwood asked whether, since the expectation of life of three score years and ten derived from the old Testament and Kosher Jewish diets, other religious dietary recommendations were equated with a different life expectation in the writings of those religions.

Professor Kritchevsky interpolated that subsistence on a Jewish diet makes it seem that you live longer!

Dr Reeds commented that Harper's work shows that in the USA in the last 100 years the age at death of those who have survived to the age of 40 has advanced by only two years. This work also shows that the standard deviation of the age at death is surprisingly small. It appears that there is a time at which bodily systems start failing and that is that.

Sir Christopher Booth closed the discussion on a lighter note by saying that it was the Americans who first suggested in the Declaration of Independence that the pursuit of happiness is an inalienable right of men. Until 1776 life was considered a duty; after that date it was considered a pleasure and that is why we eat and drink too much!

List of participants

Professor D. G. ARMSTRONG: Department of Agricultural Biochemistry and Nutrition, University of Newcastle-upon-Tyne, Newcastle-upon-Tyne, NE1 7RU, UK.

Dr J. M. BASSETT: Growth & Development Unit, University Field Laboratory, Wytham, Oxford, OX2 8RJ, UK.

Professor A. C. BEYNEN: Department of Laboratory Animal Science, State University, P.O. Box 80.166, 3508 TD Utrecht, The Netherlands.

Sir Kenneth BLAXTER: Stradbroke Hall, Stradbroke, near Eye, Suffolk, IP21 5HH, UK.

Sir Christopher BOOTH: Clinical Research Centre, Watford Road, Harrow, Middlesex, HA1 3UJ, UK.

Professor P. J. BUTTERY: Department of Applied Biochemistry and Food Science, University of Nottingham, Sutton Bonington, Loughborough, LE12 5RD, UK.

Dr B. M. CAMPBELL BROWN: QGPC (Onshore), P.O. Box 70, Doha, Qatar, Arabian Gulf.

Professor A. D. CARE: Department of Animal Physiology and Nutrition, The University of Leeds, Leeds, LS2 9JT, UK.

Dr M. E. COATES: The Robens Institute, University of Surrey, Guildford, Surrey, GU2 5XH, UK.

Professor D. M. CONNING: The British Nutrition Foundation, 15 Belgrave Square, London, SW1X 8PS, UK.

Dr C. B. COWEY: NERC Institute of Marine Biochemistry, St. Fittick's Road, Torry, Aberdeen, AB1 3RA, UK.

Dr M. J. DAUNCEY: Department of Cell Biology, AFRC Institute of Animal Physiology & Genetics Research, Babraham, Cambridge, CB2 4AT, UK.

Dr M. A. EASTWOOD: Gastrointestinal Unit, Wolfson Laboratories, Western General Hospital, Edinburgh, EH4 2XU, UK.

Dr J. EDELMAN: Marlow Foods, P. O. Box 127, Lancaster House, Lincoln Road, High Wycombe, HP12 3RL, UK.

Dr M. ELIA: Dunn Clinical Nutrition Centre, 100 Tennis Court Road, Cambridge, CB2 1QL, UK.

Dr S. K. ELTRINGHAM: Department of Applied Biology, University of Cambridge, Pembroke Street, Cambridge, CB2 3DX, UK.

Dr S. J. FAIRWEATHER-TAIT: AFRC Institute of Food Research, Colney Lane, Norwich, NR4 7UA, UK.

Professor, J. M. FORBES: Department of Animal Physiology and Nutrition, The University of Leeds, Leeds, LS2 9JT, UK.

Professor D. R. FRASER: Department of Animal Husbandry, University of Sydney, New South Wales 2006, Australia.

Dr M. F. FULLER: Rowett Research Institute, Greenburn Lane, Bucksburn, Aberdeen, AB2 9SB, UK.

Professor L. E. GARBY: Department of Physiology, Odense University, Campusvej 55, Odense, Denmark.

Professor J. S. GARROW: Department of Human Nutrition, Medical College of St. Bartholomew's Hospital, Charterhouse Square, London, EC1M 6BQ, UK.

Dr D. F. GOLDSPINK: Department of Physiology, Medical Biology Centre, The Queen's University, 97 Lisburn Road, Belfast, BT9 7BL, UK.

Professor G. GOLDSPINK: Molecular and Cell Biology, The Royal Veterinary College, Royal College Street, London, NW1 0TU, UK.

Dr R. F. GRIMBLE: Department of Nutrition, University of Southampton, Bassett Crescent East, Southampton, S09 3TU, UK.

Professor M. I. GURR: Milk Marketing Board, Thames Ditton, Surrey, KT7 0EL, UK.

Dr D. HALLIDAY: Nutrition Research Group, MRC Clinical Research Centre, Watford Road, Harrow, Middlesex, HA1 3UJ, UK.

Dr C. J. K. HENRY: Department of Food Studies, Oxford Polytechnic, Headington, Oxford, OX3 0BP, UK.

Professor D. L. INGRAM: Department of Cell Biology, AFRC Institute of Animal Physiology & Genetics Research, Babraham, Cambridge, CB2 4AT, UK.

Professor A. A. JACKSON: Department of Nutrition, University of Southampton, Bassett Crescent East, Southampton, SO9 3TU, UK.

Professor W. P. T. JAMES: The Rowett Research Institute, Greenburn Road, Bucksburn, Aberdeen, AB2 9SB, UK.

Professor D. KRITCHEVSKY: The Wistar Institute, 3601 Spruce Street, Philadelphia, Pa 19104, USA.

Dr D. E. M. LAWSON: AFRC Institute of Animal Physiology and Genetics Research, Babraham, Cambridge, CB2 4AT, UK.

Dr G. E. LOBLEY: Rowett Research Institute, Greenburn Road, Bucksburn, Aberdeen, AB2 9SB, UK.

Professor I. MACDONALD: Department of Physiology, Guy's Hospital Medical and Dental Schools, London, SE1 9RT, UK.

Dr K. J. McCRACKEN: Agricultural & Food Chemistry Research Division, Queen's University of Belfast, Newforge Lane, Belfast, BT9 5PX, UK.

Dr D. J. MELLOR: Moredun Research Institute, 408 Gilmerton Road, Edinburgh, Scotland, EH17 7JH, UK.

Dr B. J. MERRY: Wolfson Institute, University of Hull, Hull, HU6 7RX, UK.

Dr D. J. MILLWARD: Nutrition Research Unit, London School of Hygiene & Tropical Medicine, 4 St. Pancras Way, London, NW1 2PE, UK.

Dr R. J. NEALE: Department of Applied Biochemistry & Food Science, University of Nottingham, Sutton Bonington, Loughborough, LE12 5RD, UK.

Miss A. A. PAUL: Dunn Nutrition Unit, Downhams Lane, Milton Road, Cambridge, CB4 1XJ, UK.

P. R. PAYNE Esq: Department of Human Nutrition, London School of Hygiene & Tropical Medicine, Keppel Street, London, WC1E 7HT, UK.

Professor M. PEAKER: Hannah Research Institute, Ayr, Scotland, KA6 5HL, UK.

Professor R. H. PETERS: Strada Valle, Corconio (Frazione Ameno), Novara 28010, Italy.

Dr A. PRENTICE: M.R.C. Dunn Nutrition Unit, Downhams Lane, Milton Road, Cambridge, CB4 1XJ, UK.

Dr A. M. PRENTICE: Dunn Clinical Nutrition Centre, 100 Tennis Court Road, Cambridge, CB2 1QL, UK.

Dr P. J. REEDS: Department of Pediatrics, Baylor College of Medicine, Medical Towers Building, 6608 Fannin Houston, Texas 77030, USA.

Sir Ralph RILEY: 16 Gog Magog Way, Stapleford, Cambridge, CB2 5BQ, UK.

Dr T. SANDERS: Department of Nutrition, King's College London, Campden Hill Road, Kensington, London, W8 7AH, UK.

Dr B. SCHURCH: The Nestlé Foundation, P.O. Box 581, 1001 Lausanne, Switzerland.

Dr P. S. SHETTY: Nutrition Research Centre, Department of Physiology, St. John's Medical College, Bangalore 560034, India.

Dr M. SILVER: Physiological Laboratory, Downing Street, Cambridge, CB2 3EG, UK.

Dr J. R. SPEAKMAN: Department of Zoology, University of Aberdeen, Aberdeen, AB9 2TN, UK.

Dr C. E. STEVENS: School of Veterinary Medicine, North Carolina State University, 4700 Hillsborough Street, Raleigh, NC27606, USA.

Professor M. J. STOCK: Department of Physiology, St George's Hospital Med. School, Cranmer Terrace, London, SW17 ORE, UK.

Dr D. I. THURNHAM: Dunn Nutritional Laboratories, Downham's Lane, Milton Road, Cambridge, CB4 1XJ, UK.

Dr A. M. TOMKINS: Department of Human Nutrition, London School of Hygiene & Tropical Medicine, Keppel Street, London, WC1E 7HT, UK.

Sir Richard TREHANE: Hampreston Manor Farm, Wimborne, Dorset, UK.

Professor P. J. VAN SOEST, 324 Morrison Hall, Cornell University, Ithaca, New York 14853, USA.

Professor J. C. WATERLOW: 15, Hillgate Street, London, W8 7SP, UK.

Professor A. J. WEBSTER: Department of Animal Husbandry, University of Bristol School of Veterinary Science, Langford, Bristol, BS18 7DU, UK.

Dr R. G. WHITEHEAD: Dunn Nutrition Unit, Downhams Lane, Milton Road, Cambridge, CB4 1XJ, UK.

Dr E. M. WIDDOWSON: Department of Medicine, Level 5, Addenbrooke's Hospital, Hills Road, Cambridge, CB2 2QQ, UK.

Professor R. YAGIL: Faculty of Health Sciences, Ben-Gurion University of the Negev, Beersheva 84105, Israel.

Dr D. A. YORK: Department of Nutrition, University of Southampton, Bassett Crescent East, Southampton, SO9 3TU, UK.

Professor M. YOUNG: 4 Preston Close, Miller's Road, Toft, Cambridge, CB3 7RU, UK.

Index